Golden Notes for
Community Health Nursing-II

Golden Notes for Community Health Nursing-II

As per the Revised Syllabus

Parimal Patel
MD (Gold Medalist) DNB (Gold Medalist) PGDMRCH
Faculty
Department of Community Medicine
BJ Medical College
Ahmedabad, Gujarat, India

Khushbu Makadia
MD PGDMRCH
Faculty
Department of Community Medicine
GMERS Medical College
Himmatnagar, Gujarat, India

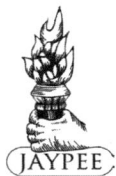

JAYPEE BROTHERS MEDICAL PUBLISHERS
The Health Sciences Publisher
New Delhi | London

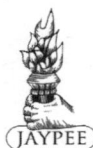

Jaypee Brothers Medical Publishers (P) Ltd

Headquarter
Jaypee Brothers Medical Publishers (P) Ltd
EMCA House, 23/23-B
Ansari Road, Daryaganj
New Delhi 110 002, India
Landline: +91-11-23272143, +91-11-23272703
+91-11-23282021, +91-11-23245672
Email: jaypee@jaypeebrothers.com

Corporate Office
Jaypee Brothers Medical Publishers (P) Ltd
4838/24, Ansari Road, Daryaganj
New Delhi 110 002, India
Phone: +91-11-43574357
Fax: +91-11-43574314
Email: jaypee@jaypeebrothers.com

Overseas Office
J.P. Medical Ltd
83 Victoria Street, London
SW1H 0HW (UK)
Phone: +44 20 3170 8910
Fax: +44 (0)20 3008 6180
Email: info@jpmedpub.com

Website: www.jaypeebrothers.com
Website: www.jaypeedigital.com

© 2023, Jaypee Brothers Medical Publishers

The views and opinions expressed in this book are solely those of the original contributor(s)/author(s) and do not necessarily represent those of editor(s) and publisher of the book.

All rights reserved. No part of this publication may be reproduced, stored or transmitted in any form or by any means, electronic, mechanical, photocopying, recording or otherwise, without the prior permission in writing of the publishers.

All brand names and product names used in this book are trade names, service marks, trademarks or registered trademarks of their respective owners. The publisher is not associated with any product or vendor mentioned in this book.

Medical knowledge and practice change constantly. This book is designed to provide accurate, authoritative information about the subject matter in question. However, readers are advised to check the most current information available on procedures included and check information from the manufacturer of each product to be administered, to verify the recommended dose, formula, method and duration of administration, adverse effects and contraindications. It is the responsibility of the practitioner to take all appropriate safety precautions. Neither the publisher nor the author(s)/editor(s) assume any liability for any injury and/or damage to persons or property arising from or related to use of material in this book.

This book is sold on the understanding that the publisher is not engaged in providing professional medical services. If such advice or services are required, the services of a competent medical professional should be sought.

Every effort has been made where necessary to contact holders of copyright to obtain permission to reproduce copyright material. If any have been inadvertently overlooked, the publisher will be pleased to make the necessary arrangements at the first opportunity.

Inquiries for bulk sales may be solicited at: jaypee@jaypeebrothers.com

Golden Notes for Community Health Nursing-II

First Edition: **2023**
ISBN: 978-93-5696-276-7

Printed at: Sterling Graphics Pvt. Ltd. India.

Dedicated to

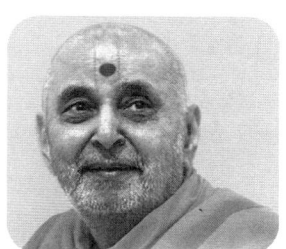

"In the joy of others, lies our own"
Brahmaswarup Shri Pramukh Swami Maharaj

All students S.t.s. are blessed by Pramukh Swami Maharaj

Pragat Brahmaswarup Shri Mahant Swami Maharaj

and
Our Parents

Preface

विद्या नाम नरस्य कीर्तिरतुला भाग्यक्षये चाश्रयो
धेनुः कामदुधा रतिश्य विरहे नेत्रं तृतीयं च सा।।
सत्कारायतनं कुलस्य महिमा रत्नैर्विना भूषणम्
तस्मादन्यमुपेक्ष्य सर्वविषयं विद्याधिकारं कुरू।।

Community Health Nursing is a vital subject for all frontline healthcare workers. It encompasses all the competencies needed to perform the activities of the healthcare delivery system, particularly, National Health Programs. So, this book; **Golden Notes for Community Health Nursing** is our genuine attempt to provide competency-based knowledge of the subject.

This book is designed as per the revised nursing syllabus. This will eliminate the need to refer to any other supplementary books to learn the subject.

Each chapter contains updated information. This book would be the first of its kind as it is written by subject matter experts who have vast experience in academics as well as fieldwork. All the chapters are written in bullet point format along with flowcharts and tables to make it easy for students to learn.

The major extent of *Community Health Nursing-II* is reproductive and child health (RCH) which have been covered extensively in this book. This book is not only for theory purposes but also covers practical aspects of the subject. All chapters of this book is prepared based on the latest information from the Ministry of Health and Family Welfare (MOHFW) guidelines, advisories, and program modules.

Community Health Nursing is a pertinent subject not only from an academic point of view but also from a career point of view, especially for those interested in joining the government sector. We can assure you that this book will help all the students not only to secure good marks in exams but also excel in professional life also.

We are confident that our book **"Golden Notes for Community Health Nursing"** will enable students to function in a variety of settings in either public/government or private healthcare settings.

We always welcome constructive criticism!

Parimal Patel (drparimalpsm3787@gmail.com)
Khushbu Makadia (khushbu20makadia@gmail.com)

Acknowledgments

First of all, we would like to thank Almighty God and our parents for giving us an opportunity to serve society and for placing us where we are today.

We would also like to thank all the nursing college faculties and all nursing students who have helped us in understanding the need of such book and also helping us by reviewing the chapters that helped in improving the content of the book.

Last but not the least; we would like to thank and appreciate Shri Jitendar P Vij (Group Chairman), Mr Ankit Vij (Managing Director), Mr MS Mani (Group President), Dr Madhu Choudhary (Director–Educational Publishing), Ms Pooja Bhandari [Director–Production (Books and Journals)], Ms Sunita Katla (Executive Assistant to Group Chairman and Publishing Manager), Ms Samina Khan (Executive Assistant to Director–Educational Publishing), Ms Alisha Talwar (Content Strategist), Mr Rajesh Sharma (Production Coordinator), Ms Seema Dogra (Cover Visualizer), Mr Deep Dogra (Typesetter), Ms Geeta Barik (Proofreader), Mr Pappu Yadav (Graphic Designer), and all the staff of the M/s Jaypee Brothers Medical Publishers (P) Ltd, New Delhi, India, for doing appreciable work in their respective field of printing and publishing.

I also thank Manager and staff of Ahmedabad branch of M/s Jaypee Brothers Medical Publishers (P) Ltd.

Contents

CHAPTER 1: Role of Community Health Nurse in Management of Emergencies and Common Disorders — 1
- 1.1 Fundamentals of Health Assessment and Examination — 1
- 1.2 Management of Common Emergencies including First Aid — 11
- 1.3 Basics of Primary Care of Common Disorders — 22

CHAPTER 2: Reproductive, Maternal, Newborn, Child, and Adolescent Health — 30
- 2.1 History and Current Status of Reproductive, Maternal and Child Health in India — 30
- 2.2 Basics of Antenatal Care — 33
- 2.3 Basics of Intranatal Care — 43
- 2.4 Basic of Postnatal Care — 48
- 2.5 Basics of Newborn and Child Care along with Related Programs and Guidelines — 52
- 2.6 Basics of Adolescent Health along with related Programs and Guidelines — 58
- 2.7 Reproductive Maternal Newborn Child Adolescent Health Plus Nutrition (RMNCAH + N) — 64
- 2.8 Universal Immunization Program (UIP) — 68

CHAPTER 3: Demography, Surveillance, and Data — 78
- 3.1 Demography: Background, Scope and Definition — 78
- 3.2 Demography Cycle — 81
- 3.3 Population Pyramid, Dependency Ratio and Other Important Definitions — 81
- 3.4 Sex Ratio — 84
- 3.5 Important Vital Statistics Indicators — 84
- 3.6 Sources of Vital Statistics — 88
- 3.8 Data: Source, Methods of Collection, Analysis and Interpretation — 95
- 3.9 National Population Policy — 109
- 3.10 Basics of Surveillance Including IDSP and IHIP — 110

CHAPTER 4: Population and Family Welfare — 113
- 4.1 Population Explosion: Reasons, Impact and Population Control — 113
- 4.2 Basics of Family Planning and Different Family Planning Measures — 115
- 4.3 Emergency Contraception — 124
- 4.4 The Medical Termination of Pregnancy (MTP) Act, 1971 — 125
- 4.5 National Family Welfare Program — 126
- 4.6 Population Stabilization Fund/Jansankhya Sthirata Kosh — 127
- 4.7 Mission Parivar Vikas — 128
- 4.8 National Family Planning Indemnity Scheme (NFPIS) — 130
- 4.9 Counseling in Reproductive and Sexual Health Problems of Adolescents — 131
- 4.10 Family Planning 2020 and 2030 — 133
- 4.11 Miscellaneous — 137

CHAPTER 5: Occupational Health — 139
- 5.1 Occupational Health Hazards — 139
- 5.2 Occupational Diseases — 141
- 5.3 The Factory Act, 1948 — 145
- 5.4 The Employees State Insurance (ESI) Act, 1948 — 147

Contents

    5.5   National Program for Control and Treatment of Occupational Diseases   150
    5.6   Role of Nurse in Occupational Health Services   151

CHAPTER 6: Geriatric Health — 152

    6.1   Health Problems of Older Adults   152
    6.2   National Program for Health Care of Elderly (NPHCE)   155
    6.3   Schemes for Welfare of Older Adults   158
    6.4   Role of Frontline Healthcare Workers in Geriatric Health   161

CHAPTER 7: Mental Health — 163

    7.1   Anxiety Disorders   163
    7.2   Depression   165
    7.3   Psychosis including Schizophrenia   167
    7.4   Dementia   170
    7.5   Suicide   171
    7.6   Alcohol and Other Common Substance Abuse   173
    7.7   Drug Deaddiction Programs   175
    7.8   National Mental Health Policy   177
    7.9   National Mental Health Program   178
    7.10   The Mental Healthcare Act, 2017   180
    7.11   Role of a Community Health Nurse in Mental Health   182

CHAPTER 8: E-Health Including HMIS — 185

    8.1   Basics of E-Health and National Digital Health Mission   185
    8.2   E-Health: Reproductive and Child Health (RCH)   188
    8.3   E-Health: Communicable Diseases   191
    8.4   E-Health: Noncommunicable Diseases   192
    8.5   Drugs and Logistics   193
    8.6   Management including Health Management Information System (HMIS)   196

CHAPTER 9: Delivery Mechanism of Community Health Services — 199

    9.1   Rural Healthcare Delivery System   199
    9.2   Urban Healthcare Delivery System   206
    9.3   IPHS for SC/HWC, PHC and CHC   209
    9.4   Financial and Inventory Management at Public Health Facilities   217
    9.5   Summary of Different Indian Systems of Medicine (AYUSH)   223

CHAPTER 10: Fundamentals of Leadership, Supervision, and Monitoring — 230

    10.1   Leadership   230
    10.2   Supervision   233
    10.3   Monitoring   235

CHAPTER 11: Disaster Management — 238

    11.1   Introduction to Disaster Management   240
    11.2   Disaster Management Cycle   241
    11.3   Disaster Impact and Rescue   241
    11.4   Epidemiologic Surveillance and Disease Control   242

CHAPTER 12: Biomedical Waste Management — 246

- 12.1 Overview of Biomedical Waste 246
- 12.2 Biomedical Waste Management at Community Level and Health Facility Level 249
- 12.3 Biomedical Waste Management Act 251

CHAPTER 13: National and International Agencies Related to Health — 257

- 13.1 World Health Organization (WHO) 257
- 13.2 United Nations Children's Fund (UNICEF) 259
- 13.3 Important UN Agencies (UNDP, UNFPA), World Bank, FAO and ILOs 261
- 13.4 International Bilateral Agencies or NGOs (CARE, Ford Foundation, Rockefeller Foundation, SIDA, DANIDA, Colombo Plan) 263
- 13.5 National Health Agencies 265

Annexures — *271*
Index — *299*

Syllabus (BSc Nursing)

COMMUNITY HEALTH NURSING—II

Placement: VII SEMESTER

Theory: 5 Credits (100 hours)—includes lab hours also

Practicum: Clinical: 2 Credit (160 hours)

Description: This course is designed to help students gain broad perspective of specialized roles and responsibilities of community health nurses and to practice in various specialized health care settings. It helps students to develop knowledge and competencies required for assessment, diagnosis, treatment, and nursing management of individuals and families within the community in wellness and illness continuum.

Competencies: On completion of the course, the students will be able to:
- Demonstrate beginning practice competencies/skills relevant to provide comprehensive primary health care/community-based care to clients with common diseases and disorders including emergency and first aid care at home/clinics/centres as per predetermined protocols/drug standing orders approved by MOHandFW
- Provide maternal, newborn and child care, and reproductive health including adolescent care in the urban and rural health care settings
- Describe the methods of collection and interpretation of demographic data
- Explain population control and its impact on the society and describe the approaches towards limiting family size
- Describe occupational health hazards, occupational diseases and the role of nurses in occupational health programs
- Identify health problems of older adults and provide primary care, counseling and supportive health services
- Participate in screening for mental health problems in the community and providing appropriate referral services
- Discuss the methods of data collection for HMIS, analysis and interpretation of data
- Discuss about effective management of health information in community diagnosis and intervention
- Describe the management system of delivery of community health services in rural and urban areas
- Describe the leadership role in guiding, supervising, and monitoring the health services and the personnel at the PHCs, SCs and community level including financial management and maintenance of records and reports
- Describe the roles and responsibilities of Mid-Level Health Care Providers (MHCPs) in Health Wellness Centers (HWCs)
- Identify the roles and responsibilities of health team members and explain their job description
- Demonstrate initiative in preparing themselves and the community for disaster preparedness and management
- Demonstrate skills in proper biomedical waste management as per protocols
- Explain the roles and functions of various national and international health agencies

COURSE OUTLINE

T–Theory

Unit	Time (Hrs)	Learning outcomes	Content	Teaching/learning activities	Assessment methods
I	10 (T)	Explain nurses' role in identification, primary management and referral of clients with common disorders/ conditions and emergencies including first aid	**Management of Common Conditions and Emergencies Including First Aid** • Standing orders: Definition, uses **Screening, diagnosing/identification, primary care and referral of gastrointestinal system** • Abdominal pain • Nausea and vomiting • Diarrhea • Constipation • Jaundice • GI bleeding • Abdominal distension • Dysphagia and dyspepsia • Aphthous ulcers **Respiratory System** • Acute upper respiratory infections – rhinitis, sinusitis, pharyngitis, laryngitis, tonsillitis • Acute lower respiratory infections—bronchitis, pneumonia and bronchial asthma • Hemoptysis, acute chest pain **Heart and Blood** • Common heart diseases: Heart attack/coronary artery disease, heart failure, arrhythmia • Blood anemia, blood cancers, bleeding disorders **Eye and ENT conditions** • Eye–local infections, redness of eye, conjunctivitis, stye, trachoma and refractive errors • ENT–Epistaxis, ASOM, sore throat, deafness **Urinary System** • Urinary tract infections—cystitis, pyelonephritis, prostatitis, UTIs in children **First aid in common emergency conditions–Review** • High fever, low blood sugar, minor injuries, fractures, fainting, bleeding, shock, stroke, bites, burns, choking, seizures, RTAs, poisoning, drowning and foreign bodies	• Lecture • Discussion • Demonstration • Role play • Suggested field visits • Field practice • Assessment of clients with common conditions and provide referral	• Short answer • Essay • Field visit reports • OSCE assessment

Syllabus (BSc Nursing)

Unit	Time (Hrs)	Learning outcomes	Content	Teaching/learning activities	Assessment methods
II	20 (T)	Provide reproductive, maternal, newborn and childcare, including adolescent care in the urban and rural health care settings	**Reproductive, maternal, newborn, child and adolescent Health (Review from OBG Nursing and application in community setting)** • Present situation of reproductive, maternal and child health in India **Antenatal care** • Objectives, antenatal visits and examination, nutrition during pregnancy, counseling • Calcium and iron supplementation in pregnancy • Antenatal care at health centre level • Birth preparedness • High risk approach–screening/early identification and primary management of complications–antepartum hemorrhage, pre-eclampsia, eclampsia, anemia, gestational diabetes mellitus, hypothyroidism, syphilis • Referral, follow-up and maintenance of records and reports **Intranatal care** • Normal labor–process, onset, stages of labor • Monitoring and active management of different stages of labor • Care of women after labor • Early identification, primary management, referral and follow-up—preterm labor, fetal distress, prolonged and obstructed labour, vaginal and perennial tears, ruptured uterus • Care of newborn immediately after birth • Maintenance of records and reports • Use of safe child birth checklist • SBA module–Review • Organization of labor room **Postpartum care** • Objectives, postnatal visits, care of mother and baby, breastfeeding, diet during lactation, and health counseling	• Lecture • Discussion • Demonstration • Role play • Suggested field visits and field practice • Assessment of antenatal, postnatal, newborn, infant, preschool child, school child, and adolescent health	• Short answer • Essay • OSCE assessment

Syllabus (BSc Nursing)

Unit	Time (Hrs)	Learning outcomes	Content	Teaching/learning activities	Assessment methods

			• Early identification, primary management, referral and follow up of complications, Danger signs—postpartum hemorrhage, shock, puerperal sepsis, breast conditions, postpartum depression
			• Postpartum visit by health care provider
			Newborn and child care
			• *Review:* Essential newborn care
			• Management of common neonatal problems
			• Management of common child health problems: Pneumonia, diarrhoea, sepsis, screening for congenital anomalies and referral
			• *Review:* IMNCI module
			• Under five clinics
			Adolescent Health
			• Common health problems and risk factors in adolescent girls and boys
			• Common gynecological conditions–dysmenorrhea, Premenstrual syndrome (PMS), Vaginal discharge, Mastitis, Breast lump, pelvic pain, pelvic organ prolapse
			• Teenage pregnancy, awareness about legal age of marriage, nutritional status of adolescents National Menstrual Hygiene scheme
			• Youth friendly services:
			  ▪ SRH Service needs
			  ▪ Role and attitude of nurses: Privacy, confidentiality, non judgemental attitude, client autonomy, respectful care and communication
			• Counseling for parents and teenagers (BCS – balanced counseling strategy)
			National Programs
			• RMNCH + A Approach: Aims, Health systems strengthening, RMNCH + A strategies, interventions across life stages, program management, monitoring and evaluation systems
			• Universal Immunization Program (UIP) as per Government of India guidelines – Review		

		Promote adolescent health and youth friendly services		• Screen, manage and refer adolescents • Counsel adolescents	

Syllabus (BSc Nursing)

Unit	Time (Hrs)	Learning outcomes	Content	Teaching/learning activities	Assessment methods
			• Rashtriya Bal Swasthya Karyakaram (RSBK)—children • Rashtriya Kishor Swasthya Karyakram (RKSK)—adolscents Any other new programs		
III	4 (T)	Discuss the concepts and scope of demography	**Demography, Surveillance and Interpretation of Data** • *Demography and vital statistics*: Demographic cycle, world population trends, vital statistics • Sex ratio and child sex ratio, trends of sex ratio in India, the causes and social implications • *Sources of vital statistics:* Census, registration of vital events, sample registration system • *Morbidity and mortality indicators:* Definition, calculation and interpretation • Surveillance, Integrated disease surveillance project (IDSP), Organization of IDSP, flow of information and mother and child tracking system (MCTS) in India • Collection, analysis, interpretation, use of data • *Review:* Common sampling techniques – random and nonrandom techniques • Disaggregation of data	• Lecture • Discussion • Demonstration • Role play • Suggested field visits • Field practice	• Short answer • Essay
IV	6 (T)	Discuss population explosion and its impact on social and economic development of India	**Population and its Control** • Population explosion and its impact on social, economic development of individual, society and country. • Population control: Women empowerment; social, economic and educational development • Limiting family size: promotion of small family norm, temporary spacing methods (natural, biological, chemical, mechanical methods, etc.), terminal methods (tubectomy, vasectomy) • Emergency contraception • Counseling in reproductive, sexual health including problems of adolescents • Medical Termination of pregnancy and MTP Act • National Population Stabilization Fund/JSK (Jansankhya Sthirata Kosh)	• Lecture • Discussion • Demonstration • Role play • Suggested field visits • Field practice	• Short answer • Essay • OSCE assessment • Counseling on family planning

Syllabus (BSc Nursing)

Unit	Time (Hrs)	Learning outcomes	Content	Teaching/learning activities	Assessment methods
		Describe the various methods of population control	• Family planning 2020 • National Family Welfare Program • Role of a nurse in Family Welfare Program		
V	5 (T)	Describe occupational health hazards, occupational diseases and the role of nurses in occupational health programs	**Occupational Health** Occupational health hazards Occupational diseases ESI Act National/ State Occupational Health Programs Role of a nurse in occupational health services: Screening, diagnosing, management and referral of clients with occupational health problems	• Lecture • Discussion • Demonstration • Role play • Suggested field visits • Field practice	Essay Short answer Clinical performance evaluation
VI	6 (T)	Identify health problems of older adults and provide primary care, counseling and supportive health services	**Geriatric Health Care** • Health problems of older adults • Management of common geriatric ailments: counseling, supportive treatment of older adults • Organization of geriatric health services • National program for health care of elderly (NPHCE) • State level programs/Schemes for older adults • Role of a community health nurse in geriatric health services: Screening, diagnosing, management and referral of older adults with health problems	• Lecture • Discussion • Demonstration	• Visit report on elderly home • Essay • Short answer

VII	6 (T)	Describe screening for mental health problems in the community, take preventive measures and provide appropriate referral services	**Mental Health Disorders**
			• Screening, management, prevention and referral for mental health disorders
			• *Review:*
			  ▪ Depression, anxiety, acute psychosis,
			  ▪ Schizophrenia
			  ▪ Dementia
			  ▪ Suicide
			  ▪ Alcohol and substance abuse
			  ▪ Drug deaddiction program
			  ▪ National Mental Health Program
			  ▪ National Mental Health Policy
			  ▪ National Mental Health Act
			• Role of a community health nurse in screening, initiation of treatment and follow up of mentally ill clients
				• Lecture
				• Discussion
				• Demonstration
				• Role play
				• Health counseling on promotion of mental health
				• Suggested field visits
				• Field practice
					• Essay
					• Short answer
					• Counseling report

Syllabus (BSc Nursing)

Unit	Time (Hrs)	Learning outcomes	Content	Teaching/learning activities	Assessment methods

VIII	4 (T)	Discuss about effective management of health information in community diagnosis and intervention	**Health Management Information System (HMIS)**
			• Introduction to health management system: data elements, recording and reporting formats, data quality issues
			• *Review:*
			  ▪ Basic demography and vital statistics
			  ▪ Sources of vital statistics
			  ▪ Common sampling techniques, frequency distribution
			  ▪ Collection, analysis, interpretation of data
			• Analysis of data for community needs assessment and preparation of health action plan
				• Lecture
				• Discussion
				• Demonstration
				• Role play
				• Suggested field visits
				• Field practice
				• Group project on community diagnosis–data management
					• Group project report
					• Essay
					• Short answer

IX	12 (T)	Describe the system management of delivery of community health services in rural and urban areas	**Management of Delivery of Community Health Services:** • Planning, budgeting and material management of CHC, PHC, SC/HWC • **Manpower planning as per IPHS standards** • **Rural:** Organization, staffing and material management of rural health services provided by Government at village, SC/HWC, PHC, CHC, hospitals—district, state and central • **Urban:** Organization, staffing, and functions of urban health services provided by Government at slums, dispensaries, special clinics, municipal and corporate hospitals • Defense services • Institutional services • Other systems of medicine and health: Indian system of medicine, AYUSH clinics, Alternative health care system referral systems, Indigenous health services	▪ Lecture ▪ Discussion ▪ Visits to various health care delivery systems ▪ Supervised field practice	• Essay • Short answer • Filed visit reports
X	15 (T)	Describe the leadership role in guiding, supervising, and monitoring the health services and the personnel at the PHCs, SCs and community level including financial management	**Leadership, Supervision and Monitoring** • Understanding work responsibilities/job description of DPHN, Health Visitor, PHN, MPHW (Female), Multipurpose health Worker (Male), AWWs and ASHA • Roles and responsibilities of Mid-Level Health Care Providers (MLHPs)	• Lecture • Discussion • Demonstration • Role play • Suggested field visits • Field practice	• Report on interaction with MPHWs, HVs, ASHA, AWWs • Participation in training programs • Essay • Short answer

Unit	Time (Hrs)	Learning outcomes	Content	Teaching/learning activities	Assessment methods
		Describe the roles and responsibilities of Mid-Level Health Care Providers (MHCPs) in Health Wellness Centers (HWCs)	• Village Health Sanitation and Nutrition Committees (VHSNC): objectives, composition and roles and responsibilities • Health team management • *Review*: Leadership and supervision – concepts, principles and methods • Leadership in health: Leadership approaches in healthcare setting, taking control of health of community and organizing health camps, village clinics • Training, supportive supervision and monitoring–concepts, principles and process, e.g. performance of frontline health workers **Financial Management and Accounting and Computing at Health Centers (SC)** • Activities for which funds are received • Accounting and book keeping requirements—accounting principles and policies, book of accounts to be maintained, basic accounting entries, accounting process, payments and expenditure, fixed asset, SOE reporting format, utilization certificate (UC) reporting • Preparing a budget • Audit **Records and Reports:** • *Concepts of records and reports*—importance, legal implications, purposes, use of records, principles of record writing, filing of records • *Types of records*—community related records, registers, guidelines for maintaining • *Report writing*—purposes, documentation of activities, types of reports • *Medical Records Department*—functions, filing and retention of medical records		

Syllabus (BSc Nursing)

Unit	Time (Hrs)	Learning outcomes	Content	Teaching/learning activities	Assessment methods
			• *Electronic Medical Records (EMR)*—capabilities and components of EMR, electronic health record (EHR), levels of automation, attributes, benefits and disadvantages of HER • **Nurses' responsibility in record keeping and reporting**		
XI	6 (T)	Demonstrate initiative in preparing themselves and the community for disaster preparedness and management	**Disaster Management** • Disaster types and magnitude • Disaster preparedness • Emergency preparedness • Common problems during disasters and methods to overcome • Basic disaster supplies kit • Disaster response including emergency relief measures and Life saving techniques • Use disaster management module	• Lecture • Discussion • Demonstration • Role play • Suggested field visits, and field practice • Mock drills • Refer Disaster module (NDMA) National Disaster/ INC–Reaching out in emergencies	
XII	3 (T)	Describe the importance of biomedical waste management, its process and management	**Biomedical Waste Management** • Waste collection, segregation, transportation and management in the community • Waste management in health center/clinics • Biomedical waste management guidelines – 2016, 2018 (Review)	• Lecture-cum-discussion • Field visit to waste management site	• Field visit report
XIII	3 (T)	Explain the roles and functions of various national and international health agencies	**Health Agencies** • **International:** WHO, UNFPA, UNDP, World Bank, FAO, UNICEF, European Commission, Red Cross, USAID, UNESCO, ILO, CAR, CIDA, JHPIEGO, any other • **National:** Indian Red Cross, Indian Council for Child Welfare, Family Planning Association of India, Tuberculosis Association of India, Central Social Welfare Board, All India Women's Conference, Blind Association of India, any other • **Voluntary Health Association of India (VHA)**	• Lecture • Discussion • Field visits	• Essay • Short answer

Syllabus (GNM)

COMMUNITY HEALTH NURSING—II

Placement: Third Year (Part – I) **Total Hours: 90**

Course Description
This course is designed to help students to practice community health nursing for the individual, family and groups at both the urban and rural settings by using concepts and principles of health and community health nursing.

General Objectives
Upon completion of this course, the students shall be able to:
- Describe the health system and health care services in India.
- Identify major health problems, national health programmes and specialized community health services.
- Explain the concept of health team and describe the nurses' role at various levels of health care setting.
- Demonstrate skills in rendering effective nursing care to the individual, family and groups in all community health settings.

Total Hours: 90

Unit	Learning objective	Contents	Hrs	Teaching/learning activities	Assessment methods
I	Explain the health system in India	**Heath System in India** Organization and administration of health system in India at: • Central level ▪ Union Ministry ▪ Directorate General of Health Services ▪ Central Council of Health • State level ▪ State Health Administration ▪ State Ministry of Health ▪ State Health Directorate • District level ▪ Sub Divisions ▪ Tehsils/ Talukas ▪ Villages ▪ Municipalities and Corporation ▪ Panchayats	10	Lecture-cum-discussion Organizational chart of various levels Visit to Municipality Office, Panchayat office, Health block office, CHC	• Short answer • Objective type • Essay type
II	Describe the health care services in India and discuss the role of the nurse in these services	**Health Care Delivery System** • Heath care concept and trends • Health care services: Public sector, Rural, Urban • Private sector • Public Private Partnership (PPP) • Other agencies • Indigenous systems of medicine Ayurvedha, yoga, unani, siddha and homeopathy (AYUSH)	8	Lecture-cum-discussion Visit to different health care agencies	• Short answer • Objective type • Essay type

Syllabus (GNM)

Unit	Learning objective	Contents	Hrs	Teaching/learning activities	Assessment methods
		• Voluntary health services • National Health Programs • Nurse role in health care services			
III	Describe health planning in India	**Health Planning in India** • National health planning • Five year plans • Health committees and reports • National health policy	10	Lecture-cum-discussion and reports	• Short answer • Essay type
IV	Describe the different specialized community health services and the nurse's role in these services	**Specialized Community Health Services and Nurse's Role** • RCH (reproductive health and child care) • National Health Mission (rural/urban) • Janani Sishu Suraksha Karaykaram (JSSK) • Emergency ambulance services. • Government health insurance schemes • School health services • Occupational health nursing (including health care providers) • Geriatric nursing • Care of differently abled-physical and mental • Rehabilitation nursing	18	Lecture-cum-discussion Visit to different agencies of specialized services, factory, Old age home, homes for the differently abled	Short answer Objective type Essay type
V	Describe the major health problems in India	**National Health Problems** • Health problems in India • Communicable diseases • Non communicable diseases • Nutritional problems • Environmental sanitation • Population	5	Lecture-cum-discussion Quiz	Short answer Objective type
VI	Describe the national health and family welfare programs in India and the role of the nurse	**National Health Program:** • National ARI program • Revised national tuberculosis control program (RNTCP) • National anti-malaria program • National filarial control program • National guinea worm eradication program • National leprosy eradication program • National AIDS control program • STD control program • National program for control of blindness • Iodine deficiency control program • Expanded program of immunization • National family welfare program • National water supply and sanitation program • Minimum needs program • National diabetes control program • Polio eradication : pulse program, NPSP • National cancer control program • Yaws eradication program • National nutritional anemia prophylaxis program • 20 point program • ICDS program • Mid-day meal program	15	Lecture-cum-discussion Government of India program flyers	Short answer Objective type

Syllabus (GNM)

Unit	Learning objective	Contents	Hrs	Teaching/learning activities	Assessment methods
		• National mental health program • Adolescent health program • Role of nurse in the national health programme			

VII	Explain the meaning of demography and describe the national family welfare programs	**Demography and Family Welfare**
		• Demography
		  ▪ Concept
		  ▪ Trends in the world and in India
		  ▪ Concept of fertility and infertility
		  ▪ Small family norm
		• Family Welfare
		  ▪ Concept, importance, aims and objectives
		  ▪ Family planning methods
		  ▪ Family planning counseling
		  ▪ National family Welfare Policy
		  ▪ National family Welfare Programme
		  ▪ Role of a nurse in the family planning programme
			18	• Lecture-cum-discussion
				• Show and explain family planning devices
				• Role play
				• Demonstration
					• Short answer
					• Objective type
					• Essay type

VIII	Describe the concept and functions of health team and the role of nursing personnel at various levels	**Health Team**
		• Concept
		  ▪ Composition
		  ▪ Functions
		• Role of Nursing personnel at various levels:
		  ▪ District Public Health Nursing Officer
		  ▪ Block health Nurse
		  ▪ Public Health Nurse
		  ▪ Lady Health Visitor/health supervisor
		  ▪ Health worker female/ANM
			7	Lecture-cum-discussion
				
				Interaction with health team members: Job description as per the Indian Public Health Standards (IPHS)
					• Short answer
					• Objective type
					• Essay type

IX	Explain the concept and uses of health information system	**Health Information System** • Concepts, components, uses, sources. • Vital statistics: ▪ Important rates and indicators • Vital health records and their uses. • Basic statistical methods • Descriptive statistics	6	Lecture-cum-discussion Exercises	• Short answer • Objective type • Exercises

X	Describe the national and international health agencies	**Health Agencies**
		• International:
		  ▪ WHO
		  ▪ UNFPA
		  ▪ UNDP
		  ▪ World bank
		  ▪ FAO
		  ▪ UNICEF
		  ▪ DANIDA
		  ▪ European commission (EU)
		  ▪ Red cross
		  ▪ USAID
		  ▪ UNESCO
		  ▪ ILO
		  ▪ CARE
		• National:
		  ▪ Indian Red Cross
		  ▪ Indian Council for child welfare
		  ▪ Family Planning association of India
		  ▪ Other NGOs
			3	Lecture-cum-discussion
				
				Seminar
					• Short answer
					• Objective type

CHAPTER 1

Role of Community Health Nurse in Management of Emergencies and Common Disorders

CHAPTER OUTLINE

1.1 Fundamentals of health assessment and examination
1.2 Management of common emergencies including first aid
1.3 Basics of primary care of common disorders

1.1 FUNDAMENTALS OF HEALTH ASSESSMENT AND EXAMINATION

GENERAL SCREENING

Health assessment is the evaluation of the health status by performing a physical examination after taking a health history.

Purposes of Health Assessment

- To identify the patient's response to health and illness
- To determine the nursing care needs of the patient
- To evaluate outcomes of healthcare and patient progress
- To screen for presence of risk factors.

Preparation for health assessment: It includes infection control, preparation of environment, equipment and patient.

Infection Control

- Use standard precautions as appropriate
- Use personal protective equipment (gloves, mask, etc.)
- Perform hand hygiene
- Utilize clean instruments.

Preparation of Environment
- Ensure adequate lighting and no noise inside the examination room
- Use special examination tables as needed
- Ensure adequate privacy (curtains).

Preparation of Equipment
- Collect and arrange all functional equipment
- Warm equipment before use, if required
- Equipment usually collected are thermometer, sphygmomanometer, stethoscope, cotton balls, tongue depressor, reflex hammer, swab stick, tuning fork, etc.

Preparation of the Patient
- Ensure physical comfort and proper position
- Dress and drape patient appropriately
- Explain the procedure
- Clarify doubts to reduce anxiety
- Provide chaperone when the patient is of the opposite gender of the nurse
- Assist patient to restroom prior to examination and collect samples (urine/stool) if required.

Methods of Physical Assessment
- **Inspection:** It is the use of vision and hearing to detect normal and abnormal findings. It provides so many useful information of different system like shape, position, size, and symmetry of the body parts.
- **Palpation:**
  - It is the use of the hands and the sense of touch to get the information. The purpose is to assess the texture, tenderness, temperature, size, distention, pulsation, and mobility of organs or masses.
  - **Types of palpation**: Light palpation (<1 cm), Moderate palpation (1-2 cm) and Deep palpation (2 cm) and Bimanual Palpation and palpation with single hand.
- **Percussion:**
  - It means tapping of various body organs and structures to produce vibration and sound.
  - **Types of percussion:** Direct percussion and Indirect (use of plexor and pleximeter) percussion.
  - **The purpose** is to determine the location, size and density of underlying tissue structures and if tissue is fluid filled, air filled or solid.
  - **Sounds heard:** Dullness (organs), resonance (lungs filled with air), hyper-resonance (emphysematous lung), tympany (air filled stomach), flatness (muscle or bone).
- **Auscultation:**
  - The act of listening to sounds within the body to evaluate the condition of body organs can be performed with stethoscope.
  - Sounds:
    - *Pitch:* The frequency of the vibrations (ranging from high to low)
    - *Intensity:* The loudness or softness of a sound
    - *Duration:* The sound length (short, medium, or long)
    - *Quality:* Subjective description of sounds (gurgling, swishing)

- **Olfaction:** It is the use of sense of smell to perceive and differentiate odors. Example: Acetone breath in diabetic ketoacidosis.

GENERAL EXAMINATION

Built
- It is the skeletal structure in relation to age and gender of the individual as compared to a normal person.
- Tall child means when the height is greater than 2 standard deviations above the mean for the age.
- Dwarfism is the term applied when the patient's height is less than 2 standard deviations for the age.
- Anthropometric measurements: Measurement of height, weight and BMI.

Cyanosis
- It is a bluish discoloration of the nails due to increased amount of deoxygenated hemoglobin (more than 5 mg%) in capillary blood.
- **Types:** Central, peripheral and cyanosis due to abnormal pigments.
- Causes of cyanosis
  - **Central:**
    - *Cardiac:* Congenital, cyanotic heart disease, congestive cardiac failure.
    - *Pulmonary:* Chronic obstructive lung disease, collapse and fibrosis of lung, pulmonary AV fistula.
    - Abdominal hepatopulmonary syndrome.
    - High altitude due to low partial pressure of oxygen.
  - **Peripheral:** Cold (local vasoconstriction), increased viscosity of blood, shock.

Jaundice
- It is characterized by yellow coloration of tissues and body fluids due to an increase in bile pigments. It may arise due to increased bile pigment load to the liver, bilirubin diffusion into the liver cells, defective conjugation, defective excretion.
- **Cause:** Cirrhosis, viral hepatitis, Weil's disease, etc.

Pallor
- Paleness of skin and mucous membrane either as a result of diminished circulating red blood cells or diminished blood supply.
- **Cause:** Deficiency of iron, folic acid or vitamin B_{12}, chronic infection, malignancies, anemia.

Lymphadenopathy
- It is inflammatory or non-inflammatory enlargement of lymph nodes.
- **Cause:** Tuberculosis, lymphadenitis, Hodgkin's disease, non-Hodgkin's lymphoma.

Edema

It is the collection of fluid in the interstitial spaces or serous cavities.

Causes
- **Bilateral edema:**
  - Cardiac: CCF, LVF, pericarditis
  - Renal: Acute nephritis, nephrotic syndrome
  - Hepatic: Cirrhosis of liver, portal hypertension
  - Venous: Inferior vena cava obstruction
  - Endocrine: Myxedema
- **Unilateral edema:**
  - Lymphatic: Filariasis, pressure by new growth, metastasis, radiation
  - Traumatic: Bruises, sprains, fractures
  - Infections: Cellulitis, boils, carbuncle
  - Metabolic: Gout
  - Venous: Venous thrombosis, varicose veins

Skin

- Dry skin is seen in myxedema and dehydration.
- Moist skin occurs when there is profuse perspiration as in shock, following myocardial infarction and thyrotoxicosis.
- Pinched skin suggests dehydration.
- Thick skin occurs in myxedema, acromegaly and scleroderma.
- Thin skin occurs in old age.

Hair

- Loss of outer third of the eyebrows: Leprosy, myxedema.
- Falling of hair: Following any infectious disease, nutritional deficiency.
- Patchy hair loss: Alopecia areata, syphilis.
- Absence of axillary, pubic and facial hair: Hypopituitarism, hypogonadism.
- Excessive hair growth in women: Cushing's syndrome, adrenocortical syndrome.

Nails

- Pallor
- Koilonychia: Spoon-shaped deformity in iron deficiency anemia.
- Onychia: Deformity of the nail, e.g. following fungal or tuberculous infection.
- Discoloration occurs in Raynaud's disease and silver and mercury poisoning.

Clubbing: Bulbous enlargement of soft parts of the terminal phalanges with both transverse and longitudinal curving of the nails.

Causes of clubbing
- Pulmonary: Bronchogenic carcinoma, bronchiectasis, mesothelioma, empyema, lung abscess, diffuse fibrosing alveolitis
- Cardiac: Cyanotic congenital heart diseases, infective endocarditis

- Alimentary: Crohn's disease, ulcerative colitis, cirrhosis
- Endocrine: Thyroid acropachy, myxedema.

Vitals Sign

Temperature
- The body temperature is kept within the normal level by maintaining a balance between the heat gain and heat loss, which is regulated by the hypothalamus. The normal body temperature varies from 36°C–37.5°C.
- Recorded with a mercury thermometer in the axilla or oral. However, if there is a lot of perspiration, oral temperature should be taken.

Pulse
It is a wave which is felt by the finger, produced by cardiac systole travelling in the peripheral direction in the arterial tree at a rate faster than the column of blood. Normal range 60–90 per min.

Respiratory Rate
The normal rate in adults is 16–20 respirations per minute.

Blood Pressure
Systolic BP is controlled by the stroke volume of the heart and the stiffness of the arterial vessels. Diastolic BP is controlled by the peripheral resistance. Normal range 120–80 mm Hg. Measured by mercury sphygmomanometer.

Examination of Head and Neck
- **Face and skull**
  - Inspection: The size, shape and symmetry of the face and skull, facial movements.
  - Palpation: The presence of any lumps, soreness, and masses are assessed.
- **Eyes**
  - Conjunctiva color, any visible capillaries, any ulcer
  - Sclera any discoloration, pigmentation
  - Cornea is transparent, any irregularities, check for corneal reflex
  - Pupils in reference to their bilateral equality, reaction to light and accommodation, the presence of any discharge, irritation, redness and abnormal eye movement are assessed.
  - Eyelid symmetrical or not, observe for ptosis
  - Use the snellen chart for visual acuity.
- **Ears**
  - The auricles are inspected in terms of color, symmetry, and any tenderness or lesions;
  - The external ear canal is inspected for color and the presence of any discharge and ear wax; and
  - The tympanic membrane in terms of color, and the lack of any bulging is also assessed through otoscope.
  - Standardized testing: The rinne test and the weber test for the assessment of hearing can be done using a tuning fork.

- **Nose**
  - Inspection: The color, size, shape, symmetry, and presence of any discharge, flaring, tenderness, and masses are assessed; nasal septum
  - Palpation: The sinuses are assessed for any signs of tenderness.
- **Mouth and throat**
  - The lips, the buccal membranes, the gums and the tongue are inspected for color, any lesions and their level of dryness or moisture; presence of teeth or missing teeth, dental carries; the uvula is assessed for movement, position; the oropharynx, tonsils, hard and soft palates are also inspected for redness and any lesions.
- **Neck**
  - Inspection: The neck and head movement; the thyroid gland is inspected for any swelling and also for normal movement during swallowing. Jugular venous distension
  - Palpation: Trachea, thyroid gland and lymph nodes.

SYSTEMIC EXAMINATION

Cardiovascular System Examination

Inspection
- **Precordium**
- **Flattened** precordium found if congenital deformity or pulmonary fibrosis.
- **Bulging** precordium present during pleural effusion, tumor, cardiomegaly, pericardial effusion.
- **Apex beat:** It is present in fifth left intercostal space inside the midclavicular line.
- Scars of any surgery.

Palpation
- Apex beat
- Thrills are associated heart murmur.

Percussion
It is done to determine the heart border of cardiac dullness. It may be changed or shifted during pulmonary effusion, cardiac enlargement.

Auscultation
- It is done for heart sounds and cardiac murmur (abnormal heart sound) in all anatomical areas aortic, pulmonic, mitral and tricuspid.
- Aortic valve (right 2nd ICS sternal border), pulmonary valve (left 2nd ICS sternal border), tricuspid valve (left 5th ICS sternal border), mitral valve (left 5th ICS midclavicular line)
- First heart sound S1 is loud and single. It occurs due to closure of mitral and tricuspid valve. Loudest at the apex.
- Second heart sound S2 produced by closure of aortic and pulmonary valve.

- Third heart sound S3 is low frequency sound and produced by rapid filling phase blood flows from atria to ventricle.
- Fourth heart sound S4 produced by rapid emptying of atrium into ventricle but inaudible.

Respiratory System Examination

Inspection
- Shape of chest: The anterior and posterior thorax and transverse diameters: Normally bilaterally symmetrical shape. Abnormal shape like barrel shaped chest (in emphysema), funnel shaped (pectus excavatum), etc.
- Observe subcostal angle, shoulders, misalignment of the spine, presence of any lesion, bulging or flattening of chest wall, position of mediastinum
- Respiratory movements, respiratory rate, rhythm
- Character: Abdominal, thoracic, thoracoabdominal or abdominothoracic
- Intercostal retraction
- Apex pulsation, scar, dilated vein.

Palpation
- The posterior thorax is assessed for respiratory excursion and tactile vocal fremitus (perception of vibration during act of phonation).
- Check tenderness.

Percussion
- It is done to assess normal (resonance note) and abnormal sounds over the thorax
- It is done in anterior region for intercostal resonance, clavicular percussion, liver dullness, cardiac dullness and in posterior region over suprascapular, interscapular and infrascapular region
- Impaired note and dull note is found when pulmonary fibrosis, consolidation. Hyperresonance note is occurred in emphysema, pneumothorax.

Auscultation
- The assessment of normal and abnormal breath sounds.
- Normal breath sounds like vesicular breath sounds, bronchial breath sounds, bronchovesicular breath sounds.
- Rales, rhonchi or wheezes, pleural friction rubs, stridor and abnormal bronchophony, egophony, and whispered pectoriloquy are auscultated.
- Vocal resonance (laryngeal vibration audible through stethoscope).

Alimentary System Examination
- **Oral cavity:** Teeth, tongue, tonsils, oropharynx

- **Abdomen:**

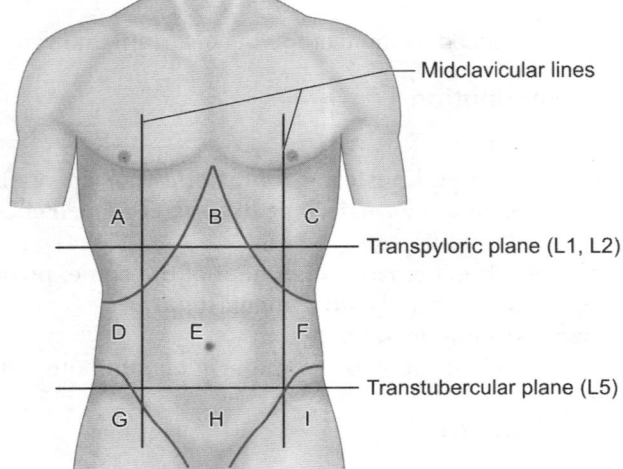

Fig. 1.1: Abdominal region.

- A-Right hypochondriac region: Liver, gallbladder, right kidney
- B-Epigastric region: Liver, stomach, duodenum, pancreas
- C-Left hypochondriac region: Spleen, stomach (fundus), tip of liver, left kidney, pancreas
- D-Right lumbar region: Ascending colon, right kidney, small intestine
- E-Umbilical region: Small intestine, transverse colon, duodenum
- F-Left lumbar region: Left kidney, small intestine, descending colon
- G-Right iliac region: Appendix, cecum, ascending colon, small intestine
- H-Hypogastric region: Bladder, small intestine, uterus (pregnant)
- I-Left iliac region: Sigmoid colon, descending colon, small intestine

Inspection

- Shape of abdomen: Normally scaphoid or boat shaped.
- Variation can be found when there is fluid, fat, full bladder, feces, fetus, fatal new growth.
- Umbilicus: Centrally situated and inverted.
- Pulsation: Normally not present. It is present during aortic aneurysm and some transmitted pulsation from tumor
- Abdominal movement: During inspiration bulges and during expiration fall.
- Observe hernia site and any peristalsis movement
- Dilated vein visible during venous obstruction.
- Observe abdominal skin for scar of previous surgery.

Palpation

- **Tenderness:** Pain when affected area is touched.
- It is commonly found when inflammation is present.
- For purpose of diagnosis, check the site o tenderness like appendicitis (right iliac fossa), peptic ulcer (epigastrium), hepatitis (right hypochondrium).
- Check the guarding and rigidity. Both are due to muscular contraction but rigidity cannot be voluntarily relaxed.
- Palpation of enlargement of spleen, liver and kidney.

Percussion
Fluid thrill and dullness is found during ascities. Dull sound on liver and spleen.

Auscultation
Bowel sound (peristalsis) and arterial bruit sound (in atherosclersosis).

Miscellaneous
Abdominal girth, per rectal examination, proctoscopy.

Central Nervous System Examination
- **Neurological assessment**
- **Consciousness:** It is a state of awareness of one's self and one's environment.
- Pathological state like drowsiness, stupor, semicoma, coma
- Observe delusion (false beliefs), delirium (confusion state), insight, dementia, hallucination (false perception)
- Balance and gait
- Speech or language disorder (due to lesion in dominant hemisphere)
- Tone of muscle (muscle resistance)
- Rigidity and spasticity
- Reflex is an automatic muscular response to the stimulus. Superficial reflexes and deep reflexes
- Example: Pupil reflex, blinking reflex, gag reflex, abdominal reflex, plantar reflex and crematic reflex, biceps reflex, triceps reflex, brachioradialis reflex, quadriceps reflex and Achilles reflex (calcaneal), knee jerk reflex
- Gross and fine motor function
- Sensory function (touch, temperature), kinesthetic sensations
- **Cranial nerve examination:**

Cranial nerve		Major functions		Assessment
Cranial nerve I	Olfactory	Sensory	Smell	Smell—coffee, cloves, peppermint
Cranial nerve II	Optic	Sensory	Vision	• Visual acuity—Snellen chart (cover eye not being examined) • Test for visual fields • Examine with ophthalmoscope
Cranial nerve III	Oculomotor	Primarily motor	Eyelid and eyeball movement	• Move eye up, down, and peripherally • Test for accommodation • Pupillary constriction • Observe for ptosis of upper eyelid
Cranial nerve IV	Trochlear	Primarily motor	• Innervates superior oblique eye muscle • Turns eye downward and laterally	Inferior lateral movement of the eye

Cranial nerve		Major functions		Assessment
Cranial nerve V	Trigeminal	Sensory and motor	Chewing Face and mouth Touch and pain	• Corneal reflex • Sensation of skin of the face (eyebrow, cheeks and chin) by using a wisp of cotton • Chewing, biting, lateral jaw movements (move jaw side to side)
Cranial nerve VI	Abducens	Primarily motor	• Turns eye laterally • Proprioception (sensory awareness of part of the body)	Inferior lateral eye movements
Cranial nerve VII	Facial	Sensory and motor	• Controls most facial expressions • Secretion of ears and saliva	• Taste—anterior two-thirds of tongue; sweet—sugar; salty; sour—lemon; bitter (rinse mouth between applications) • Movement of forehead and mouth • Raise eyebrows, show teeth, smile, and puff out cheeks
Cranial nerve VIII	Vestibulocochlear (auditory)	Sensory	• Hearing • Equilibrium sensation	• Hearing, balance • Weber and Rinne tests • Otoscope
Cranial nerve IX	Glossopharyngeal	Sensory and motor	• Taste • Senses carotid blood pressure • Muscle sense – proprioception, sensory awareness of the body	• Swallowing and phonation • Taste—posterior one third of tongue; (see cranial nerve VII)
Cranial nerve X	Vagus	Sensory and motor	• Senses aortic blood pressure • Slows heart rate • Stimulates digestive organs • Taste	• Sensations of posterior one-third of tongue, throat. • Gag reflex (stimulate back of pharynx with a tongue blade) • Swallowing and phonation
Cranial nerve XI	Spinal accessory	Primarily motor	• Controls trapezius and sternoclei-domastoid controls swallowing movements • Muscle sense - proprioception	Shoulder movement, shoulder shrug, head rotation—push against examiner's hand
Cranial nerve XII	Hypoglossal	Primarily motor	• Controls tongue movements • Muscle sense-proprioception	Tongue movement—protrude tongue, push tongue into the cheek

BIBLIOGRAPHY

1. https://www.indiannursingcouncil.org/uploads/pdf/1653647581794.pdf
2. https://lms.rn.com/courses/2051/presentation_content/external_files/Cranial%20Nerve%20Chart.pdf

Role of Community Health Nurse in Management of Emergencies and Common Disorders

1.2 MANAGEMENT OF COMMON EMERGENCIES INCLUDING FIRST AID

- Nurses play an important role in early identification of life-threatening situations, assist Medical Officer in providing advanced care management.
- In cases which need to be referred to a higher facility, provide first aid and stabilize the victim before referring to a higher center.
- Medical emergencies often require urgent interventions even before a specific diagnosis is made and a presentation-based approach is essential. So, knowledge about a general approach that can be used for every medical emergency which would rapidly assess and manage immediate life threats which would allow for a safer transfer of patient.

GENERAL APPROACH TO ANY EMERGENCY

AVPU Scale

- Check the responsiveness of the patient (unconscious or altered mental status or hyperactive delirium or comatose)
- For evaluation of critical illness, **AVPU scale** is used. It gives you an idea how serious the condition of the patient is.
- **A: Alert**: The person is aware and is responding to the surrounding on their own. The person will also be able to follow instructions, open eyes spontaneously, and track objects.
- **V: Verbally responsive**: The person is not alert. On calling the person's name or on trying to talk to the person, they will respond by opening eyes, may talk few words. They close eyes and then stop responding. They are responding to 'VERBAL' stimuli.
- **P: Responsive to pain**: The person's eyes do not open on their own and will only respond if a painful stimulus is given by pinching the shoulder muscles (do not poke or put pressure to the chest). The victim may move or cry out directly in response to the painful stimuli for a moment and then closes eyes.
- **U: Unresponsive/unconscious**: The victim does not respond spontaneously and does not respond to verbal or painful stimuli.

ABCDE Approach

- This approach helps in rapid assessment and recognition of critical illness.
- This standard protocol offers a consistent and reproducible framework for evaluation and management of the critically ill patient.
- This sequence has minor variations in certain scenarios as follows:
  - **ABC** in non-trauma medical emergencies.
  - **CAB** in patients with cardiac arrest where addressing C is a priority. CAB is the standard sequence recommended for CPR.
  - **(H) ABCDE** only in trauma cases where H stands for management of life-threatening Hemorrhage.

(H) Hemorrhage

- **Controllable:** Usually in the extremities in leg and hands and it can be controlled with compression (pressure) which prevents further blood loss.

- **Internal bleeding**: Abdomen, chest and pelvis. It cannot be controlled with pressure. This uncontrollable bleeding can only be stopped by a surgery. So stabilize the patients and immediately refer.

A: AIRWAY

Assessment
- Can the patient talk normally? If YES, the airway is open
- If the patient cannot talk: Assess if the chest wall is moving and listen to see if there is air movement from the mouth or nose
- Listen for abnormal sounds (stridor/grunting) or a hoarseness of voice that indicates a partial airway obstruction.
- Look and listen for fluid (such as blood, vomit) in the airway and look for foreign body.
- Check for cervical spine injury.

Management
- If the airway is not patent (patient is unconscious and not normally breathing): Open the airway using the head-tilt and chin-lift maneuver. Place an oropharyngeal or nasopharyngeal airway to maintain the airway.
- If a foreign body is suspected:
  - If the object is visible, remove it
  - Be careful not to push the object any deeper and encourage coughing
  - If the patient is unable to cough, not making sounds (choking), use age-appropriate chest thrusts/ abdominal thrusts/back blows.
  - If the patient becomes unconscious while choking, start BLS (Basic Life Support)
- If secretions or vomit are present, suction when available, or wipe clean.
- Placing the patient in the recovery position.
- If the patient has swelling, rashes, consider severe allergic reaction (anaphylaxis), and give intramuscular adrenaline (0.3–0.5 mg, 1:1000).

B: BREATHING

Assessment
- Look, listen and feel to see if the patient is breathing.
- Assess if breathing is very fast, very slow, or very shallow and with any abnormal sound.
- Asses for signs of increased work of breathing (such as accessory muscle use, chest indrawing/retractions, nasal flaring) or abnormal chest wall movement.
- Listen to see if breath sounds are equal on both sides.
- Check for the absence of breath sounds and dull sounds with percussion on one side then it may be due to large pleural effusion and if no breath sounds on one side and distended neck veins or a shifted trachea then it may be due to tension pneumothorax.
- Check oxygen saturation with a pulse oximeter when available.

Management

- If unconscious with abnormal breathing, start bag-valve-mask ventilation and check for pulse.
- If not breathing adequately (too slow for age or too shallow), begin bag-valve-mask ventilation with oxygen. If oxygen not immediately available, DO NOT DELAY ventilation. Start ventilation while oxygen is being prepared
- If severe allergic reaction (anaphylaxis), give intramuscular adrenaline (0.3–0.5 mg, 1:1000)
- If concern for large pleural effusion or hemothorax, give oxygen and refer.

C: CIRCULATION

Assessment

- Look and feel for signs of poor perfusion or shock [cool extremities, delayed capillary refill (greater than 3 seconds), low blood pressure, tachypnea, tachycardia, absent pulses].
- Check and record heart rate and blood pressure and listen heart sounds.
- Look for both external and internal bleeding.

Management

- If signs of poor perfusion, give IV fluids and oxygen.
- For external bleeding, apply direct pressure or use other technique to control.
- If internal bleeding or pericardial tamponade are suspected then transfer patient rapidly to nearby center where surgical facilities are available.
- If cause unknown, remember the possibility of occult bleeding like gastrointestinal bleed or ectopic pregnancy in female patients.

D: DISABILITY

Assessment

- Assess level of consciousness with the AVPU scale (Alert, Voice, Pain, Unresponsive)
- Assess pupillary size and reaction
- Check blood glucose level
- Check movement and sensation in all four limbs
- Look for abnormal repetitive movements or seizure/convulsion.

Management

- If altered mental status, place the patient in recovery position and take care of the airway while transportation.
- If blood glucose is low (<50 mg/dL) or glucose test not available and patient has altered mental status, give intravenous 25% dextrose 100 mL.
- For active seizures, place the patient in recovery position, prevent trauma and after teleconsult give a benzodiazepine.
- If pregnant and having seizures, after teleconsult give magnesium sulfate.
- If pupils are not equal, consider increased pressure on the brain and raise head of bed 30° and rapid transfer to nearest center with facility for neurosurgical care.

E: EXPOSURE

To examine the patient full exposure of the body is necessary (along with ensuring the prevention of hypothermia) as it makes easier to know the extent of injury, any fracture or any bleeding areas. If referral is required then put the patient is in recovery position.

BASICS OF COMMON MEDICAL/SURGICAL EMERGENCIES

Trauma and Accidents

- Trauma or accident is the **most common** type of emergency. There are two modes of stabilization for prevention of death.
  1. Immobilization
  2. Control of bleeding
- **Major bleeding wounds:**
  - Find the source of bleeding, if the bleeding is near the area of the mouth or neck, it is possible that it could cause airway blockage.
  - Expose the area: Open or remove the clothing over the wound.
  - Bleeding may be controlled by applying direct pressure, applying pressure bandage, elevation of the body part above level of heart, pressure over the major arteries (pressure points).
  - Do not move the limb if you suspect any fractures.
  - As soon as bleeding is controlled, apply dressing and observe for shock.
  - Secure IV access and IV fluids.
- **Minor wounds:**
  - If a patient with a minor cut or wound, ensure the safety of the victim and wash your hands well before touching the injured area of the victim.
  - If the wound is dirty, wash it thoroughly with soap and sterile normal saline, then apply firm pressure for around 5 minutes. This will stop most bleeding.
  - Elevate the wound, above the level of the heart if possible. When bleeding has reduced, clean the area with the antiseptic lotion and keep it dry.
  - Use a sterile dressing to avoid touching the wound directly
  - Administer a dose of Td injection.
  - Give antibiotic such as amoxicillin 500 mg, 8 hourly for 5 days if needed.
  - If at risk of infection administer IV Penicillin G and metronidazole as per instructions by PHC medical officer.
  - Deep gaped wound with exposed fat or muscle will need to be sutured. If gap is more refer as soon as possible.
  - Whenever head injury, spinal injury, fracture or any severe condition then provide first aid and refer the patient to higher center.

Fracture

- Common signs of a fracture are:
  - Painful and difficult or impossible normal movement of the limb.
  - Deformity, abnormal twist or shortening of limb.
  - Tenderness at the site of fracture and swelling over and around the fracture.
  - Bruising at the site of fracture.
  - Crepitation sound if one end of the bone moves against the other.

Role of Community Health Nurse in Management of Emergencies and Common Disorders

- **Management: RICER (Rest, Ice, Compression, Elevation and Referral).** It is a first aid technique used within first 48 hours after fracture or sprain or strain. It limits swelling and help in fast recovery.
- **Example:** Here in cases of any trauma/accidents/fracture wound assessment and need of TT/Td vaccine can be decided based on **Figure 1.2**.

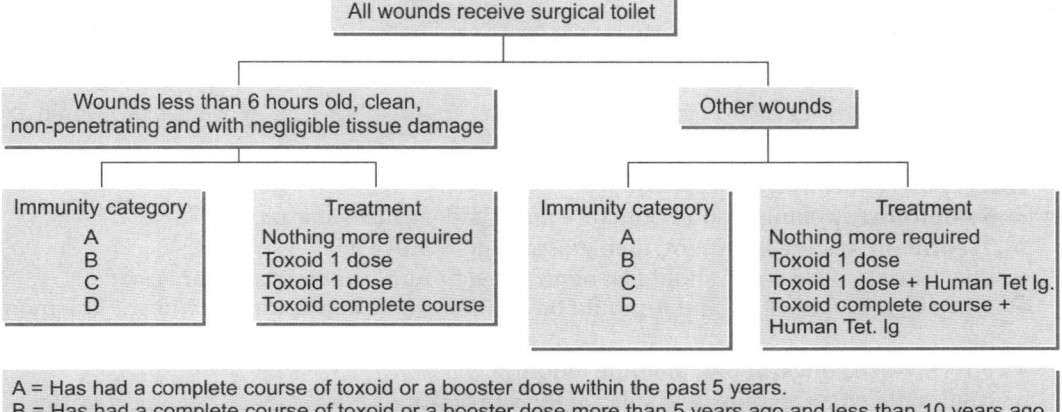

Fig. 1.2: Wound management with the context of TT/Td.

Bite

- **Scorpion bite:**
  - **Mild form**: Burning pain or numbness, itching and swelling near the site of bite
  - **Severe form:** Restlessness, lacrimation, nausea, vomiting, sweating, chest pain, palpitation, difficulty in breathing.
  - **Treatment:** Apply a tourniquet proximal to the site of sting and release it every 5–10 minutes for a few seconds to prevent gangrene formation. Apply ice packs/cold compress on the region to slow down the absorption of poison.
  - Give ibuprofen tablet to relieve pain and swelling and antihistamine for allergy.
  - Give 'Ring Block' at site of bite to decrease the pain. Give inj. lignocaine 2% (without adrenaline) locally surrounding the bite site from all sides. Assess for sign of shock and if condition worsens then refer to higher center.
- **Animal bite (dog, cat, monkey and wild animals):**
  - Thoroughly wound toileting (at least for 15 minutes) with soap and water as soap has very good effect against rabies virus as it contains lipid layer.
  - Nothing should be applied over wound like cow dung or chilly.
  - Apply antiseptic solution, such as povidone iodine.
  - There should be no suture of wound.
  - Give Td injection, analgesic and anti-inflammatory medicine
  - Administer antirabies vaccine and rabies immune globulin based on wound category.

- Example: Animal bite categories for PEP-ARV:

Category	Type of contact	Type of exposure	Management
I	Touching or feeding of animals, licks on intact skin	None	None, if reliable history is available
II	Nibbling of uncovered skin, minor scratches or abrasions without bleeding	Minor	• Wound management • Antirabies vaccine
III	• Single or multiple transdermal bites or scratches • Licks on broken skin • Contamination of mucous membrane with saliva	Severe	• Wound management • Rabies immunoglobulins • Antirabies vaccine

- **Insect bites (Bee/wasp, jelly fish):**
  - **Symptoms**: Swelling around puncture point and it causes sharp pain.
  - **Treatment**: If sting is present, then grasp it and remove it.
  - Bee venom is acid and it should be neutralized by application of ammonia, soda.
  - Wasp venom is alkaline and it should be neutralized by application of vinegar or lemon juice.
  - For jelly-fish stings, apply calamine lotion.
  - Apply cold compressions and spirit at the site of sting.
  - Give antihistamine (avil/pheniramine tablet/injection) for allergy.
  - Give ibuprofen tablet to relieve pain and swelling.
- **Snake-bite:**
  - Two puncture wound indicates bite mark of snake.
  - Snake bite leads to burning and throbbing pain. Local swelling develops immediately and sometimes spread to the whole limb which may sometimes lead to necrosis.
  - **Treatment:** Administer antivenom to the victim. Keep under observation for 24 hours.
  - **RIGHT** approach:
    - **R**: Reassure the person (70% of snakebites are from non-poisonous snakes and only 50% poisonous snakes inject poison).
    - **I**: Immobilize the affected body part of the person.
    - **GH**: Get to the hospital immediately.
    - **T**: Tell the doctor about presence of any symptoms (pain, weakness, bleeding, etc.).

Stroke

- **Symptoms (NEW FAST):**
  - **N:** Nausea, vomiting
  - **E:** Eyes—double vision, field cut, neglect, nystagmus
  - **W:** Walking—difficulty in walking
  - **F:** Facial droop—one side of the face is droopy
  - **A:** Arm weakness—especially one side being weak
  - **S:** Speech—slurred, confused, absent speech
  - **T:** Terrible headache, dizziness
- **Management (Fig. 1.3)**

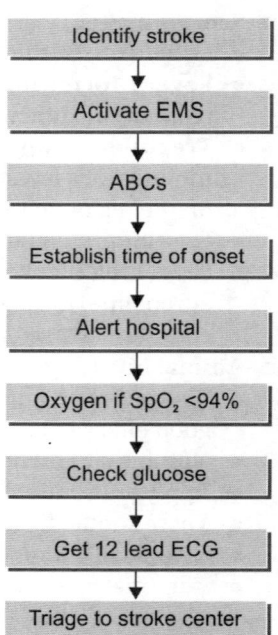

Fig. 1.3: Prehospital stroke management.

Burn

- Burn is the second most common injuries after road accidents.
- Nearly 10% burn injuries are life-threatening and require hospitalization.
- **Types:**
  - **Flame burns**: Mostly accidental, they are frequently due to leaking gas pipe or cylinder and sometimes due to use of kerosene pressure stove.
  - **Scald** is the most common cause of burns in children due to negligence by the caregiver when a small child ventures near a vessel containing hot liquid and spills it on himself or herself.
  - **Chemical burns:** They are often seen as accidental burns due to spillage of strong sulfuric acid or nitric acid.
  - **Electrical burns:** Mostly accidental, they are most commonly seen with illegal electrical wiring, defective electrical sockets, etc.
- **Rule of nine** is most popular method of describing the surface area affected by burn. In this method, body is divided into 11 equal parts making this 99% and 1% is given to perineum as shown in **Figure 1.4.**

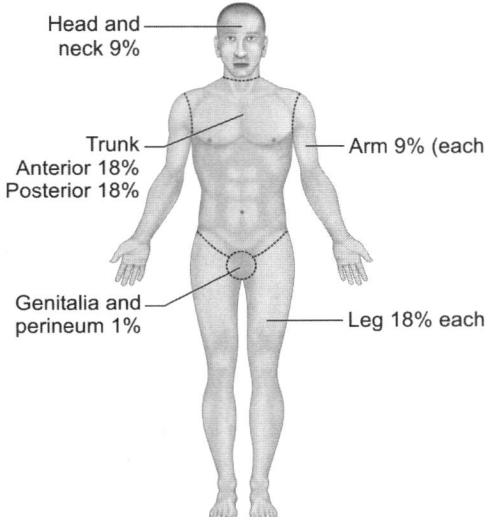

Fig. 1.4: Distribution of body parts in percentage for assessment of burn area.

- **Degree of burn:**
  - 1st degree burn is epidermal burn only–does not require treatment, heals with no scarring.
  - 2nd degree superficial burn: It is very painful. It heals in less than 2 weeks.
  - 2nd degree deep burn: It heals in 3 weeks and have less pain.
  - 3rd degree burn or full thickness burn does not heal by itself. It requires skin replacement.
- **Management:**
  - Always take the victim away from site of burns.
  - Electrical injury patients require close monitoring for cardiac arrhythmias.
  - Ensure A-Airway, B-Breathing and C-Circulation before transportation to higher center.
  - Always rule out head and cervical spinal injury before transportation.
  - In case of chemical burns, wash the wound with copious saline.

- After burns, there is massive increase in capillary permeability causing rapid escape of fluid and electrolytes into extravascular space. So, primary treatment of burns is fluid, fluid and fluid.
    - No role of colloid in first 24 hours, Ringer lactate is the intravenous fluid of choice.
    - Parkland formula most widely accepted for calculating burn resuscitation fluid is 4 X wt.(kg) X % TBSA burns.
    - Record hourly urine output, pulse rate, blood pressure.
    - Fluid to be given parenterally till patient starts taking orally adequately.
    - All burn areas are cleaned and loose dead skin is removed. Blisters are deroofed, collected plasma removed and an appropriate dressing is applied.
- All burn patients should be given tetanus prophylaxis.
- Collagen is cheap and good skin substitute for partial thickness burns. If this is not available then a non-adhesive dressing in the form of paraffin gauze impregnated with 1% Silver Sulfadiazine (SSD), colloidal silver, ionic silver cream or silver nitrate cream is applied.
- Early change of dressing is advised if dressing becomes wet, smelly, contaminated with urine or stool, any signs of infection like fever, vomiting
- Topical antibiotic creams like SSD, Soframycin, Neosporin should be used
- Biological dressings should be reserved for superficial burns especially in small children
- For full thickness burns, sequential excision and skin grafting should be done.

Acute Abdomen

- It refers to sudden, severe abdominal pain requiring immediate diagnosis and often urgent surgical intervention.
- Diagnosis is based on the location of the pain in quadrant shown in **Figure 1.5**.
- According to diagnosis provide care and refer urgently.

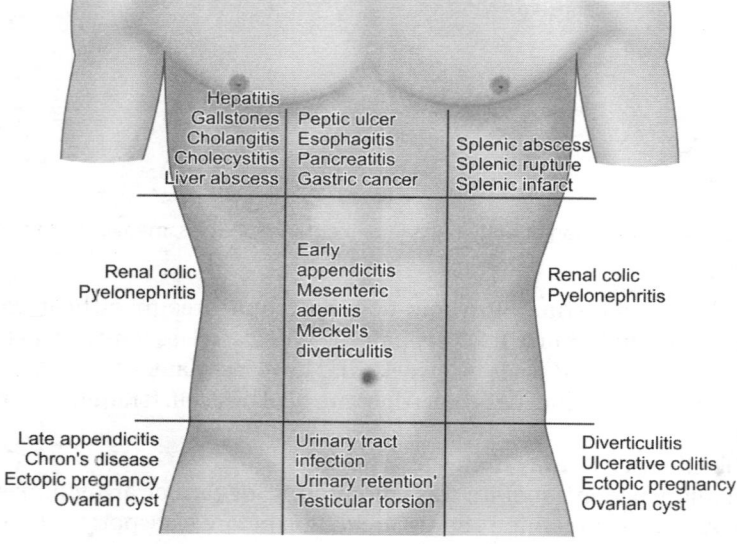

Fig. 1.5: Differential diagnosis of acute abdominal pain based on the location.

Role of Community Health Nurse in Management of Emergencies and Common Disorders

Near Drowning

- Drowning is the process of experiencing respiratory impairment from submersion/immersion in liquid.
- **Near drowning**: A person almost died from not being able to breathe (suffocating) under water.
- **Signs and symptoms of drowning victim:** No breathing, no pulse, cold and clammy skin, nail beds—slow or no circulation, mouth, nose or skin turning blue.
- Quick first aid and medical attention are very important. If no pulse and breathing: Do CPR if present, then manage accordingly.

Seizures

- **Seizures (fits):** It can occur due to many underlying medical causes.
  - **Generalized fits** involves shaking of the whole body (the person is on the floor and vigorously shaking, he/she may appear confused or may lose consciousness).
  - **Focal fits** involve only some parts of the body (the person may have repetitive movements like chewing/blinking or rhythmic twitching of any body part).
  - **Assure the following measure at the time of seizure**:
    - Keep the surrounding safe (e.g., keep pillows to avoid injury from surrounding objects).
    - To prevent tongue bite, place a clean cloth between the teeth of the patient
    - Place patient in recovery position after the fits stop and according to history manage patient shown in the following Table.

History	Possible diagnosis	Management
Head injury, history of fall down	Brain injury, intracranial hemorrhage	Manage ABCD stabilize patient and refer
History of delayed cry at the time of birth, or history of similar episodes of seizures	Congenital defects	Manage ABCDE, rule out any infection, hypoglycemia and assist doctor in treatment plan
Fever since few hours to days, with or without headache, vomiting and skin rash, with one or more episodes of seizures	Infections: • Cerebral malaria • Meningitis (Virus/bacteria/others)	• Manage ABCDE, rule out any infection, malaria and hypoglycemia. • Give first dose of IV antibiotic and refer
Additional history of common symptoms of pulmonary TB in patient or family	TB meningitis	Manage ABCDE rule out malaria and refer
Person with or without any of the above symptoms and history, and additional history of recent lethargy, sweating and palpitations or poor feeding and poor cry in children	Hypoglycemia • Mild: If RBS <70 mg/dL • Severe: If RBS <40 mg/dL	• Give Inj. Dextrose 25% 2 mL/kg IV bolus • Repeat dose if necessary, after check of RBS

Foreign Body Ingestion/Choking

- In cases of choking, the initially conduct ABCDE assessment
- There is a high risk of these objects to descend down into airway or esophagus and stomach.
- The airway may get blocked and patient could die within minutes due to choking.

- In adults, most commonly observed foreign objects stuck in throat are food particles while coins, bottle caps, batteries, etc. are commonly noted among children.
- These foreign bodies can be managed with following techniques:
  - Give 5 back blows. First, deliver five back blows between the person's shoulder blades with the heel of your hand.
  - Give 5 abdominal thrusts. Perform five abdominal thrusts (also known as the Heimlich maneuver).
  - Alternate between 5 back blows and 5 abdominal thrusts until the blockage is dislodged.
  - If the person becomes unconscious, do CPR.
  - Check the mouth for any object and if visible remove it.
  - Do not perform a blind finger sweep because this could push an object farther into the airway.

Steps to Perform the Heimlich Maneuver

- Stand behind the person. Wrap your arms around the waist of the person and tip the forward slightly.
- Make a fist with one hand. Position it slightly above the person's navel.
- Grasp the fist with the other hand. Press hard into the abdomen with a quick, upward thrust, as if trying to lift the person up.
- Perform a total of 5 abdominal thrusts, if needed. If the blockage still is not dislodged, repeat the five-and-five cycle.

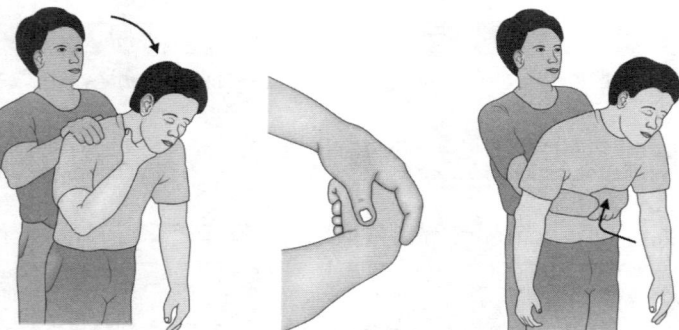

Fig. 1.6: Heimlich maneuver.

Foreign Body in the Esophagus and Stomach

If smooth objects like coins, buttons swallowed then the stomach and intestines most often adjust themselves in a way so as to expel them spontaneously. But if sharp object like pin, needle then urgent intervention required.

CARDIOPULMONARY RESUSCITATION (CPR)

CPR in Adults: Hands-only CPR

Steps	Description
Step 1	Kneel by the side of the victim
Step 2	Place the heel of one hand in the center of victim's chest
Step 3	Place the heel of your other hand on top of the first hand
Step 4	Interlock the fingers of your hands and ensure that pressure is not applied over the victim's ribs
Step 5	Position yourself vertically above the victim's chest and with your arms straight, press down on the sternum 4–5 cm
Step 6	After each compression release all the pressure on the chest without losing contact between your hands and sternum
Step 7	Repeat at the rate of minimum 100 to 120 compressions per minute (a little less than 2 compression a second)
Step 8	Compression and release should take equal amount of time.

CPR in adults with rescue breaths

- Use the heel of one or two hands for chest compression.
- Press the sternum approximately one-third the depth of the chest (about 2 inches) at the rate of least 100–120/minute.

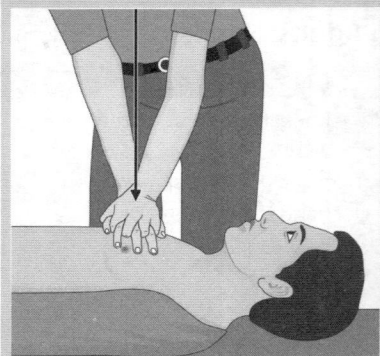

- Tilt the head back and listen for breathing. If not breathing normally, pinch nose and cover the mouth with yours and blow until you see the chest rise. Give 2 breaths. Each breath should take 1 second.

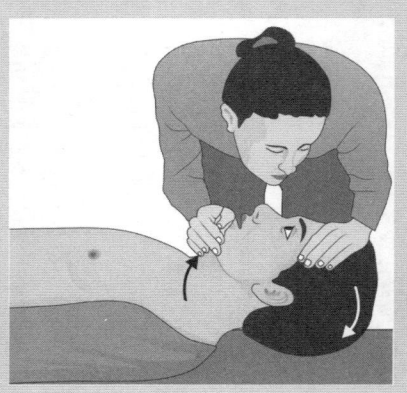

BIBLIOGRAPHY

1. https://dghs.gov.in/WriteReadData/userfiles/file/Practical_handbook-revised_Karoon.pdf
2. https://nhsrcindia.org/sites/default/files/202205/Emergency%20Module%20Staff%20Nurse_Inside_23%20March%202022.pdf
3. Supplemenatry Module on Management of Acute Simple Illnesses for Community Health Officers, MOHFW

1.3 BASICS OF PRIMARY CARE OF COMMON DISORDERS

FEVER

- Fever is technically an increased body temperature above normal (98.6°F or 37°C).
- Take history in details ask for any other complain like, chills, rigor, weakness, diarrhea, headache, cough, etc.
- Assess sign and check vital
- Take blood smear

Causes:

Short duration	
Rigors	Malaria, filariasis (lymphedema), septicemia, UTI (burning micturition), kala-azar
Chest pain, cough	Pneumonia
Rash	Chickenpox, measles, rubella, dengue hemorrhagic fever
Throat pain	Tonsillitis, diphtheria, pharyngitis
Long duration	
Cough, weight loss	Tuberculosis
Abdominal pain, rash	Typhoid
Lymphadenopathy, liver and spleen enlargement	Leukemia, lymphoma
With delirium	Meningitis, encephalitis

- **Treatment:**
  - Advise antipyretic: Tab. Paracetamol 500–650 mg oral stat; may be repeated 6–8th hourly. For children give syrup paracetamol 15 mg/kg/dose 6–8 hourly.
  - Advise cold sponging and bed rest.
  - Advise for more fluid
  - If high grade, then refer

SORE THROAT

- Take history
- Examine throat and check for redness, tonsil enlargement, white patches, ulcer, etc.
- Advise for gargle with salt and warm water
- Advise for take more fluids
- Assess for other complain and treat accordingly.
- If persist then refer to higher level.

COUGH

- Cough occurs due to inflammation of respiratory system due to allergy or infection.
- Sometimes it occurs as a defensive reflex that enhance the clearance of secretion and foreign materials.
- **Types:** Acute (up to 3 weeks), subacute (3–8 weeks), chronic (more than 8 weeks)
- **Cause:** Viral and bacterial infection, asthma, COPD, tuberculosis, foreign body, irritants
- Take coughing history: time, type, affect with position/posture
- Sputum color, amount, time
- History of difficulty in breathing, throat pain, difficulty in deglutination
- Examine throat and check for redness, tonsil enlargement, white patches, ulcer, etc.

Assessment of coughing in children:

Signs	Classify as	Management
• Genral danger signs (inability to breastfeed or drink, lethargy or reduced level of consciousness, convulsions) • Stridor in calm child	Severe pneumonia or Very severe disease	• Hospitalize • Give oxygen if saturation <90% • Manage airway • Give recommended antibiotics

• Chest indrawing
Or
• Fast breathing (respiratory rates):
  ▪ 2–11 months ≥50/min
  ▪ 12–59 months ≥40/min
	Pneumonia	• Give oral amoxicillin for 5 days
		• Treat wheeze* if present
		• Advise home care for cough and cold
		• Advise mother when to return immediately
		• Follw-up after 2 days

No signs of severe PNEUMONIA or PNEUMONIA	No pneumonia	• Advise home care for cough and cold • If coughing for more than 14 days refer for assessment • Follow-up after 5 days if not improving

* If the child has wheezing, give 3 doses of nebulized salbutamol for 20 minutes; of 2–4 puffs of salbutamol MDI (at a gap of 2–3 min between each puff) with spacer repeated every 20 minutes and reassess.

Treatment:
- Advise for gargle with salt and warm water and steam inhalation.
- Advise for take more fluids.
- Antihistaminic tab like cetirizine, levocetrizine, chlorpheniramine maleate.
- If bacterial then give antibiotics.
- If fever, then give antipyretic.
- If persist then refer to higher level for further management. Advise for sputum microscopy, CBNAAT, chest X-ray.

DYSPNEA

Causes:
- **Respiratory:** Bronchial asthma, chronic obstructive lung disease, airway obstruction, pulmonary infections, pulmonary edema, bronchogenic carcinoma, etc.
- **Cardiac:** Acute myocardial infarction, congenital cyanotic heart disease, etc.
- **Physiological:** Exercise, hyperpyrexia, mountaineers, anemia and psychogenic, anxiety
- **Treatment:** Bronchodilator, avoid overexertion and address underlying condition

EPISTAXIS

- **Causes:** Nasal trauma, tumor, sinusitis, high altitude, platelet disorder, coagulation disorder, hypertension, dry air, cold, inserting object in nose.
- Direct compression of nostril, nasal spray, nasal packing if severe then refer
- Treat according to underlying condition.

ANEMIA

- When Hb concentration decreased than normal level in red blood cell presented as anemia.

Table 1.1: Hemoglobin levels to diagnose anemia (g/dL).

Population	Anemia		
	Mild	Moderate	Severe
Children 6–59 months of age	10–10.9	7–9.9	< 7
Children 5–11 years of age	11–11.4	8–10.9	< 8
Children 12–14 years of age	11–11.9	8–10.9	< 8
Non-pregnant women (15 years of age and above)	11–11.9	8–10.9	< 8
Pregnant women	10–10.9	7–9.9	< 7
Men (15 years of age and above)	11–12.9	8–10.9	< 8

Source: WHO-Nutritional anemia: Tools for effective prevention and control, 2017

- **Cause**: Decreased RBC production, early destruction, underlying chronic disease
- Ask for other associated condition like blood in stool, blood in sputum, blood in vomitus, blood in urine, vaginal bleeding, bleeding from nose.

Treatment

- If bleeding is ongoing or frequent or in larger amounts, then:
  - Assess hemodynamic status and A-B-C
  - Give necessary resuscitation
  - Refer to CHC/DH
- If no history of bleeding, then give OPD based treatment as:
  - For intestinal worms: Albendazole 400 mg single dose
  - Antacids for gastric ulcer
  - Examine and treat simple wounds
  - Splenomegaly with anemia advice for blood tests for malaria
  - Tab. vitamin C for better absorption of iron
  - History of UTI, decreased urine output, swelling over face (Refer for further assessment of renal function)
  - Give iron supplements to treat anemia.

Treatment of Iron Deficiency Anemia among Pregnant Women

Hb level	First level of treatment	Follow-up and referral
10–10.9 g/dL (mild anemia)	Two tablets of iron and folic acid tablet (60 mg elemental iron and 500 mcg folic acid) daily, orally	• Every 2 months • 1 g/dL increase per month in Hb is expected
7–9.9 g/dL (moderate anemia)	Two tablets of iron and folic acid tablet (60 mg elemental iron and 500 mcg folic acid) daily, orally Parental iron (IV iron sucrose or fcm) may be considered (if compliance is low)	• Follow-up every two months. • If no improvement in hemoglobin (<1 g/dL increase) after two month of treatment, refer

Hb level	First level of treatment	Follow-up and referral
5.0–6.9 g/dL (severe anemia)	IV Iron sucrose/ferric carboxy maltose (FCM)	Follow-up will be on monthly basis. Severely anemic pregnant women with hemoglobin less than 5 g/dL, immediate hospitalization

Prevention of Anemia

Table 1.2: Prophylactic dose and regime for iron folic acid supplementation.

Age group	Dose and regime
Children 6–59 months of age	• Biweekly 1 mL iron and folic acid syrup. • Each mL Iron and folic acid syrup containing 20 mg elemental Iron + 100 mcg of folic acid. • Bottle (50 mL) to have an 'auto-dispenser' and information leaflet as per MoHFW guidelines in the mono-carton
Children 5–9 years of age	• Weekly, 1 iron and folic acid tablet. • Each tablet containing 45 mg elemental Iron + 400 mcg folic acid, sugar-coated, pink-color.
School-going adolescent girls and boys, 10–19 years of age Out-of-school adolescent girls, 10–19 years of age	• Weekly, 1 Iron and folic acid tablet. • Each tablet containing 60 mg elemental Iron + 500 mcg folic acid, sugar-coated, blue-color
Women of Reproductive Age (non-pregnant, non-lactating) 20-49 years (Under Mission Parivar Vikas)	Weekly, 1 Iron and Folic Acid tablet. Each tablet containing 60 mg elemental Iron + 500 mcg Folic Acid, sugar-coated and red-color
Pregnant Women and Lactating Mothers (of 0-6 months child)	• Daily, 1 iron and folic acid tablet starting from the fourth month of pregnancy (that is from the second trimester), continued throughout pregnancy (minimum 180 days during pregnancy) and to be continued for 180 days, postpartum • Each tablet containing 60 mg elemental Iron + 500 mcg folic acid, sugar-coated and red-color.

NAUSEA AND VOMITING

- Gastrointestinal causes, (e.g. peptic ulcer, infection, gastroesophageal reflux), abdominal colic, pregnancy
- Central causes (e.g. headache, motion sickness, raised intracranial pressure, inner ear problems)
- Pregnancy (hormone changes, pressure on stomach by the uterus)
- Other illnesses, (e.g. appendicitis, hepatitis, myocardial infarction, meningitis, intestinal obstruction). Drugs side effect

Treatment

Treat according to underlying cause:

Role of Community Health Nurse in Management of Emergencies and Common Disorders

❑ **If vomiting with:**
  - History of ingestion of contaminated food/water/milk: antiemetic and maintain hydration. If severe then give IV fluid for prevention of shock
  - History of abdominal pain, abdominal distension, constipation suggestive of intestinal obstruction. History of shock start IV fluid and plan urgent surgery.
  - History of accident/fell down then it is a sign of raised intracranial pressure give first aid and refer patient.
  - History of vomitus with blood, abdominal pain last 1 week suggestive of gastric ulcer: Avoid hot fluids, spicy food, advise for antacid, give more fluids if severe then refer
  - History of fever and rice water stool, blood in stool suggestive of cholera, dysentery
  - History of travel then motion sickness give T. Promethazine before travelling
  - History of pain in loin, dysuria, fever suggestive of UTI
  - History of headache, neck rigidity, fever, altered sensorium suggestive of meningitis
  - If recurrent history of then rule out pregnancy.

CONSTIPATION

❑ Take history: Since how many days, diet pattern, transportation pattern
❑ Assess any other complain like piles or anal fissure (break in anal canal skin)
❑ Advise for fiber rich foods like fruit and vegetable, drink plenty of water
❑ Mild laxative like liquid paraffin
❑ If history of pain in anal region, blood lost through stool suggestive of piles or hemorrhoids: advise for sitz bath, topical pain relievers, maintain hygiene
❑ If chronic history then rule out hypothyroidism, neurological disorder.

DIARRHEA

❑ Take history: when occurred, reason, frequency, type, watery, semisolid, stain with blood.
❑ Any associated complain like fever, vomiting, abdominal pain.
❑ Assess sign of dehydration.
❑ Advise for ORS and zinc.
❑ Advise for extra fluid like, lemon water, coconut water, juice.
❑ May advise for probiotics.
❑ If severe then admit and give injectable fluid or refer.
❑ **Types:**
  - Acute watery diarrhea—lasts several hours or days,
  - Acute bloody diarrhea—also called dysentery; and
  - Persistent diarrhea—lasts 14 days or longer.
❑ **Causes:**
  - Viruses: Rotavirus, astrovirus, adenovirus, etc.
  - Bacteria: *E. coli, Vibrio cholera, Salmonella typhi, Shigella*, etc.
  - Parasites: *E. Histolytica* (causes amoebiasis), *Giardia*
  - Chronic diseases condition also cause diarrhea like HIV/AIDS, inflammatory bowel diseases and cancers.

Assessment of Dehydration in Children

Two of the following signs:
• Movement only when stimulated or no movement even when stimulated
• Sunken eyes
• Skin pinch goes back very slowly
	Severe dehydration	• If infant does not have very severe disease:
		  ▪ Give fluid for severe dehydration (Plan C)
		  OR
		• If infant also has very severe disease:
		  ▪ Refer URGENTLY to hospital with mother giving frequent sips of ORS on the way.
		  ▪ Advise the mother to continue breastfeeding

Two of the following signs:
• Restless, irritable
• Sunken eyes
• Skin pinch goes back slowly
	Some dehydration	• Give fluid, and food for some dehydration (Plan B)
		• If infant also has very severe disease:
		  ▪ Refer URGENTLY to hospital with mother giving frequent sips of ORS on the way
		  ▪ Advise the mother to continue breast feeding
		• Advise mother when to return immediately.
		• Follow-up in 2 days if not improving

• Not enough signs to classify as some or severe dehydration	No dehydration	• Give fluids to treat diarrhea at home (Plan A) • Advise mother when to return immediately • Follow-up in 2 days if not improving

Management
❑ Oral rehydration solutions and zinc (20 mg per day for children >6 months for a period of 14 days).
❑ Early recognition of danger signs and treatment of complications.
❑ Rehydration and maintaining hydration.
❑ Ensuring adequate feeding.

Plan A: Treatment of diarrhea with no dehydration
❑ Give WHO ORS at home.
❑ ORS, home remedies like nimbu paani, dalpani, soups, juice, etc. can be used. After every episode of loose stools give fluids as given below:

Age	Amount of ORS or other culturally appropriate ORT fluids to give after each loose stool	Minimum amount of ORS to provide for use at home per day for diarrhea patient with no dehydration
<2 years	50–100 mL	500 mL/day
2–10 years	100–200 mL	1000 mL/day
>10 years	>200 mL and as required	2000 mL/day

If danger signs like refusal to feed, diarrhea beyond 3 days, increased volume/ frequency of stools, repeated vomiting, fever or blood in stools appear consult physician.

Plan B: Treatment of diarrhea with some dehydration
❑ Rehydration therapy is calculated as 75 mL/kg of ORS, to be given over 4 hr.
❑ If there is no improvement in 4 hours after 1st bolus of replacement, then repeat this amount of oral fluids again. If ORS cannot be taken orally then nasogastric tube can be used.

Plan C: Treatment of diarrhea with severe dehydration
- Ringer lactate: Dose is 100 mL/kg and out of that 30 mL/kg of IV fluids should be given over 1 hour for infants (age <12 months) and over 30 minutes for all children above age of 12 months and in adults. And rest 70 mL/kg to be given over 5 hour period in <12 months old and over 2.5 hours in children >1 year of age.

SCABIES

- It is a type of skin infection caused by small mites.
- Symptoms are severe itching, rash
- Application of permethrin cream (5%) in whole body at bed time and should be washed off next morning.
- Bedding, clothing, and towels used by infested persons be decontaminated by washing in hot water and drying.

BIBLIOGRAPHY

1. https://nhm.gov.in/index1.php?lang=1&level=1&sublinkid=197&lid=136
2. https://nhsrcindia.org/sites/default/files/202205/Emergency%20Module%20Staff%20Nurse_Inside_23%20March%202022.pdf
3. Supplementary Module on Management of Acute Simple Illnesses for Community Health Officers, MOHFW

CHAPTER 2

Reproductive, Maternal, Newborn, Child, and Adolescent Health

CHAPTER OUTLINE

- 2.1 History and current status of reproductive, maternal and child health in India
- 2.2 Basics of antenatal care
- 2.3 Basics of intranatal care
- 2.4 Basics of postnatal care
- 2.5 Basics of newborn and child care along with related programs and guidelines
- 2.6 Basics of adolescent health along with related programs and guidelines
- 2.7 Reproductive maternal newborn child adolescent health plus nutrition (RMNCAH + N)
- 2.8 Universal Immunization Program (UIP)

2.1 HISTORY AND CURRENT STATUS OF REPRODUCTIVE, MATERNAL AND CHILD HEALTH IN INDIA

HISTORY OF VARIOUS PROGRAMS/STRATEGIES/ ACTS FOR THE MATERNAL AND CHILD HEALTH

Year	Act/program/plan/other
1951	• National Family Planning Program
1956	• The Immoral Traffic Act
1961	• Dowry Prohibition Act • Maternity Benefit Act
1962	• School Health Program
1966	• Department of Family Planning Constituted
1969	• The Central Birth and Death Registration Act (1969)
1970	• All India Hospital (Postpartum) Family Planning Program

Reproductive, Maternal, Newborn, Child, and Adolescent Health

Year	Act/program/plan/other
1971	- The Medical Termination of Pregnancy
1975	- ICDS
1978	- Expanded Program for Immunization
1985	- Universal Immunization Program
1991	- Baby Friendly Hospital Initiative
1992	- CSSM - The Infant Milk Substitute, Feeding Bottles and Infant Foods (Regulation of Production, Supply and Distribution Act)
1994	- PNDT (Came into Force in 1996) - ICPD conference at Cairo, Egypt
1995	- Pulse Polio Immunization (First Round: 9th Dec 1995, 20th Jan 1996)
1997	- RCH-I Launched
2000	- National Population Policy
2001	- National Policy for Empowerment of Women
2002	- National Health Policy
2004	- Launching of Vandemataram Scheme - Low Dose Osmolarity ORS
2005	- RCH-II - JSY - NRHM
2006	- New Growth Chart (WHO) - IMNCI
2012	- Protection of Children of POCSO Act
2013	- RMNCH+A - NHM
2014	- Indian Newborn Action Plan (27th March) - Mission Indradhanush (25th December)
2015	- Introduction of IPV
2016	- Introduction of bOPV (Switch)
2017	- National Nutrition Mission - National Health Policy, 2017
2019	- IDCF (28th May–8th June 2019) - SUMAN (October 2019) - SAANS (November 2019) - IMI 2.0 (1st Round)—December 2019
2020	- IMI 2.0 (4th Round)—March 2020
2021	- Nationwide expansion of Pneumococcal Conjugate Vaccine (PCV) under the Universal Immunization Program (UIP) on 29th October 2021. - IMI 3.0 (November 2021) - RMNCAH+N

Year	Act/program/plan/other
2022	IMI 4.0 (Feb-April 2022)
	IDCF-2022 launched on 13th June 2022
2023	Introduction of Third dose of fIPV to be given at 9 months of age

CURRENT STATUS OF MATERNAL AND CHILD HEALTH

Table 2.1: Status of key vital statistics (SRS 2022 report).

Birth rate	19.5 per 1,000 live birth
Death rate	6 per 1,000 live birth
Infant mortality rate	28 per 1,000 live birth
Maternal mortality ratio	97 per 1,00,000 live birth

Table 2.2: Comparison of key RCH and Nutrition related indicators as per NFHS-4 and NFHS-5.

Indicators	NFHS-4	NFHS-5
Total fertility rate (TFR)	2.2	2.0
Contraceptive prevalence rate (CPR)	53.5%	66.7%
Unmet needs of family planning	12.9%	9.4%
Proportion of ANC visit in the first trimester	58.6%	70%
At least 4 ANC visit	51.2%	58.1%
Institutional births	78.9%	88.6%
Children age 12–23 months fully immunized	62%	76.4%
Sex ratio at birth (female per 1,000 male)	919	929
Anemia prevalence (%)		
All women (15–49 years)	53.1	57
Pregnant women (15–49 years)	50.4	52.2
Adolescent girls (15–19 years)	54.1	59.1
Children (6–59 months)	58.6	67.1
Adolescent boys (15–19 years)	29.2	31.1
Nutritional status of children under 5 years of age (%)		
Stunting	38.4	35.5
Wasting	21.0	19.3
Severely wasted	7.5	7.7
Overweight	2.1	3.4
Infant and child mortality rate		
Neonatal mortality rate per 1,000 live birth	29.5	24.9
Infant mortality rate per 1,000 live birth	40.7	35.2
Under 5 mortality rate per 1,000 live birth	49.7	41.9

BIBLIOGRAPHY

1. http://rchiips.org/nfhs/NFHS-5_FCTS/India.pdf
2. https://censusindia.gov.in/census.website/data/SRSB
3. https://censusindia.gov.in/census.website/data/SRSMMB

2.2 BASICS OF ANTENATAL CARE

- Antenatal care is the systemic supervision of women during pregnancy to monitor the progress of fetal growth and to ascertain the well-being of the mother and the fetus.
- A proper antenatal check-up provides necessary care to the mother and helps identify any complications of pregnancy such as anemia, pre-eclampsia and hypertension, etc., in the mother and slow/inadequate growth of the fetus.
- Antenatal care allows for the timely management of complications through referral to an appropriate facility for further treatment.
- It also provides an opportunity to prepare a birth plan and identify the facility for delivery and referral in case of complications.
- However, one must realize that even with the most effective screening tools, one cannot predict which woman will develop pregnancy-related complications during and immediately after childbirth.
- You must therefore:
  - Recognize that 'Every pregnancy is special and every pregnant woman must receive special care'.
  - Complications being unpredictable may happen in any pregnancy/childbirth and we should be ready to deal with them if and whenever they happen. Ensure that ANC is used as an opportunity to detect and treat existing problems, e.g., essential hypertension.
  - Prepare the woman and her family for the eventuality of an emergency.
  - Make sure that services to manage obstetric emergencies are available on time.

Essential Components of Antenatal Care

- Early registration
- History taking
- Physical examination (weight, BP, pallor, respiratory rate, edema)
- Abdominal palpation
- Vaginal examination
- Laboratory investigations—Hb, urine for sugar and proteins, rapid testing for syphilis screening, rapid testing kits for HIV screening and referral and management of +ve cases, OGTT testing for gestational diabetes, ultrasound, etc.
- Optional investigations: Hepatitis B and Thyroid Stimulating Hormone
- Tetanus and Adult Diphtheria (Td) Vaccine
- Folic acid supplementation in the first 3 months followed by IFA supplementation throughout pregnancy
- Calcium supplementation: Two tablet of Calcium after first trimester for next six months

- Deworming
- Malaria prophylaxis and treatment (wherever applicable)
- Nutritional counseling
- Micro birth planning

These can be remembered with the help of acronym **"ABCCDDEFGHII"** (Fig. 2.1).

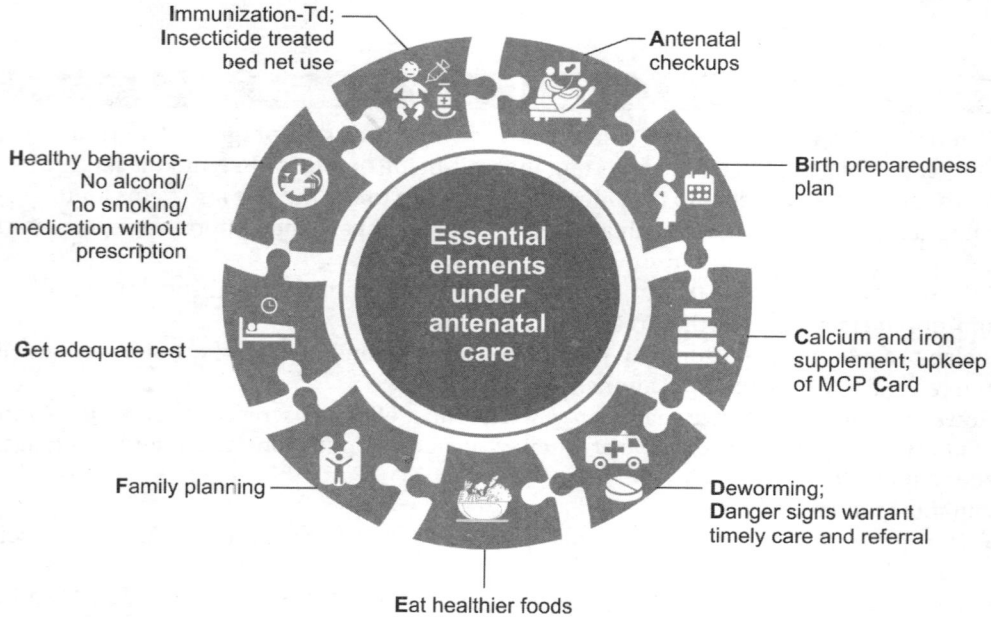

Fig. 2.1: Essential elements of antenatal care.

Confirmation of Pregnancy

With the help of 'Nishchay' pregnancy test kit, confirmation of pregnancy is done **(Fig. 2.2)**. It should be done as early as possible after the first missed period.

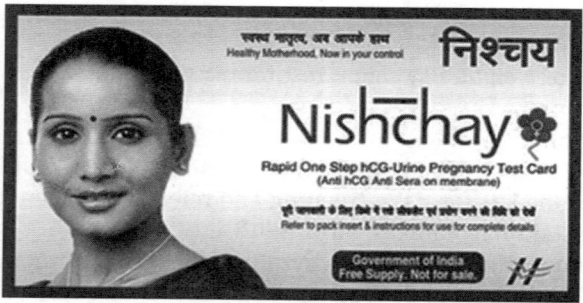

Fig. 2.2: Nishchay pregnancy test kit.

Early Registration of Pregnancy

- Ensure early registration and first check-up is conducted within 12 weeks.
- Early registration helps in planning, to calculate the EDD (EDD = Date of LMP + 9 months + 7 days), to know any existing illness and even abortion under the purview of MTP Act also can be offered.
- Early interaction between healthcare workers and pregnant lady helps in developing good rapport which helps in overall provision of services throughout the pregnancy.

Suggested Schedule for Antenatal Visits (Minimum Visits)

- **1st visit:** Within 12 weeks—preferably as soon as pregnancy is suspected—for registration of pregnancy and first antenatal check-up
- **2nd visit:** Between 14 and 26 weeks
- **3rd visit:** Between 28 and 34 weeks (usually at PHC level with MO)
- **4th visit:** Between 36 weeks and term
- **PMSMA visit:** in 2nd or 3rd trimester

Essential Components of Every Antenatal Check-Up

- Take the patient's history: Mainly about previous pregnancy (if any) related information and other relevant information which can affect the current pregnancy.
- Conduct a physical examination–measure the weight, blood pressure and respiratory rate and check for pallor and edema (which appears in the evening and disappears in the morning after a full night's sleep, could be a normal manifestation of pregnancy).
- Blood pressure and weight to be measured during every visit.
- If the woman has high blood pressure, check her urine for the presence of albumin. The presence of albumin (+2) together with high blood pressure means having pre-eclampsia. So, need to refer her to the PHC-MO immediately. Whenever the diastolic blood pressure reaches 110 mmHg then its sign of imminent eclampsia and refer her to FRU.
- Normally, a woman should gain 9–11 kg during her pregnancy. Ideally after the first trimester, a pregnant woman gains around 2 kg every month. An inadequate dietary intake can be suspected if the woman gains less than 2 kg per month while Excessive weight gain (more than 3 kg in a month) should raise suspicion of pre-eclampsia, twins (multiple pregnancy) or diabetes.
- Conduct abdominal palpation for fetal growth, fetal lie and auscultation of fetal heart sound (FHS) according to the stage of pregnancy.
- If the fetal heart rate (FHR) is between 120 and 160 beats per minute, it is normal. If it is less than 120 beats per minute or more than 160 beats per minute, the woman should be referred to the MO checking for the FHS should start only when the gestational age is more than 24 weeks.
- Fetal movements are a reliable sign of fetal well-being. Fetal movements, also called 'quickening', begin at around 18–22 weeks of pregnancy. They are felt earlier in a multigravida and later in a primigravida. Decreased movements (<10 movements in an hour) may be an indication of fetal distress and need to be referred to the FRU.

Determining the Fetal Lie and Presentation is Relevant Only in Late Pregnancy (32 Weeks Onwards)

A. Fundal palpation/fundal grip	B. Lateral palpation/lateral grip
This maneuver helps determine the lie and presentation of the fetus.	This maneuver is used to locate the fetal back.

C. First pelvic grip/superficial pelvic grip	D. Second pelvic grip/deep pelvic grip
The third maneuver must be performed gently. It helps to determine whether the head or the breech is present at the pelvic brim. If the head cannot be moved, it indicates that the head is engaged. In the case of a transverse lie, the third grip will be empty.	This maneuver, in experienced hands, will be able to tell us about the degree of flexion of the head.

The gestational age (in weeks) corresponds to the fundal height (in cm) after 24 weeks of gestation.

Measurement of fundal height:

At 12th week	Just palpable above the symphysis pubis
At 16th week	At lower one-third of the distance between the symphysis pubis and umbilicus
At 20th week	At two-thirds of the distance between the symphysis pubis and umbilicus
At 24th week	At the level of the umbilicus
At 28th week	At lower one-third of the distance between the umbilicus and xiphisternum
At 32nd week	At two-thirds of the distance between the umbilicus and xiphisternum
At 36th week	At the level of the xiphisternum
At 40th week	Sinks back to the level of the 32nd week, but the flanks are full, unlike that in the 32nd week

Reproductive, Maternal, Newborn, Child, and Adolescent Health

☐ Carry out laboratory investigations, such as hemoglobin estimation and urine tests (for sugar and proteins).

Prophylaxis During Pregnancy

Intervention	Composition	Dose regime	Timing and duration	Prevention
Tablet folic acid	500 µg	One tablet once a day	1st trimester (once pregnancy confirmed)	Neural tube defects in fetus
Tablet iron folic acid (IFA)	60 mg Iron and 0.5 mg (500 µg) folic acid	One tablet once a day	In the second and third trimester of pregnancy for 6 months (180 tablets) and continued for 6 months after delivery (180 tablets). Though the tablets should be taken preferably early in the morning on an empty stomach, she may take the tablets with meals or at night. This will help avoid nausea	Anemia
Tetanus toxoid (TT)/ tetanus adult diphtheria (Td)	0.5 mL tetanus toxoid	2 injections one month apart OR one booster (I/M in upper arm)	1st dose at ANC registration, followed by 2nd dose after one month. Give only Booster if immunized with 2 injections in previous pregnancy within last 3 years	Maternal and neonatal tetanus
Tablet calcium	500 mg calcium and 250 IU vitamin D3	One tablet twice a day (total 1 g calcium daily)	From the second trimester (14 weeks) onwards throughout pregnancy for 6 months (360 tablets) and continued for 6 months after delivery (360 tablets) taken in between meals. Iron folic acid tablets and calcium tablets should not be taken together at the same time. There should be a gap of at least 2 hours between IFA and calcium for better absorption of both. Calcium should not be taken immediately after a meal	Pregnancy induced hypertension and preterm births
Tablet albendazole (deworming)	400 mg	One tablet once only (under observation)	After 1st trimester (after 12 weeks)	Worm infestation, anemia, malnutrition
Insecticide treated bed-nets (ITN)	—	—	At 1st ANC visit	Malaria

Counseling

☐ Help the woman to plan and prepare for birth (birth preparedness/micro birth plan). This should include deciding on the place of delivery and the presence of an attendant at the time of the delivery.

- Inform the advantages of institutional deliveries and risks involved in home deliveries.
- Advise the woman on where to go if an emergency arises, and how to arrange for transportation, money and blood donors in case of an emergency.
- Educate the woman and her family members on signs of labor and danger signs of obstetric complications.
- Emphasize the importance of seeking ANC and PNC.
- Advise on diet (nutrition) and rest. During Pregnancy 350 kcal and during lactation women need 600 kcal requires extra calorie so they need to consume more food. They should take rest for at least for 2 hours in daytime also.
- Inform the woman about breastfeeding, including exclusive breastfeeding.
- Warn against domestic violence (explain the consequences of violence on a pregnant woman and her fetus).
- Promote family planning.
- Inform the woman about the Janani Suraksha Yojana (JSY)/any other incentives offered by the state.

Micro birth planning: 5 Is of micro-birth planning:
- **I**nform about the essential antenatal and intranatal care components, signs of labor and danger signs
- **I**nform expected date of delivery
- **I**temize the essentials that will be required at the time of delivery (e.g.: money, towel, cloths, transportation, etc.)
- **I**dentify the place of delivery
- **I**dentify the referral facility.

Home Delivery

- If in spite of all your efforts the pregnant woman decides to go for a home delivery, tell her that there are situations when complications arise and a home delivery may be risky and potentially life-threatening.
- Disposable Delivery Kits (DDKs) are to be supplied to those pregnant women in your community who insist on having a home delivery.
- Explain the **'six cleans'** to such women. **These are clean surface, clean hands, clean cord cut, clean cord tie, clean umbilical stump and clean perineum**. Counsel and help them to maintain the 'six cleans' during delivery at home.
- Female health worker should prepare herself to attend to such women at their home during delivery.

Important Programs and Schemes for Care During Antenatal Period
- PMSMA
- JSY
- JSSK
- SUMAN
- PMVVY

PRADHAN MANTRI SURAKSHIT MATRITVA ABHIYAN (PMSMA)

- Ministry: Ministry of Health and Family Welfare
- Launched date: 9 June 2016
- **Goal:** To improve the quality and coverage of Antenatal Care (ANC), including diagnostics and counseling services as part of the Reproductive Maternal Neonatal Child and Adolescent Health (RMNCH+A) Strategy.
- **Objectives:**
    - Ensure at least one antenatal check-up for all pregnant women in their second or third trimester by a physician/specialist.
    - Improve the quality of care during antenatal visits. This includes ensuring provision of the following services:
        - All applicable diagnostic services
        - Screening for the applicable clinical conditions
        - Appropriate management of any existing clinical condition such as Anemia, Pregnancy induced hypertension, Gestational Diabetes, etc.
        - Appropriate counseling services and proper documentation of services rendered
        - Additional service opportunity to pregnant women who have missed antenatal visits
- Identification and line-listing of high-risk pregnancies based on obstetric/medical history and existing clinical conditions.
- Appropriate birth planning and complication readiness for each pregnant woman especially those identified with any risk factor or comorbid condition.
- Special emphasis on early diagnosis, adequate and appropriate management of women with malnutrition.
- Special focus on adolescent and early pregnancies as these pregnancies need extra and specialized care.

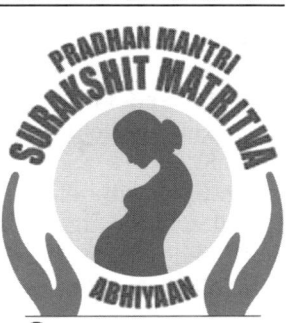

9th of Every Month

Strategy

- On the 5th day of every month ANMs/ASHAs will make line list of all pregnant women in 2nd and 3rd trimester of pregnancy.
- On **the 9th day of every month**, a minimum package of antenatal care services would be provided at the Pradhan Mantri Surakshit Matritva Clinics.
- PMSMA is to ensure that every pregnant woman receives at least one antenatal check-up in the 2nd and 3rd trimester of pregnancy.
- Using the principles of a single window system, it is envisaged that a minimum package of investigations (including one ultrasound during the 2nd trimester of pregnancy) and medicines such as IFA supplements, calcium supplements, etc. would be provided to all pregnant women attending the PMSMA clinics.
- If the 9th day of the month is a Sunday/a holiday, then the Clinic should be organized on the next working day.
- These services will be provided by the Medical Officer and/OBGY specialist but if such trained manpower is not available then services from Private Practitioners (OBGY) on voluntary basis should be arranged.
- It will be ensured that before reaching to the Medical Officer and/OBGY specialist all basic laboratory investigations will be done and reported within one hour.

Reproductive, Maternal, Newborn, Child, and Adolescent Health

- Sticker indicating the condition and risk factor of the pregnant women should be added onto MCP card for each visit:
  - **Green sticker:** For women with no risk factor detected
  - **Red sticker:** For women with high-risk pregnancy
  - **Blue sticker:** For women with pregnancy induced hypertension
  - **Yellow sticker:** Pregnancy with comorbid conditions such as diabetes, hypothyroidism, STIs.
- PMSMA will help in providing quality ANC and also detection, referral, treatment and follow-up of high-risk pregnancies and women having complications.
- 'I Pledge For 9' Achievers Awards have been devised to celebrate individual and team achievements and acknowledge voluntary contributions for PMSMA in states and districts across India.

JANANI SURAKSHA YOJANA

- Janani Suraksha Yojana (JSY) is a safe motherhood intervention under the National Health Mission which was launched on 12 April 2005 by the Hon'ble Prime Minister.
- It is being implemented with the objective of reducing maternal and neonatal mortality by promoting institutional delivery among poor pregnant women.
- JSY is a centrally sponsored scheme, which integrates cash assistance with delivery and post-delivery care.
- The Yojana has identified Accredited Social Health Activist (ASHA) as an effective link between the government and pregnant women.
- The scheme focuses on poor pregnant woman with a special dispensation for states that have low institutional delivery rates and these states have been named Low Performing States (LPS), the remaining states have been named High Performing States (HPS).

The Eligibility for Cash Assistance Under the JSY

LPS	All pregnant women delivering in government health centers, such as subcenters (SCs)/ Primary Health Centers (PHCs)/Community Health Centers (CHCs)/First Referral Units (FRUs)/general wards of district or state hospitals
HPS	All BPL/Scheduled Caste/Scheduled Tribe (SC/ST) women delivering in a government health center, such as SC/PHC/CHC/FRU/general wards of district or state hospital
LPS and HPS	BPL/SC/ST women in accredited private institutions.

Cash assistance for institutional delivery (in ₹): The cash entitlement for different categories of mothers is as follows:

Category	Rural area			Urban area		
	Mother's package	ASHA's package*	Total (Amount in ₹)	Mother's package	ASHA's package**	Total (Amount in ₹)
LPS	1400	600	2000	1000	400	1400
HPS	700	600	1300	600	400	1000

*ASHA package of ₹ 600 in rural areas include ₹ 300 for ANC component and ₹ 300 for facilitating institutional delivery.
**ASHA package of ₹ 400 in urban areas include ₹ 200 for ANC component and ₹ 200 for facilitating institutional delivery.

JANANI-SHISHU SURAKSHA KARYAKRAM (JSSK)

- Institutional deliveries in India increased substantially after launched of Janani Suraksha Yojana (JSY).
- However, 25% women still hesitate to access health facilities for delivery due to out of pocket expenditure during stay at health facilities on drugs, diet, and diagnosis and arrangement blood, etc.
- Janani Shishu Suraksha Karyakaram (JSSK) launched on 1st June 2011 entitles all pregnant women delivering in public health institutions to absolutely free and no expense delivery, including cesarean section.
- Janani Shishu Suraksha Karyakaram (JSSK) was launched to eliminate out-of-pocket expenses for both pregnant women and sick infants.
- Essential care is provided to the mother and her neonate within 48 hours. This postnatal period is critical for identification and management of complication of post-delivery.
- In the case of institutional delivery, accessing availing this care is a little easier.
- In 2014, the Program was extended to all antenatal and postnatal complications of pregnancy and similar entitlements have been put in place for all sick newborns and infants (up to one year of age) accessing public health institutions for treatment.
- The initiative entitles all pregnant women delivering in public health institutions to absolutely free and no expense delivery, including cesarean section.
- The entitlements include free drugs and consumables, free diagnostics, free blood wherever required, and free diet for 3 days during normal delivery and 7 days for C-section.
- This initiative also provides for free transport from home to institution, between facilities in case of a referral and drop back home.

SURAKSHIT MATRITVA AASHWASAN (SUMAN)

Introduction

- Surakshit Matritva Aashwasan is **'An Initiative for Zero Preventable Maternal and Newborn Deaths'**.
- It is launched on October 10, 2019.
- Under surakshit matritva aashwasan scheme, pregnant women, mothers up to 6 months after delivery, and all sick newborns will be able to avail free healthcare benefits.

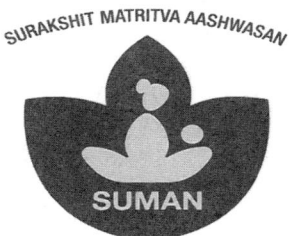

Objectives

- To provide assured, dignified and respectful delivery of quality healthcare services at no cost.
- To ensure zero tolerance for denial of services to any woman and newborn visiting a public health facility.
- To end all preventable maternal and newborn deaths and morbidities
- To provide a positive birthing experience.

All Pregnant Women/Newborns visiting public health facilities are entitled to the following free services:
- At least four antenatal check-ups
- At least one check-up under Pradhan Mantri Surakshit Matritva Abhiyan,
- Iron folic acid supplementation
- Tetanus Diphtheria injection and other components of comprehensive Ante-Natal Care (ANC) package

- Elimination of mother to child transmission of HIV, HBV and syphilis.
- Six home-based newborn care visits.
- Early initiation of breastfeeding and zero dose vaccination
- Zero expense delivery and C-section facility
- Zero expense care facility after or during the pregnancy, in case of complications
- Management of sick neonates and infants.
- Free transport to pregnant women from home to the health facility and drop back after discharge
- Conditional cash transfer/direct benefit transfer under various schemes
- Postpartum counseling on family planning.

Service guarantee Enablers:
- Zero tolerance for any negligence
- Integrates existing initiatives (JSSK, PMSMA, Lakshya, FRUs, etc.)
- Respect for Women's Autonomy, Dignity, Feelings and Choices
- 100% Maternal Death Reporting and Reviews
- Grievance redressal mechanism
- Client feedback mechanism
- Awards to champions
- Community level maternal death reporting
- Community engagement and mega IEC/BCC
- Intersectoral convergence.

PRADHAN MANTRI MATRU VANDANA YOJANA (PMMVY)

- **Ministry**: Women and child development
  - **Launched date**: 01.01.2017
  - Initially this scheme was launched as Indira Gandhi Matritva Sahyog Yojana (IGMSY)—a Conditional Maternity Benefit Scheme in 2010-2011.
  - It's centrally sponsored scheme.
- **Objectives**:
  - To improve the health and nutrition status of Pregnant and Lactating women and their young infants thus provide partial compensation for the wage loss so that the woman is not under compulsion to work till the last stage of pregnancy and can take adequate rest before and after delivery.
  - To improve health seeking behavior amongst the pregnant women and lactating mothers.

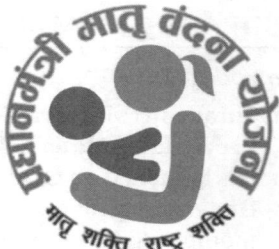

- **Beneficiaries:**
  - Under PMMVY, a cash incentive of Rs. 5000*/- is provided directly to the Bank/Post Office Account of Pregnant Women and Lactating Mothers for **first living child** of the family subject to fulfilling specific conditions relating to Maternal and Child Health.
  - Women who are either employee of state/central government or receiving benefits of any such other scheme would not be eligible for the PMMVY.
  - Private hospitals directly cannot avail the benefit of the scheme. However, if the requisite conditions are duly certified by a government doctor or officer/functionary of the Health Department not below the rank of ANM, the beneficiary can claim maternity benefit under PMVVY.

Reproductive, Maternal, Newborn, Child, and Adolescent Health

❏ **Benefits under the Scheme:**

Instalment	Conditions	Documents required	Amount
First instalment	• Register her pregnancy in the MCP card along with required documents within 150 days from LMP	• Duly filled application Form 1A • Copy of MCP card • Copy of Identity proof • Copy of Bank/Post-office Account Passbook	₹ 1,000
Second instalment	• At least one antenatal check-up • Can be claimed post 180 days of Pregnancy	• Duly filled Application Form 1 B • Copy of MCP Card	₹ 2,000
Third instalment	• Childbirth is registered • Child has received first cycle of immunizations of Hepatitis B Birth dose, BCG, OPV (0 and 1,2 and 3, DPT and Hepatitis B or Pentavalent 1,2 and 3 • Aadhaar is mandatory in all states except for J and K, Assam, Meghalaya	• Duly filled Application Form 1C • Copy of MCP Card • Copy of Aadhaar ID • Copy of Childbirth Registration Certificate	₹ 2,000

*Additional ₹ 1000 given if childbirth takes place at hospital and mother is beneficiary of JSY scheme.

❏ In Gujarat State, there is one more similar scheme known as Kasturba Poshan Sahay Yojna (KPSY), in which ₹ 6,000 is given to the beneficiaries when they fulfilled almost same criteria which are applicable in PMMVY. As they are similar schemes, benefit of both schemes would not be given and so, at the time of first child, 5,000 ₹ from PMMVY and 1,000 ₹ from KPSY will be given to all BPL families while for non-BPL families at the time of first child, benefits of only PMMVY as ₹ 5,000 will be given. Benefits of KPSY will continue to only BPL families as ₹ 6000 for second and third childbirth.
❏ Pradhan Mantri Matru Vandana Yojana Common Application Software (PMMVY- CAS) is used to maintain all the details of the beneficiaries and for DBT as well.

BIBLIOGRAPHY

1. https://nhm.gov.in/images/pdf/Programs/maternalhealth/guidelines/sba_guidelines_for_skilled_attendance_at_birth.pdf
2. https://wcd.nic.in/schemes/pradhan-mantri-matru-vandana-yojana
3. https://wcd.nic.in/sites/default/files/PMMVY%20Scheme%20Implementati n%20Guidelines%20-%20 MWCD%20%281%29_0.pdf
4. https://pmsma.mohfw.gov.in/about-scheme/#about

2.3 BASICS OF INTRANATAL CARE

❏ Intermittent contractions after 22 weeks of gestation, contractions associated with blood-stained discharge or watery vaginal discharge should raise a suspicion of the onset of labor.
❏ **The onset of labor can be confirmed by the following:**
  • Cervical effacement—progressive shortening and thinning of the cervix during labor
  • Cervical dilatation

- **Stages of labor:**
  - **The first stage** of labor starts with the onset of labor pains to full dilatation of the cervix. This stage takes about 12 hours in primigravida's and half that time for subsequent deliveries.
  - **The second stage** starts from full dilatation of the cervix to the delivery of the baby. This stage takes about 2 hours for primigravida,s and only about half an hour for subsequent deliveries.
  - **The third stage** starts after the delivery of the baby and ends with the delivery of the placenta. This stage takes about 15 minutes to half an hour, irrespective of whether the woman is a primigravida or multigravida.
  - **The fourth stage:** Frequent monitoring for one hour immediately after delivery to detect PPH.
- **Assessment of the progress of labor:** The progress of labor is assessed by:
  - Assessing the changes in cervical effacement and dilatation (by conducting a P/V examination)
  - Assessing the progress in fetal descent (by conducting an abdominal and/or a P/V examination).
- **Supportive care to the woman during labor:**
  - Explain all the procedures, seek permission for examination and carrying out the procedures with ensuring privacy and dignity and discuss the findings with the woman.
  - Keep the woman informed about the progress of labor.
  - Praise the woman, encourage her and reassure her that things are going well.
  - Encourage the woman to keep clean her genitals at the onset of labor.
  - Always wash your hands with soap and water before examining the woman.
  - Ensure cleanliness of the birthing area.
  - Enema should NOT be routinely given during labor.
- Encourage the woman to empty her bladder frequently (every 2 hours).
- The presence of a birth companion of the woman's choice in addition to an SBA is beneficial. Birth companions provide comfort, emotional support, reassurance, encouragement and praise.
- Women should be allowed to remain mobile during labor, especially the first stage, as this helps in having a shorter and less painful labor.
- The woman should be free to choose any position she desires and feels comfortable in during labor and delivery. She may choose from the left lateral, squatting, kneeling, or even standing (supported by the birth companion) positions.
- Other non-pharmacological methods of relieving pain during labor include:
  - Calm and gentle voice of the birth attendant
  - Offering the woman encouragement, reassurance and praise
  - Relaxation techniques performed by the woman such as deep breathing exercises and massage
  - Placing a cool cloth on the woman's forehead
  - Assisting the woman in voiding urine and in changing her position.
- Women who are not at risk of requiring general anesthesia can have light, easily digested, low-fat food during labor, if they wish. This is because labor requires large amounts of energy.

Management of the Different Stages of the Normal Delivery

Management of the first stage of labor: Usually to be done once the cervix is dilated 3 cm or more:

- Monitor the following every 30 minutes:
  - Frequency, intensity and duration of the contractions
  - FHR
  - Presence of any emergency sign
- Monitor the following every 4 hours:
  - Cervical dilatation (in cm)
  - Temperature
  - Pulse
  - BP
- Start maintaining a partograph once the woman is in active labor.

Partograph

- The partograph is a graphic recording of the progress of labor and salient features of the mother and fetus.
- It is a tool to assess the progress of labor and recognize the need for action and referral at the appropriate time.
- **The instructions for filling the partograph are given below:**
- **Fetal condition**
  - The FHR should be counted and recorded every half-an-hour. Count the FHR for one full minute.
  - The rate should preferably be counted immediately following a uterine contraction. An FHR of >160 beats/minute or <120 beats/minute indicates fetal distress.
- Simultaneously record the condition of the membranes and **color of the amniotic fluid** as visible at the vulva every 30 minutes as:
  - Intact membranes (mark 'I')
  - Clear liquor (mark 'C')
  - Meconium stained (mark 'M')
  - No liquor (mark 'A').
- **Labor:**
  - Start plotting on the labor graph only after the woman is in active labor. The woman is said to be in active labor when the cervical dilatation is more than 3 cm and at least 2 good contractions (i.e., each lasting for more than 20 seconds) occur in 10 minutes.
  - Start recording the cervical dilatation (in cm) when the woman first reports in labor and then every four hours.
  - The initial recording is placed to the left of the alert line. Normally the line should continue to remain to the left of the alert line. Write the time accordingly in the row for time.
  - If the alert line is crossed (the graph moves to the right of the alert line), it indicates prolonged labor, and you should be alert that labor is not progressing as it should. Note the time when the alert line is crossed. Start preparing for referral to an FRU.
  - Crossing of the action line (the graph moves to the right of the action line) indicates the need for intervention and referral. There is a difference of 4 hours between the alert and the action line. By the time the action line is crossed, the woman should ideally have reached the FRU for receiving appropriate and timely intervention.

- Record the number of good contractions (lasting more than 20 seconds) in 10 minutes every half-an-hour and accordingly, blacken the boxes on the partograph.

Maternal Condition
- Record the maternal pulse and BP every half-an-hour and plot them on the graph.
- Record both the systolic and the diastolic BP using a vertical arrow, with the upper end of the arrow representing the systolic BP and the lower end indicating the diastolic BP.
- Use crosses to mark the pulse.

Note: Partograph is attached as *Annexure 4*.

Intervention
- Mention here any drug that you have administered during labor, including the dose and route of administration, and when.
- Also include the food items and liquids consumed by the woman during that period.

Management of the Second Stage of Labor
- Monitor the following every 5 minutes:
  - Frequency, duration and intensity of contractions
  - FHR
  - Perineal thinning and bulging
  - Visible descent of the fetal head during contractions
  - Presence of any signs indicating an emergency
- The upright positions such as standing, sitting, squatting and being on all fours makes pushing easier.
- The woman should be allowed to push down when she has contractions if she has the urge to do so during the second stage of labor.
- Bearing down efforts are required after the cervix is fully dilated, and even more so when the head is distending the perineum.
- Occasionally, the woman feels the urge to push before the cervix is fully dilated. This should be discouraged as it can result in edema of the cervix which may delay the progress of labor.
- **Things to be avoided during second stage of labor:**
  - Asking the woman to hold her breath and bear down in the second stage of labor should NOT be done. Holding the breath is potentially harmful. It may reduce the quantity of blood reaching the uterus and placenta. It may also reduce the supply of oxygen to the fetus.
  - Giving the woman oxytocics to shorten the second stage of labor is NOT advisable.
  - Avoid ironing the perineum (or using the "Sweep and stretch" technique) to hasten delivery.
- **Episiotomy:** There is no evidence that routine episiotomy decreases perineal damage, future vaginal prolapse or urinary incontinence. Remember, whenever an episiotomy is required, a **right paramedian episiotomy** is preferred.
- **Indications for conducting an episiotomy:**
  - Complicated vaginal delivery (refer to a higher health facility in case of a malpresentation)
  - History of third- or fourth-degree perineal tears
  - Fetal distress
  - Instrumental/assisted delivery

- **Ensure a controlled delivery of the head by taking the following precautions:**
  - Encourage the woman to push only during pains (a contraction).
  - Keep one hand gently on the head as it advances with the contractions.
  - Support the perineum with the other hand during delivery and cover the anus with a pad held in position by the side of the hand.
  - Leave the perineum visible (between the thumb and the index finger).
  - Ask the mother to breathe steadily and to not push during delivery of the head.
  - Encourage rapid breathing with the mouth open.
  - Do NOT apply fundal pressure to hasten delivery of the head.
  - Note the time of delivery.
  - Cutting the cord: Tie and cut the cord after 2–3 minutes of delivery, during which time the cord will normally stop pulsating. This will result in an increased amount of blood being transfused into the fetal circulation, and thus help in avoiding neonatal anemia.
  - Put ties tightly around the cord at 2 cm and 5 cm from the baby's abdomen.
  - Cut between the ties with a sterile blade.
  - Look for oozing of blood from the stump. If there is oozing, place a second tie between the baby's skin and the first tie.

Immediate Newborn Care

- If the baby does not cry in 30 seconds, take steps to resuscitate the baby.
- Ensure warmth to the baby to prevent hypothermia.
- It is recommended that the umbilical cord stump be left dry, and only routine daily care be given with clean safe water. Do not apply any substance to the stump.
- Note the apgar score of the baby at 1 minute and at 5 minutes after delivery.
- Leave the baby on the mother's chest for skin-to-skin contact.
- Cover the baby to prevent loss of body heat. If the room is cool, use additional blankets to cover the mother and the baby.
- Encourage the mother to initiate breastfeeding.

Care of the Newborn: Elements of Essential Newborn Care

- Maintain the body temperature and prevent hypothermia
- Maintain the airway and breathing
- Breastfeed the newborn
- Take care of the cord
- Take care of the eyes

Active management of the third stage of labor: It consists of the following three activities:

- **Uterotonic drug:** Giving a uterotonic drug (one that enhances the contraction of the uterine muscles) has been shown to be effective in preventing PPH. Although Inj. Oxytocin (in a dose of 10 IU IM) is the drug of choice for preventing PPH, due to administrative difficulties, Misoprostol can now be used for the same purpose. Three tablets of 200 mcg each of Misoprostol (a total dose of 600 mcg) should be given immediately after delivery of the baby.
- **Controlled cord traction (CCT):** This is a technique to assist the expulsion of the placenta and helps to reduce the chances of a retained placenta and subsequent PPH.

- **Uterine massage:** This technique helps in contraction of the uterus and thus prevents PPH immediately after delivery of the baby, massage the uterus by placing your hand on the woman's abdomen until it is well contracted. Repeat the massage every 15 minutes for the first 2 hours. Ensure that the uterus does not become relaxed (soft) after the massage is stopped.

Family Planning

PPIUCD: The PPIUCD can be placed immediately following delivery of the placenta, during cesarean section or within 48 hours following childbirth. The IUCD should NOT be inserted from 48 hours to 6 weeks following delivery because there is an increased risk of infection and expulsion.

PAIUCD: Insertion of IUCD following an abortion, if there is no infection, bleeding or any other contraindications.

BIBLIOGRAPHY

1. http://www.nrhmorissa.gov.in/writereaddata/upload/documents/normal_delivery_and_management_of_obstetric_complications_.pdf

2.4 BASIC OF POSTNATAL CARE

Background
- Conventionally, the first 42 days (6 weeks) after delivery are taken as the postpartum period.
- First 48 hours and the first one week are the most crucial periods for the health and survival of both the mother and her newborn.
- More than 60% of maternal deaths take place during the postpartum period.

Immediate Postpartum Care
- The first one hour after delivery of the placenta is sometimes referred to as the fourth stage of labor.
- After delivery of the placenta, check that the uterus is well contracted, i.e., it is hard and round, and there is no heavy bleeding.
- Repeat the check every 5 minutes. If the uterus is not well contracted, massage the uterus and expel the clots. If bleeding continues even after 10 minutes, manage as "Postpartum hemorrhage".
- Examine the perineum, lower vagina and vulva for tears. If present, manage as "Vaginal and perineal tears".
- Estimate and record the amount of blood lost throughout the third stage and immediately afterwards. If the loss is around 250 mL, but the bleeding has stopped, observe the woman for the next 24 hours.

- Monitor the following every 10 minutes for the first 30 minutes, then every 15 minutes for the next 30 minutes, and then every 30 minutes for the next three hours:
  - BP, pulse, temperature
  - Vaginal bleeding
  - Uterus, to make sure that it is well contracted.
- Clean the woman and the area beneath her. Put a sanitary pad or a folded cloth under her buttocks to collect blood. This will also help in estimating the amount of blood lost, by counting the number of pads/cloths soaked. Help her change her clothes, if necessary.
- Ensure that the mother has enough sanitary napkins or clean cloths to collect the vaginal blood.
- Dispose of the placenta in the correct, safe and culturally appropriate manner. Use gloves while handling the placenta. Put the placenta into a leak-proof bag. Incinerate the placenta or bury it at least 10 m away from a water source, in a 2 m deep pit.
- Keep the mother and the baby together; do not separate them. Encourage early breastfeeding.
- Encourage the woman to eat and drink and rest.
- Encourage the woman to pass urine. If the woman has difficulty in passing urine, or the bladder is full (as evidenced by a swelling over the lower abdomen) and she is uncomfortable, help her pass urine by gently pouring water over her vulva
- Weigh the baby.
- Ask the birth companion to stay with the mother. Do not leave the mother and the newborn alone. Ask the companion to watch the woman and call for help if any of the following occurs:
  - The bleeding increases
  - The woman feels dizzy
  - The woman has severe headache
  - The woman has visual disturbance
  - The woman has epigastric distress
  - The woman complains of breathlessness.
  - The woman complains of increased abdominal or perineal pain.
- Enter the following information in the labor register:
  - Name of the woman
  - Age of the woman
  - Parity
  - ANC received (or not): mention the number of ANC visits received
  - Mode of delivery (normal or assisted)
  - Birth weight of the baby
  - Apgar score of the baby at 1 minute and 5 minutes after delivery.

Counseling: Counsel the woman regarding the aspects discussed below.

Postpartum Care and Hygiene

- To always have someone near her for the first 24 hours after delivery to respond to any change in her condition.
- Not to insert anything into the vagina.
- To wash the perineum daily and after passing stools. Wash in an anteroposterior direction from the vulva to the anus.

- To change the perineal pads every 4–6 hours, or more frequently, if there is heavy lochia.
- To wash cloth pads, if used, with plenty of soap and water and dry them in the sun.
- To bathe daily.
- To have enough rest and sleep. For the first 6 weeks postpartum, advise the woman to not do anything except look after herself and her baby.
- To avoid sexual intercourse for the first six weeks or until the perineal wound heals, whichever is later.
- To wash her hands before handling the baby.

Nutrition

- Advise the woman to eat a greater amount and variety of healthy foods. Give her examples of the types of food and how much to eat.
- Reassure the mother that she can eat normal food; these will not harm the breastfed baby.
- Spend more time on nutrition counseling with very thin women and adolescents.
- Determine if there are important food taboos, especially against foods that are nutritionally healthy.

Contraception: Advise the woman regarding birth spacing or limiting as the case may be

Breastfeeding: Explain about the importance of breastfeeding, exclusive breastfeeding, good position and attachment for proper breastfeeding.

Registration of birth: Advise for the registration of birth to be given.

Postpartum Visits

Visits	After home delivery delivery at HWC-SC	After delivery at PHC/FRU (Woman discharged after 48 hours)
First visit	1st day (within 24 hours)	NA*
Second visit	3rd day after delivery	3rd day after delivery
Third visit	7th day after delivery	7th day after delivery
Fourth visit	6 weeks after delivery	6 weeks after delivery

Note: Under HBNC, along with newborn care maternal care is also given on 3rd, 7th, 14th, 21st, 28 th and 42 nd day.

- **The first postpartum visit:** The following questions should be asked to the woman during the first visit:
    - Where did the delivery take place?
    - Who conducted the delivery?
- **Maternal symptoms:** Ask for the following symptoms:
    - History of
        - Heavy bleeding P/V: This is important to assess the presence of immediate PPH.
        - Convulsions or loss of consciousness
        - Abdominal pain
        - Fever
- Inform the woman about the next routine postpartum visit.
- As the woman is kept under observation for the first 24 hours after delivery, the first postpartum visit is taken care of during her stay at the PHC/health facility.

- The second postpartum visit should be planned within 7–10 days after delivery. Either ask the ANM of that area to pay a visit to the woman and her baby, or ask the woman to return to the PHC for a postpartum check-up.
- If the woman misses her postpartum visits, inform her regarding the danger signs and when to return.

Danger signs: For the following symptoms and signs in the mother, advise the woman and her family to go to an FRU immediately, day or night, WITHOUT WAITING.
- Excessive vaginal bleeding, i.e. soaking more than 2 or 3 pads in 20-30 minutes after delivery, OR bleeding increases rather than decreases after the delivery
- Convulsions
- Fast or difficult breathing
- Fever and weakness; inability to get out of bed
- Severe abdominal pain

Advice about the occurrence of the following symptoms to women as it requires referral to PHC:
- Fever
- Abdominal pain
- The woman feels ill
- Swollen, red or tender breasts, or sore nipples
- Dribbling of urine or painful micturition
- Pain in the perineum, or pus draining from the perineal area
- Foul-smelling lochia.

Second and Third Visits
- Look for any delayed PPH (postpartum bleeding occurring 24 hours or more after delivery)
- Assess and ask for any foul-smelling discharge, fever, swelling in breast and any feeling like unhappiness.
- Overall examination to be done as same as done during the first visit.
- Advise related to diet to be given as calory and protein requirement increases during the lactation period.
- It is very important to advise related contraception if not done yet as whenever mother periods begin again and/or she stops exclusive breastfeeding, she can conceive even after a single act of unprotected sex.

BIBLIOGRAPHY

1. http://www.nrhmorissa.gov.in/writereaddata/upload/documents/normal_delivery_and_management_of_obstetric_complications_.pdf

2.5 BASICS OF NEWBORN AND CHILD CARE ALONG WITH RELATED PROGRAMS AND GUIDELINES

Causes of child mortality in India: The major causes of child mortality in India as per the SRS reports (2010-13) are:
- Prematurity and low birth weight (29.8%): Most common
- Pneumonia (17.1%), diarrheal diseases (8.6%), other non-communicable diseases (8.3%), birth asphyxia and birth trauma (8.2%), injuries (4.6%), congenital anomalies (4.4%), ill-defined or cause unknown (4.4%), acute bacterial sepsis and severe infections (3.6%), fever of unknown origin (2.5%) and all other remaining causes (8.4%).
- Besides these, malnutrition is a contributory factor in 45% of under-five child deaths.
  - The first hour after birth has a major influence on the survival, future health and well-being of a newly born infant.
  - The four basic needs of ALL babies at the time of birth (and for the first few weeks of life) are:
    1. Warmth
    2. Normal breathing
    3. Mother's milk
    4. Protection from infection

Immediate Care of a Normal Newborn at the Time of Birth
- Call out the time of birth.
- Deliver the baby onto a warm, clean and dry towel or cloth and keep on mother's chest and abdomen (between the breasts). If this is not possible, the baby should be kept in a clean, warm, safe place close to the mother.
- Clamp and cut the umbilical cord in 1-3 minutes using a sterile, disposable clamp or a sterile tie.
- Immediately dry the baby with a warm clean towel or piece of cloth; wipe the eyes.
- Assess the baby's breathing while drying*. A normal newborn should be crying vigorously or breathing regularly at a rate of 40–60 breaths per minute.
- Wipe both the eyes (separately) with sterile gauze. Wipe from the medial side (inner canthus) to the lateral side (outer canthus).
- Leave the baby between the mother's breasts to start skin-to-skin care.
- Place an identity label on the baby.
- Cover the baby's head with a cap. Cover the mother and baby with a warm cloth.
- Encourage the initiation of breastfeeding within one hour of birth in all babies.
- It is recommended to give BCG, zero dose of oral polio vaccine and birth dose of Hepatitis B vaccine and also injection of Vitamin K.

* if the baby is not crying or breathing well, the next steps of resuscitation have to be carried out.

Immediate Care of the Umbilical Cord
- Put the baby on mother's abdomen or on a warm, clean and dry surface close to the mother.
- Change gloves; if not possible, wash gloved hands.
- Put ties (using a sterile tie) tightly around cord at 2 cm and 5 cm from the abdomen.
- Cut between the ties with a sterile instrument (e.g., blade).
- Observe for oozing blood. If blood oozes, place a second tie between the skin and first tie.
- Do not apply any substance to the stump.

- Do not bind or bandage stump.
- Leave stump uncovered.

Prevention of Infection
- **Clean delivery (WHO six cleans): Clean Chain**
  - Clean attendant's hands (washed with soap).
  - Clean delivery surface.
  - Clean cord- cutting instrument (i.e. razor, blade).
  - Clean string to tie cord.
  - Clean cloth to wrap the baby.
  - Clean cloth to wrap the mother.
- **After delivery:**
  - All caregivers should wash hands before handling the baby.
  - Feed only breast milk.
  - Keep the cord clean and dry; do not apply anything.
  - Use a clean cloth as a diaper/napkin.
  - Wash your hands after changing diaper/napkin.

Prevention of Hypothermia 'Warm Chain'
- **At delivery:**
  - Ensure the delivery room is warm (25° C), with no draughts.
  - Dry the baby immediately; remove the wet cloth.
  - Wrap the baby with clean dry cloth.
  - Keep the baby close to the mother (ideally skin-to-skin) to stimulate early breastfeeding.
  - Postpone bathing/sponging for 24 hours.
- **After delivery:**
  - Keep the baby clothed and wrapped with the head covered.
  - Minimize bathing especially in cool weather or for small babies.
  - Keep the baby close to the mother.
  - Use kangaroo care for stable LBW babies and for re-warming stable bigger babies.

KANGAROO MOTHER CARE (KMC)

- It is a simple method of care for low-birth-weight infants that include early and prolonged skin-to-skin contact with the mother/caregiver and exclusive and frequent, breastfeeding.
- This natural form of human care stabilizes body temperature, promotes breastfeeding, and prevents infection and other morbidities.
- This also leads to early discharge, better neurodevelopment and encourages bonding between mother and infant.
- KMC is initiated in the hospital and continued at home until the needs it.
- **When should be started?**
  - If weight between: 1800–2500 g: KMC can be initiated immediately after birth
  - More than 1200 up to less than 1800 g: May take days before KMC initiated
  - Less than 1200 g: May take days to weeks before KMC can be initiated.
- **Duration of KMC:**
  - Short: 4 hours daily
  - Extended: 5–8 hours daily

- Long: 9–12 hours daily
- Continuous: More than 12 hours daily

☐ **Two components of KMC are:**
1. **Skin-to-skin contact**: Early, continuous and prolonged skin-to-skin contact between the mother and her baby is the basic component of KMC. The infant is placed on her mother's chest between the breasts.
2. **Exclusive breastfeeding**: The baby on KMC is breastfed exclusively. Skin-to-skin contact promotes lactation and thus facilitates exclusive breastfeeding.

☐ **The two prerequisites of KMC are:**
1. **Support to the mother** in hospital and at home
   A mother needs counseling, support, and supervision from healthcare providers for initiating KMC in the hospital. She would also require assistance and cooperation from her family members for continuing KMC at home.
2. **Post-discharge follow-up**
   KMC is continued at home after early discharge from the hospital. A regular follow-up and access to health providers for solving problem are crucial to ensure safe and successful KMC at home.

Benefits of KMC

☐ Temperature maintenance with a reduced risk of hypothermia
☐ Increased breastfeeding rates
☐ Early discharge from the health facility
☐ Less morbidities such as apnea and infections
☐ Less stress (for both baby and mother) and
☐ Better infant bonding.

Breastfeeding

The following are the advantages of breastfeeding:
Exclusive breastfed babies are at decreased risk of:
☐ Diarrhea
☐ Pneumonia
☐ Ear infection and
☐ Death in first year of life

The Four Key Points in Proper Positioning

1. The baby's head and body should be straight
2. The baby's face should face mother's breast
3. The baby's body should be close to her body
4. She should support the baby's whole body.

The Four Key Signs of Good Attachment

1. More areola is visible above the baby's mouth than below it
2. The baby's mouth is wide open
3. The baby's lower lip is turned outwards
4. The baby's chin is touching the breast

Effective sucking: Infant takes several slow deep sucks followed by swallowing, and then pauses.

Breastfeeding is Considered Adequate if the Baby

- Passes urine 6–8 times in 24 hours.
- Goes to sleep for 2–3 hrs after the feeds.
- Gains weight @10–15 gm/kg/day.
- Crosses birth weight by 2 weeks
- **Initiating breastfeeding within one hour of birth**: Breastfeeding must be initiated for all normal newborns as early as possible after birth, ideally within first hour for vaginal delivery and within 4 hours for cesarean section. Colostrum, the milk secreted in the first 2–3 days, must not be discarded but should be fed to newborn as it contains high concentration of protective immunoglobulins and cells. No pre-lacteal fluid should be given to the newborn.
- **Exclusive breastfeeding for the first six months of life**: It means an infant receives only breast milk from his or her mother or expressed breast milk, and no other liquids or solids, not even water. The only exceptions include administration of oral rehydration solution, oral vaccines, vitamins, minerals supplements or medicines.
- **Initiation of appropriate complementary feeding from the age of 6 months**: It means complementing breast milk with introduction of solid/semi-solid food with after child attains age of six months. It should be Timely, Adequate and Safe.

High Risk Newborn Criteria

- Babies born before full term (preterm)
- Birth weight less than 2.5 kg (low birth weight babies)
- Sick babies discharged from SNCU after treatment
- Newborns with congenital anomalies/birth defects
- Newborn whose mother is either sick/dead or cannot take care.

Continuum of Newborn Care

Facility-based Newborn Care (FBNC) along with Home Based Newborn Care (HBNC) establishes a continuum of care to ensure that every newborn receives essential services right from the time of birth and first 48 hours at the health facility and then at home during the first 42 days of life.

FACILITY-BASED NEWBORN CARE PROGRAM

Newborn Care Corner (NBCC)

- Newborn Care Corner is a designated space in the labor room and obstetric Operation Theater which is situated in draught free area, with equipments like radiant warmers, suction machines, self-inflating bag/AMBU bag including masks of size 0 and 1, oxygen availability, etc.
- NBCC is established to provide support to newborns required essential newborn care and resuscitation services.

Newborn Stabilization Unit (NBSU)

- All FRUs/CHCs must have a NBSU (within or in close proximity of the maternity ward), in addition to the newborn care corner.
- It should be for 4 bedded unit and two beds in postnatal ward for rooming-in.
- It is a unit where sick and low birth weight newborns care is provided for during short periods.

Special Newborn Care Unit (SNCU)

- Any facility (SDH/DH) with more than 3000 deliveries per year should have an SNCU.
- It provides all special care (except assisted ventilation and major surgery) for sick newborns.
- The minimum recommended number of beds in SNCU is 12.

Mother Newborn Care Unit (MNCU)

This is a new concept where the aim is 'no separation' of mother and baby including small and sick babies who require newborn care. The mother and newborn pair are to be cared for together.

HOME-BASED NEWBORN CARE (HBNC)/HOME-BASED CARE FOR YOUNG CHILD (HBYC)

- It is comprising of six home visits in case of institutional delivery (Days 3,7,14,21,28 and 42) and seven visits in case of home delivery (Day 1,3,7,14,21,28 and 42). ASHA gets INR 250/- after completing all these 6 or 7 visits with provided that baby and mother are healthy, baby's birth weight is measured and mentioned, birth registration done and vaccination of 1.5 months of age is done.
- To reduce child mortality and morbidity and improve nutrition status, growth and early childhood development of young children through additional home visits by our community health worker, the ASHA and Anganwadi worker have been incorporated in the HBYC.
- Five additional home visits by ASHA in coordination with AWW starting from 3rd months and extending into 2nd year of life (in 3rd, 6th, 9th, 12th and 15th months) will be part of HBYC. Additional incentive of INR 250/—for these five visits (Rs. 50 per visit) will be given under NHM.

NAVJAAT SHISHU SURAKSHA KARYAKRAM

The objective of this new initiative is to have a trained health personal in Basic newborn care (i.e., Prevention of Hypothermia, Prevention of infection, Early initiation of Breast-feeding and Basic Newborn Resuscitation) at every delivery point.

SOCIAL AWARENESS AND ACTIONS TO NEUTRALIZE PNEUMONIA SUCCESSFULLY (SAANS)

Goal

Reducing mortality due to childhood pneumonia in India to less than three per thousand live birth by 2025.

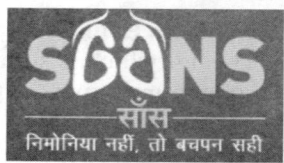

Objectives

- To create community awareness for protection and prevention against Childhood Pneumonia
- To increase awareness among caregiver to identify pneumonia early
- Dispel myths and trigger behavior change to take pneumonia seriously and seek care early.

SAANS Campaigns Requires

- Availability of amoxicillin dispersible tablet
- Severe pneumonia Inpatient care like antibiotics, pulse oximeter, oxygen

- Standard treatment protocol
- SAANS booth.

COMMUNITY-BASED PROGRAMS FOR CHILDREN

- **Mothers absolute affection (MAA) program for appropriate infant and young child feeding (IYCF)**
    - Early initiation of breastfeeding (colostrum feeding) within one hour
    - Exclusive breastfeeding for six months
    - Appropriate complementary feeding on completion of 6 months of age
    - Counseling for continued breastfeeding up to 2 years and beyond
    - Active feeding for children during and after illness.
- **Micronutrient supplementation and deworming**
    - Iron and folic acid (IFA) supplementation (from 6 month-59 month and 5-9 years)
    - Vitamin A prophylaxis Program (9 months – 59 months)
    - Deworming in children and adolescent (1–19 years)
- **Support for development care (to ensure early childhood development)**
    - Identify the interaction between a child and a parent
    - Counsel mothers/families on play and communication activities
    - Discuss age- appropriate activities for the child
- **Early detection, prevention and management of common childhood illnesses (IMNCI)**
    - Prevention and early detection of malnutrition
    - Promoting healthy practices for infant and young child feeding
    - Enabling early childhood development
    - Ensuring immunization
    - Prevention and management of common childhood illnesses (fever, jaundice, diarrhea, pneumonia, etc.)
- **Coordinating for screening and management of 4 Ds**-Developmental delays, Defects, Disease and Deficiency Disorders under RBSK, covering children at birth to 18 years of age.
- **Other national programs related to nutrition**
    - Integrated Child Development Services (ICDS) Scheme
    - National Program of Mid-Day Meal in Schools (MDMS)
    - National Iodine Deficiency Disorders Control Program (NIDDCP)

Summary of all Interventions for Newborn and Child Health

Key newborn and child intervention	Schemes/Programs under NHM
Financial incentives/entitlements for free transport and treatment of newborns and infants (up to 1 year of age) in health facilities	• Janani Suraksha Yojana (JSY) • Janani Shishu Suraksha Karyakaram (JSSK)
Care at birth, including resuscitation, at delivery points	• Newborn Care Corners • Navjaat Shishsu Suraksha Karyakarm (NSSK)
Facility-based newborn care	• Newborn Stabilization Unit (NBSU) • Special Newborn Care Unit (SNCU)
Home-based care by community health workers	• Home-based newborn care (HBNC) • Home-based care for Young Child (HBYC)

Key newborn and child intervention	Schemes/Programs under NHM
Ensuring immunization	• Universal Immunization Program (UIP) • Intensified Mission Indradhanush (IMI)
Screening and management of 4Ds—developmental delays, defects, disease and deficiency disorders	Rashtriya Bal Suraksha Karyakram (RBSK)
Facility-based management of Severe Acute Malnutrition	Nutrition Rehabilitation Centers (NRCs)
Micronutrient supplementation (Iron, Folic acid, Vitamin A)	• Anemia Mukt Bharat • Vitamin A supplementation
Deworming	• National Deworming Day (NDD)
In-patient and out-patient management of common childhood illnesses including pneumonia, diarrhea, malnutrition, etc.	• Integrated management of newborn and childhood illnesses in community (IMNCI) and Facility (F-IMNCI) • Social Awareness and Action to Neutralize Pneumonia Successfully (SAANS) • Strengthening Pediatric Care at District Hospital
Other National Programs related to Nutrition	• National Iodine Deficiency Disorders Control Program (NIDDCP)

BIBLIOGRAPHY

1. Government of India, Facility-based Newborn Care Operational Guideline, Ministry of Health and Family Welfare, New Delhi; January 2011.
2. Government of India, Navjaat Shishu Suraksha Karyakram, Basic Newborn Care and Resuscitation Program Facilitator's Guide, Ministry of Health and Family Welfare, New Delhi.
3. Government of India, Newborn Child Health Services and Programs, Supplementary Module for Community Health Officers Child Health Division, Ministry of Health and Family Welfare,
4. http://www.nrhmorissa.gov.in/writereaddata/Upload/Documents/Operational%20Guide%20IYCF.pdf

2.6 BASICS OF ADOLESCENT HEALTH ALONG WITH RELATED PROGRAMS AND GUIDELINES

- The term adolescence is derived from the Latin word "adolescere" meaning to grow and to mature.
- The term "adolescence" is applied to the lifespan, usually between 10–19 years, in which children undergo rapid changes in body size, physiology and surging hormones and social functioning.
- It is the result of the transition from childhood to adulthood.
- According to UNICEF there are 1.3 billion adolescents in the world, making up 16% of the world's total population.

Reproductive, Maternal, Newborn, Child, and Adolescent Health

- In India, Adolescents constitute about one-fifth (21.4% or 243 million) of India's population. Every fifth person in India is an adolescent. India has the largest adolescent population in the world.
- **Adolescence:** 10–19 years
- **Early adolescence:** 10–13 years
- **Mid adolescence:** 14–16 years
- **Late adolescence:** 17–19 years
- **Youth:** 15–24 years
- **Young people:** 10–24 years

The following changes are taking place during adolescent period:
- **Biological changes:** Onset of puberty
- **Cognitive changes:** Emergence of more advanced cognitive abilities
- **Emotional changes:** Self-image, intimacy, relation with adults and peers' group
- **Social changes:** Transition into new roles in the society

Group	Problems
Communicable diseases	- HIV - STIS/STDS - Tuberculosis - Hepatitis - Respiratory infections - Other infections
Non-communicable diseases	Obesity
Accidents/Injuries	- Violence - Injuries both unintentional and self injury - RTA
Addictions	- Drugs use/Abuse - Smoking/Nicotine use/Tobacco use - Alcohol use
Reproductive and sexual health problems	- Teen and unintended pregnancies - Illegal abortions - Menstrual disorders
Psychosocial problems	- Mental disorders like depression, suicide, homicide - Trafficking and prostitution - Homelessness - Academic problems and dropping out of school - Eating disorders (mental disorders are the 3rd leading cause of morbidity and mortality among adolescents)
Nutritional problems	- Nutritional anemia - Malnutrition/undernutrition

Teenage Pregnancy

- Maternal deaths are considerably higher among adolescents as compared to older women, also that the babies born to them have low birth-weight and are more likely to die at birth or in infancy.

- Early pregnancy has serious psychological, social and economic consequences also. It continues to be an impediment to improvement in the educational, economic and social status of women and is likely to have an adverse impact on the quality of life of the family.
- **Factors which lead to teenage pregnancy:**
  - Customs and traditions that lead to early marriage
  - Lack of education and information about reproductive sexual health including lack of access to tools that prevent pregnancies
  - Peer pressure to engage in sexual activity/substance misuse
  - Incorrect use of contraception
  - Exposure to abuse, violence and family strife at home
  - Low self-esteem
  - Low educational ambitions and goal.

Unsafe Abortions

- Adolescent pregnancy often leads to unsafe abortion especially if the girl is unmarried.
- The consequences of this type of abortion can be life threatening. Although abortion is legal in India (under the purview of MTP Act), it is estimated that 8 lakh Indian women a year still resort to illegal abortions because of social stigma, lack of awareness and lack of access to health facilities that offer technically competent services.

For mental health assessment among adolescents, HEADS approach could be useful:

HEADS Approach: It is very useful approach to understand the health status of adolescent age group:
- **Home**
  - Where they live, with whom?
  - Any recent changes in their home situation
  - How do they perceive their home situation
- **Education/Employment**
  - Whether they study/work, how do they perceive
  - Relationship with teachers, fellow students/employers and colleagues
  - Any recent changes
- **Eating**
  - How many meals, what they eat, what they think about their bodies
- **Activity**
  - Activities outside study/work
  - Free time activities during weekdays, holidays; spending time with family friends
- **Drugs**
  - Use of tobacco, alcohol, or other substances, injectable
  - If yes, how much, with whom, when, where
- **Sexuality**
  - Knowledge about sexual and reproductive health, menstrual hygiene
  - Sexually active, if so, nature and context

- Contraceptive use, steps to avoid SRH problems
- Problems- unwanted pregnancy, infection, sexual coercion
- Sexual orientation
☐ **Safety**-at home, road, if feel unsafe, why
☐ **Suicide/Depression:** Whether adequate sleep, do they feel unduly tiredness, whether they eat well, how do they feel emotionally, mental health problems, suicidal thoughts and attempted suicide

RASHTRIYA KISHOR SWASTHYA KARYAKARAM (RKSK)

☐ In order to respond to the health and development needs of adolescents in a holistic manner, 'Rashtriya Kishor Swasthya Karyakaram' has been lauched.
☐ This Program has shifted the focus from the existing clinic based curative services to a more comprehensive preventive and promotive care for the adolescents within their community and schools.
☐ **Target population:** Target population includes all adolescents in the age group of 10–19 years of age, Girls and boys, urban and rural, in school and out of school, married and unmarried adolescents.
☐ There is special focus on adolescents of vulnerable and marginalized population groups including urban slums, tribal areas, migrants, working adolescents and those with mental/physical disability, street children, those in care homes, and juvenile homes.

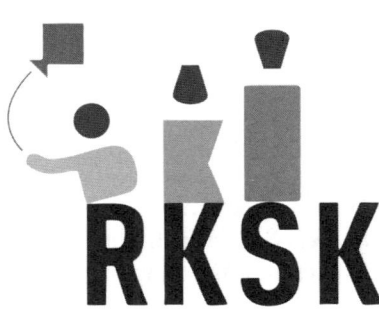

RKSK Includes Six Strategic Priorities and Objectives

Sr.	Strategic priorities	Objectives
1.	Enable sexual and reproductive health	• Improve knowledge attitude and behavior in relation to menstrual hygiene • Reducing teen age pregnancies • Improve birth preparedness and complications readiness • Provide parenting support for adolescent parents
2.	Improve nutrition	Reduce prevalence of malnutrition and iron deficiency anemia
3.	Address non-communicable diseases	Promote behavior change in adolescents to prevent NCDs
4.	Prevent substance misuse	Increase adolescent awareness on the adverse effects of substance misuse
5.	Prevent injuries and violence	Promote favorable behavior and attitudes for preventing injuries and violence including gender based violence
6.	Enhance mental health	Improve knowledge and skills on mental health issues of adolescents among health workers

Implementation Approach of RKSK

Facility-based approach	Community-based approach	School-based approach
• Adolescent friendly health • Clinics (AFHCs) providing • clinical and counseling services • Adolescent health resource center at district hospital	• Weekly Iron Folic Acid Supplementation (WIFS) • National Deworming Day (NDD) • Provision of sanitary napkins (MHS) • Peer Education Program (PE) • Quarterly Adolescent Health Days (AHD) • Adolescent Friendly Clubs (AFCs)	• Strengthening of school health activities (School Health Program) • Screening of adolescents for 4 Ds (RBSK) • National Deworming Day (NDD) • Provision of sanitary napkins (MHS) • Peer Education Program (PE)

Adolescent Friendly Health Clinics (AFHCs)

- AFHCs are established at the levels of CHC/SDH/DH and Medical College where services are provided on daily basis.
- A dedicated counsellor is available on all days at higher facilities—CHC and above.
- Sub-centers/HWC can function as walk-in-clinics for adolescents coming to these centers and services at sub-center will be provided by the CHO/ANM while the trained Medical Officer and ANM can provide Adolescent friendly services at the PHC on a weekly basis.

Package of Services at Adolescent Friendly Health Clinics

- BMI (Body Mass Index) Screening
- Hemoglobin testing
- RTI/STI management
- ANC for pregnant adolescents
- Management of menstrual problems
- Management of iron deficiency anemia
- HIV testing and counseling
- Treatment of NCDs
- Management of injuries related to accident and violence
- Counseling by counselors for common problems of adolescents.

Peer Education Program

- The adolescents in the community are covered through Peer Education (PE) Program.
- The selected Peer Educators called **Saathiya** ensure that adolescents benefit from regular and sustained peer education sessions covering all six themes of RKSK.
- This approach would facilitate the coverage of out of school adolescents in addition to the school going adolescents.
- Four peer educators (two boys and two girls) are selected per village/1000 population/ASHA habitation to reach out to adolescents.
- Each Saathiya forms a group of 15–20 boys or girls from their community and conducts weekly one to two hour participatory sessions using PE kits.

Adolescent Health Days

- The Quarterly Adolescent Health Day (AHD) is to improve coverage with preventive and promotive interventions for adolescents and to increase awareness among adolescents, parents, families and stakeholders about issues and needs related to adolescent health.
- AHDs are conducted at the village level at Anganwadi Centers or any other public place where adolescents and all stakeholders have easy accessibility.
- There is Provision of Rs.2500 for organizing quarterly AHD and incentive of Rs. 200 per ASHA for mobilization of adolescents and other stakeholders to the AHDs.

Weekly Iron Folic Acid Supplementation (WIFS)

- The Ministry of Health and Family Welfare is implementing the Weekly Iron and Folic Acid Supplementation (WIFS) Program to meet the challenge of high prevalence and incidence of anemia amongst adolescent girls and boys.
- **Intervention in schools and AWC (for out of school adolescent girls):**
  - Administration of supervised Weekly Iron-folic Acid tablet of 60 mg elemental iron and 500 ug folic acid using a fixed day approach.
  - Screening of target groups for moderate/severe anemia and referring these cases to an appropriate nearby government health facility.
  - Biannual deworming (Albendazole 400 mg) for control of helminthes infestation.
  - Information and counseling for improving dietary intake and prevention of intestinal worm infestation.

Menstrual Hygiene Scheme (MHS)

- This scheme is being implemented in majority of the States for promotion of menstrual hygiene among adolescent girls in the age group of 10–19 years living primarily in the rural areas.
- Now, the scheme is being extended to urban areas in a phased manner with implementation strategy remaining the same as for the rural areas.
- **Objectives:**
  - To increase awareness among adolescent girls on menstrual hygiene, build self-esteem, and empower girls for greater socialization.
  - To increase access to and use of high quality sanitary napkins by adolescent girls.
  - To ensure safe disposal of sanitary napkins in an environment friendly manner.
- ASHAs provide sanitary napkins to adolescent's girls in schools and within the communities at the subsidized rate of Rs. 6/- for a pack of 6 napkins and are entitled to get Rs. 1/-for every pack sold and one free pack of sanitary napkins per month for themselves.

Other Initiatives for Adolescents

- RMNCAH + N
- RKSK
- School Health and Wellness Ambassador Initiative, etc.
- RBSK
- ICDS
- Kishori Shakti Yojana
- Adolescent Girl Scheme
- Nutrition program for adolescent girls
- SABLA

BIBLIOGRAPHY

1. https://vikaspedia.in/health/nrhm/national-health-Programs-1/rashtriya-bal-swasthya-karyakram-rbsk
2. https://pib.gov.in/PressReleasePage.aspx?PRID=1744059 https://nhm.gov.in/New_Updates_2018/NHM_Components/RMNCHA/AH/Training_Materials/Curriculum-on-Health-and-Wellness-of-School-Going-Children-English.pdf

2.7 REPRODUCTIVE MATERNAL NEWBORN CHILD ADOLESCENT HEALTH PLUS NUTRITION (RMNCAH + N)

- Following the Government of India's "Call to Action (CTA) Summit" in February, 2013, the Ministry of Health and Family Welfare launched Reproductive, Maternal, Newborn, Child plus Adolescent Health (RMNCH+A) Program/strategy to ensure effective integration of these health services for reducing maternal and child morbidity and mortality.
- Due to the importance of nutrition across all life stages, the strategy now includes nutrition as one of its important pillars.
- RMNCAH+N strategy thus covers Reproductive, Maternal, Newborn, Child and Adolescent Health and the "plus" within it focuses on Nutrition, as well as important linkages between these services and with other components like family planning, adolescent health, HIV, gender, and preconception and prenatal diagnostic techniques.
- It also focuses on linkages between community-based services and facility-based services and ensures referrals, and counter-referrals between various levels of healthcare system to create a continuous care pathway.
- The RMNCAH+N Strategy is at the heart of the flagship National Health Mission.
- **Current Status:**

Indicator	National Health Policy	SDG 2030	Current Status (SRS)
Maternal mortality ratio	100 by 2020	<70	97
Neonatal mortality rate	16 by 2025	<12	20
Infant mortality rate	28 by 2019	–	28
Under 5 mortality rate	23 by 2025	≤25	32
Total fertility rate	Replacement level fertility	–	2.0

RMNCAH+N Life Cycle Approach

- Under RMNCAH+N, reproductive health and nutrition interventions are cross cutting across all life stages.
- The reproductive health forms the primary pillar of RMNCAH+N and aims at ensuring healthy reproductive practices, encouraging contraceptive use while having an effective integration of the maternal, child, adolescent health and family planning.

Reproductive, Maternal, Newborn, Child, and Adolescent Health

Both support each other

Healthy adult man
- Maintains good nutritional status
- Free from STI/RTI/HIV
- Has knowledge about contraception
- Plans with partner about when to become a parent

Healthy adult woman
- Maintains good nutritional status
- Free from anemia
- Free from STI/RTI/HIV
- Aware about contraception
- Plans with partner about when to become a parent

Becomes pregnant
- Not before 20 years of age
or
- At least 2 years after previous childbirth
or
- At least 6 months after an abortion

Healthy pregnant woman
- Takes essential ANC services
- Receives essential care at home, birth preparedness
- Takes nutritious diet, IFA and calcium supplementation
- Recognize danger signs
- Has knowledge about healthy spacing and contraception

Healthy adolescent boy/girl
- Have normal growth with good nutrition status
- Free from anemia
- Aware of body changes, functions and menstrual hygiene
- Aware about risks involved in teenage pregnancy and how to prevent it
- Aware about prevention of RTIs/STIs/HIV and is free from these infections

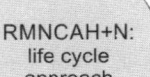

RMNCAH+N: life cycle approach

Has a safe delivery

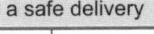

Healthy mother (postpartum)
- Receives PNC care at home
- Takes nutritious diet
- Free from complications
- Initiates breastfeeding immediately after delivery
- Adopts contraception during or just after postpartum period

Grows into

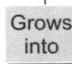

Healthy child
- Have normal growth with good nutritional status
- Free from serious illness
- Received full immunization

Grows into

Healthy infant (1 year)
- Receives exclusive breastfeeding for 6 months and complementary feeding after 6 months while continuation of breastfeeding at least till 2 years
- Receives immunization as per protocol
- Have normal growth and milestones

Grows into

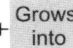

Healthy newborn baby
- Has normal birth weight
- Initiation of breastfeeding within an hour after delivery
- Free from any gross congenital anomaly
- Receives essential newborn care

Reproductive, Maternal, Newborn, Child, and Adolescent Health

❏ **Main Interventions under RMNCAH+N:**

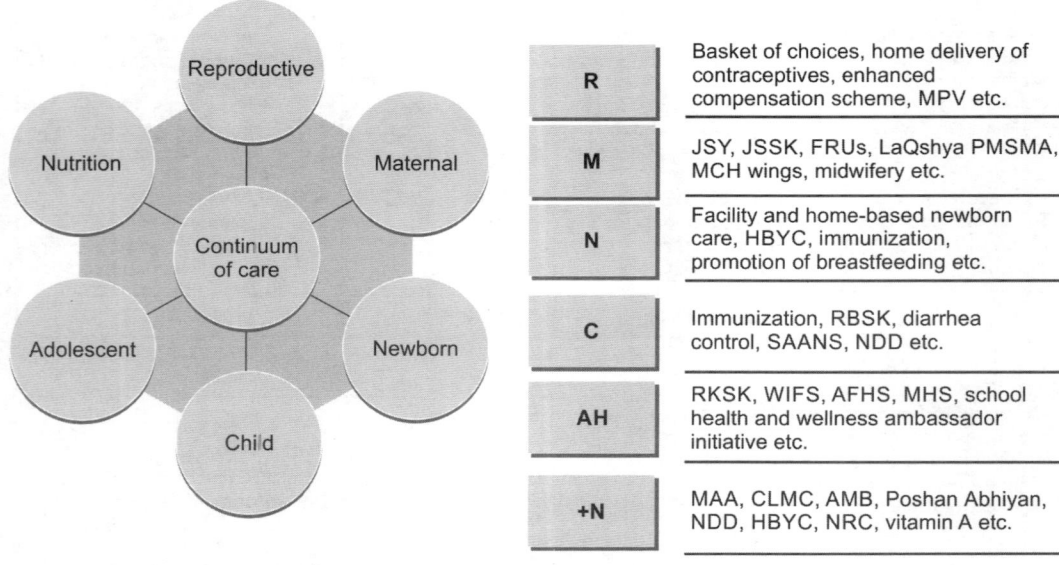

R	Basket of choices, home delivery of contraceptives, enhanced compensation scheme, MPV etc.
M	JSY, JSSK, FRUs, LaQshya PMSMA, MCH wings, midwifery etc.
N	Facility and home-based newborn care, HBYC, immunization, promotion of breastfeeding etc.
C	Immunization, RBSK, diarrhea control, SAANS, NDD etc.
AH	RKSK, WIFS, AFHS, MHS, school health and wellness ambassador initiative etc.
+N	MAA, CLMC, AMB, Poshan Abhiyan, NDD, HBYC, NRC, vitamin A etc.

❏ **Maternal Health Interventions:**

Surakshit Matritva Aashwashan (SUMAN)	Janani Shishu Suraksha Karyakram (JSSK)	Janani Suraksha Yojana (JSY)	Pradhan Mantri Surakshit Matritva Abhiyan (PMSMA)
LaQshya - labor room and maternity OT	Midwifery initiative	Comprehensive abortion care services (CAC)	Universal screening for GDM, HIV and syphilis
Strengthening first referral units (FRUS) and delivery points (DP)	MCH wings and obstetric HDUs/ ICUs	Capacity building of human resource: Dakshata, CEmONC, LSAS, SBA etc.	Maternal death surveillance and response (MDSR)

Reproductive, Maternal, Newborn, Child, and Adolescent Health

□ **Newborn and Child Health Interventions:**

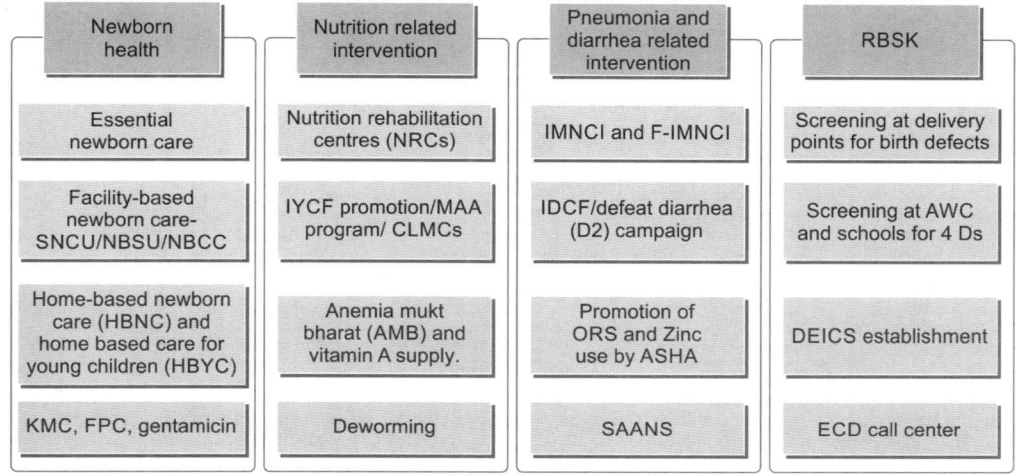

□ **Key Interventions for Child Nutrition:**

- Anemia Mukt Bharat Strategy
- National Deworming Day (NDD)
- Nutrition Rehabilitation Centres (NRCs)
- Intensified Diarrhea Control Fortnight
- Mothers Absolute Affection (MAA) Program
- Lactation Management Centers (LMCs)
- Vitamin A Supplementation
- POSHAN Abhiyaan

□ **Key Interventions for Reproductive Health:**

- Mission Parivar Vikas: Launched in 146 high fertility districts (TFR > 3.0) in seven high focus states
- New Contraceptive Choices: Injectable contraceptive (under antara program) and centchroman (Chhaya)
- Family planning logistics management information system (FP-LMIS)
- Quality assurance committees at state and district levels to monitor the quality of family planning services including adverse events
- National family planning indemnity scheme (NFPIS)
- Enhanced compensation scheme
- Scheme for home delivery of contraceptives by ASHAs at doorstep of beneficiaries.
- Vasectomy fortnight
- World population day campaign

Reproductive, Maternal, Newborn, Child, and Adolescent Health

❏ **5 × 5 Matrix for High Impact RMNCH+A Interventions (old strategy):**

Reproductive health	Maternal health	Newborn health	Child health	Adolescent health
• Focus spacing methods particularly PPIUCD at high case load facilities • Focus on interval IUCD at all facilities including subcentres on fixed days • Home delivery of contraceptives (HDC) and ensuring spacing at birth (ESB) through ASHAs • Ensuring access to pregnancy testing kits (PTK-"nischay kits") and strengthening comprehensive abortion care services. • Maintaining quality sterilization services.	• Use MCTS to ensure early registration of pregnancy and full ANC • Detect high risk pregnancies and line list including severely anemic mothers and ensure appropriate management. • Equip delivery points with highly trained HR and ensure equitable access to EmOC services through FRUs; add MCH wings as per need • Review maternal, infant and child deaths for corrective actions • Identify villages with low institutional delivery and distribute misoprostol to select women during pregnancy; incentivize ANMs for domiciliary deliveries	• Early initiation and exclusive breastfeeding • Home-based newborn care through ASHA • Essential newborn care and resuscitation services at all delivery points • Special newborn care units with highly trained human resource and other infrastructure • Community level use of gentamicin by ANM	• Complementary feeding, IFA supplementation and focus on nutrition • Diarrhea management at community level using ORS and zinc • Management of pneumonia • Full immunization coverage • Rashtriya bal swasthya karyakram (RBSK): screening of children for 4Ds' (birth defects, development delays, deficiencies and disease) and its management	• Address teenage pregnancy and increase contraceptive prevalence in adolescents • Introduce community-based services through peer educators • Strengthen ARSH clinics • Roll out national Iron plus initiative including weekly IFA supplementation • Promote menstrual hygiene

Health systems strengthening	Cross cutting interventions
• Case load based deployment of HR at all levels • Ambulances, drugs, diagnostics, reproductive health commodities • Health education, demand promotion and behavior change communication • Supportive supervision and use of data for monitoring and review including scorecards based on HMIS • Public grievances redressal mechanism; client satisfaction and patient safety through all round quality assurance	• Bring down out of pocket expenses by ensuring JSSK, RBSK and other free entitlements • ANMs and nurses to provide specialized and quality care to pregnant women and children • Address social determinants of health through convergence • Focus on unserved and underserved villages, urban slums and blocks • Introduce difficult area and performance based incentives

BIBLIOGRAPHY

1. https://nhm.gov.in/New_Update-2021-22/Presentation/PS-MD-Orientation-workshop-26-08-2021/RMNCAH+N.pdf
2. https://nhm.gov.in/images/pdf/Programs/familyplaning/guidelines/RMNCAH+N_Manual_on_Counseling_2021.pdf
3. https://nhm.gujarat.gov.in/images/pdf/High-Impact-English.pdf

2.8 UNIVERSAL IMMUNIZATION PROGRAM (UIP)

❏ Expanded program on immunization was launched in 1978. It was renamed as Universal Immunization Program in 1985 when its reach was expanded beyond urban areas.
❏ In 1992, it was included in child survival and safe motherhood program and in 1997 it became part of reproductive and child health program.
❏ UIP is one of the largest immunization programs in the world on the basis of quantities of vaccine used, number of beneficiaries (2.76 crore newborns and almost 3 crore pregnant women), number of immunization sessions organized, geographical spread and diversity of areas covered.
❏ It is one of the most cost-effective public health interventions and largely responsible for reduction of vaccine preventable under-5 mortality rate.
❏ Under UIP 12 vaccines are being provided free of cost. These are—BCG, bOPV, Hepatitis B, Pentavalent, Rotavirus, PCV, fIPV, Measles/MR, JE, DPT, and Td.
❏ Except JE vaccine, all 11 vaccines are available in all states.

Reproductive, Maternal, Newborn, Child, and Adolescent Health

Table 2.3: Milestones.

Year	Milestone
1978	Expanded Program of immunization BCG, DPT, OPV, typhoid (urban areas)
1983	TT vaccine for pregnant women
1985	Universal Immunization Program— measles added, typhoid removed., Focus on children less than 1 year of age
1990	Vitamin-A supplementation
1995	Polio National Immunization Days
1997	VVM introduced on vaccines in UIP
2002	Hep B introduced as pilot in 33 districts and cities of 10 states
2005	• National Rural Health Mission Launched • Auto Disable (AD) Syringes introduced into UIP
2006	JE vaccine introduced after campaigns in endemic districts
2007–8	Hep 13 expanded to all. districts in 10 states and schedule revised to 4 doses from 3 doses
2010	Measles 2nd dose introduced in RI and MCUP (14 states)
2011	• Hepatitis B universalized and Hemophilus influenza type b introduced as pentavalent states • Open Vial Policy for vaccines in UIP
2013	• Pentavalent expanded to 9 states • Second dose of JE vaccine
2014	India and South East Asia Region certified POLIO- FREE
2015	• India validated for Maternal and Neonatal Tetanus elimination • Pentavalent expanded to all states • IPV Introduced
2016	• Rotavirus vaccine introduced in 4 states in Phase I. • tOPV to bOPV switch • Switch to fractional IPV (Phased) • Rotavirus vaccine introduced (Phased launch)
2017	• MR Vaccine introduced • PCV (phased launch) • Use of adrenaline IM by ANM in AEFI
2019	• Tetanus and adult diphtheria (Td) introduced • RVV expanded to all states
2021	PCV expanded to all states
2022	IMI 4.0 was conducted
2023	Third dose of fIPV introduced

The Objectives of UIP

- Rapidly increase immunization coverage
- Improve the quality of services
- Establish a reliable cold chain system up to the health facility level
- Introduce a district-wise system for monitoring of performance
- Achieve self-sufficiency in vaccine production

Table 2.4: National immunization schedule.

Vaccine	Type	Schedule	Dose	Route	Site	Strain and VVM	Remarks	Images
TT-1 or Td 1	Toxoid	as Early as possible in pregnancy	0.5 mL	Intra-muscular	Upper arm	VVM 30	• Currently TT is replaced by Td • **Td**- Tetanus and adult diphtheria • **Td Booster** if pregnancy occurs within 3 years of last pregnancy and two Td dose were received.	
TT-2 or Td 2	Toxoid	4 weeks after TT-1/Td-1	0.5 mL	Intra-muscular	Upper arm			
For infant								
BCG	Live	At birth	0.1 mL (0.05 until 1 month age- because neonatal skin is too thin)	Intra-dermal	Left upper arm	• Danish 1331 Strain • **VVM 2** (VVM 2 means vaccine remain stable for 2 days at 37°C)	• **Diluent:** 1 mL sodium chloride • **Discard** 4 hour after reconstitution • Reconstituted vaccine is light sensitive and it should be protected from sun light – hence vial is amber color • **Maximum age limit:** till one year of age • If scar does not appear after vaccination, there is no need for revaccination.	
Hepatitis B-0 (Birth dose)	Recom-binant	At birth (within 24 hours)	0.5 mL	Intra-muscular	Antero lateral aspect of mid-thigh-Left	VVM 30	• It is freeze sensitive vaccine and never to be frozen • Give within 24 hours of birth	

Reproductive, Maternal, Newborn, Child, and Adolescent Health

Vaccine	Type	Schedule	Dose	Route	Site	Strain and VVM	Remarks	Images
OPV-0 (Zero dose)	Live	At birth	2 drops	Oral	Oral	Bivalent strain (Type 1 and 3) **VVM 2**	**Maximum age limit** - within 15 days of birth	
OPV-1,2,3	Live	At 6 weeks, 10 weeks, 14 weeks	2 drops	Oral	Oral	Bivalent strain Type 1 and 3) **VVM 2**	**Maximum age limit:** till five years of age	
Pentavalent 1,2,3	DPT: Diphtheria and Tetanus are toxoid, Pertussis killed, Hepatitis B recombinant	At 6 weeks, 10 weeks, 14 weeks	0.5 mL	Intra-muscular	Antero-lateral side of mid-thigh-Left	VVM 30	It contains DPT, Hepatitis B, Hi Influenza type B **Maximum age limit:** till one year of age	
fIPV (Fractional Inactivated Polio vaccine)	Killed	At 6 weeks, 14 weeks and 9 months	0.1 mL	Intra-dermal	At 6 weeks and 4 weeks at right upper arm while at 9 months on left upper arm	VVM 7 • Strains of IPV are Mahoney (type 1 poliovi-rus), MEF-1 (type 2 poliovi-rus), and Saukett (type 3 poliovirus)	**Maximum age limit:** till one year of age	

Reproductive, Maternal, Newborn, Child, and Adolescent Health

Vaccine	Type	Schedule	Dose	Route	Site	Strain and VVM	Remarks	Images
Rota virus-1,2,3 (Rotasii)	Live attenuated freeze dried vaccine	At 6 weeks, 10 weeks, 14 weeks	2.5 mL	Orals	Oral	**Rotasiil** (RV5) vaccine containing five viruses (Human and Bovine reassortant strains) of serotype G1, G2, G3, G4 and G9. **VVM 30**	**Procedure:** 2.5 mL Orally, administer slowly with the nozzle of the 6 mL oral syringe pointed towards the inner cheek (buccal cavity) of the infant. **Diluent:** Citrate bicarbonate It can be used up to maximum of 4 hours after reconstitution **Maximum age limit:** till one year of age **Now it is available in sachet form**	
Rota virus-1,2,3 (Rotavac)	Live (liquid formulation)	At 6 weeks, 10 weeks, 14 weeks	5 drops	Orals	Oral	**Rotavac** (ORV116E), a live vaccine containing suspension of Rotavirus 116E **VVM 2**	Rotavirus vaccine vial can be used up to a maximum of 4 hours after opening. **Maximum age limit:** till one year of age	
PCV-1, PCV-2, PCV B (Pneumococcal conjugate vaccine)	Conjugate vaccine	**Two primary doses:** - At 6 weeks, 14 weeks, **Booster dose:** - 9 months	0.5 mL	Intramuscular	Antero lateral side of mid-thigh-Right	PCV13 **VVM 30**	**Maximum age limit:** till one year of age	

Reproductive, Maternal, Newborn, Child, and Adolescent Health

Vaccine	Type	Schedule	Dose	Route	Site	Strain and VVM	Remarks
MR -1 (Measles, Rubella)	Live	First dose at- 9 month completed	0.5 mL	Sub-cutaneous	Right upper arm	Measles: Edmonston Zagreb strain (Most common, Schwartz strain, Moraten strain) Rubella : RA 27/3	**Diluent:** 2.5 mL double distilled water. Reconstitution vaccine should be used within 4 hour. Reconstituted vaccine looses potency on exposure to light and is very heat labile and needs to-be protected from light. Hence, the vaccine vial is available in amber colour. Diluent should be kept at 2–8°C at least 24 h before use, **Maximum age limit:** till five years of age
JE* 1st dose (Japanese Encephalitis)	Live	9–12 months	0.5 mL	Sub-cutaneous	Left supper arm	SA 14-14-2 strain **VVM 14**	**Diluent:** Phosphate buffer solution **Maximum age limit:** till fifteen years of age **JenVac** vaccine to be launched which is to be given i.e., and will be under open vial policy
Vitamin A	First dose at 9 months with measles		1 mL (1 lakh IU)	Oral	Oral		Second dose at 16th months (with 2nd dose of measles) Then after every 6 months 2 lakh IU/2 mL up to 5 years of age. If vit A is given as treatment, Administer 2,00,000 IU of vitamin A to child >1 year of age immediately after diagnosis. To be followed by 2,00,000 IU of vitamin A 1—4 weeks later vitamin A syrup should be discarded after 8 weeks of opening.

Reproductive, Maternal, Newborn, Child, and Adolescent Health

Vaccine	Type	Schedule	Dose	Route	Site	Strain and VVM	Remarks	Images
For Children								
DPT Booster-1	Formalin-inactivated diphtheria toxin (killed), with whole cell Pertussis and tetanus toxoid	16–24 months	0.5 mL	Intra-muscular	Antero-lateral side of mid-thigh-Left		Freeze sensitive and need to be protected from freezing **Maximum age limit:** till seven years of age	
OPV Booster	Live	16–24 months	2 drops	Oral	Oral		**Maximum age limit:** till five years of age	
MEASLES 2nd dose Or MR-2	Live	16–24 months	0.5 mL	Sub-cutaneous	Right upper arm		**Maximum age limit:** till five years of age	
JE 2nd dose	Live	16–24 months	0.5 mL	Sub-cutaneous	Left upper arm		**Maximum age limit:** till fifteen years of age	
5–6 years								
DPT Booster-2	As same as DPT Booster 1	5–6 years	0.5 mL	Intra-muscular	Left upper arm		**Maximum age limit:** till seven years of age	
For 10–16 years								
Td-1, Td-2	Toxoid	10 years, 16 years	0.5 mL	Intra-muscular	Upper Arms	VVM 30	Td : Tetanus and adult diphtheria **Maximum age limit:** till sixteen year of age If schedule started with TT then also Td vaccine can be given in subsequent dose.	

* JE wherever introduced

* Multiple injections can be given in the same thigh but the distance between the two injections should be at least 2.5 cm (1 inch)

*Pentavalent, IPV, PCV and Rotavirus vaccines, if at least one dose is given before one year of age, then remaining doses can be administered and schedule must be completed irrespective of the age of child. If the first dose is not administered before one year of age, then these vaccines cannot be administered to the child under UIP.

Reproductive, Maternal, Newborn, Child, and Adolescent Health

Note: If 1st dose of MR vaccine delayed beyond 12 months, then ensure minimum 1 month gap between two MR doses while JE vaccine delayed beyond 12 months then ensure minimum 3 months gap between two JE doses.

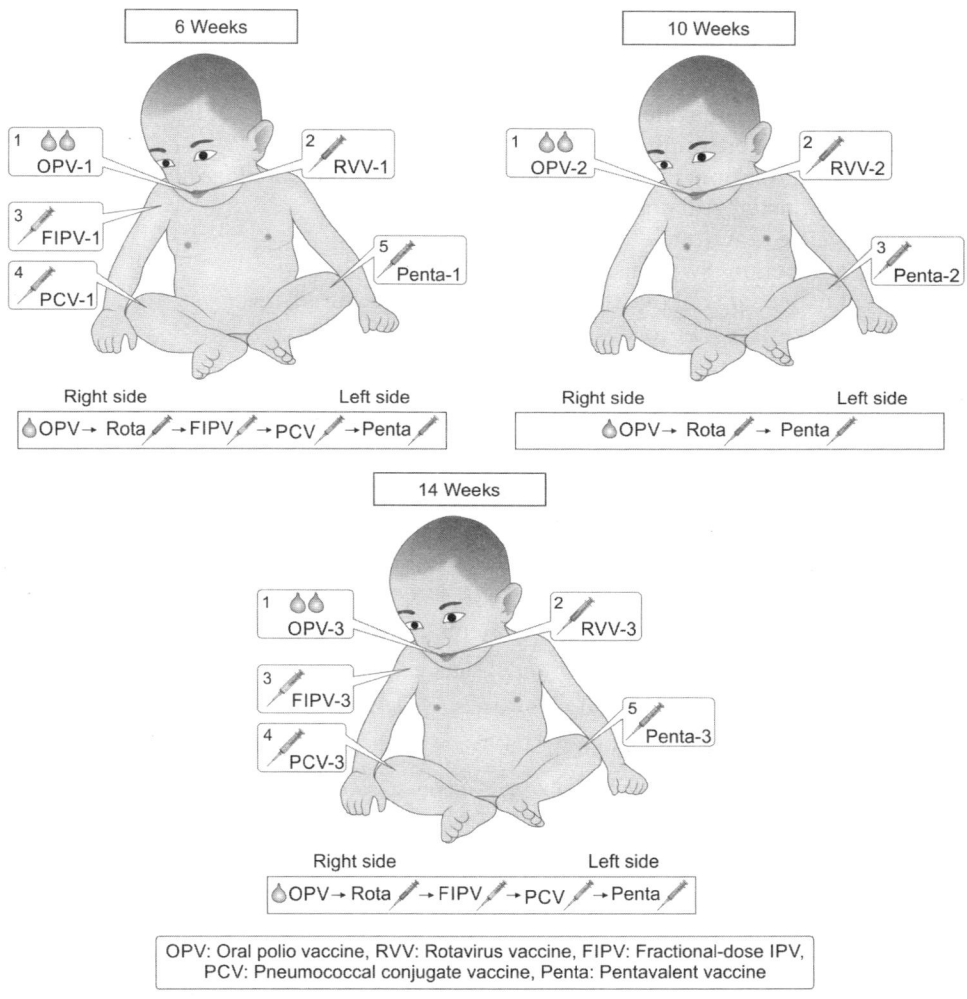

Fig. 2.3: Ideal sequence of administration of vaccines.

Some Important FAQs Regarding Due Vaccines as per Different Age Group

What vaccines should be given to a 7-months old child who has not been vaccinated?
   Answer: BCG, OPV-1, RVV-1, Penta-1, fIPV- 1, PCV-1
❑ What vaccines should be given to a 9-months old child who has received BCG, OPV-2, RVV-1, Penta-2, fIPV-1, PCV-1 only?
   Answer: Give OPV-3, RVV-2, fIPV-2, Penta-3, PCV- 2, MR-1, JE-1
❑ What vaccines should be given to 16-months old child who has never been vaccinated?
   Answer: OPV-1, DPT-1, MR-1, JE-1

- What vaccines should be given to 18-months old child who has received BCG, OPV-2, RVV-2, fIPV-1 Penta-2, PCV-1 only?
  Answer: OPV-3, RVV-3, fIPV-2, Penta-3, PCV-2, MR-1, JE-1

Definition of Full and Complete Immunization

- **Full immunization**: Before age of 1 year: one dose of BCG, 3 doses of OPV, 3 doses of rotavirus, 3 doses of pentavalent, 3 doses of fractional IPV, 3 doses of PCV, MR vaccine -1st dose, JE 1st dose (where applicable).
- **Complete immunization**: Before the age of 2 years received 2nd dose of Measles/MR, DPT booster, polio booster, 2nd dose of JE (where applicable)
- **Common vaccine reaction:**
  - BCG: Local reaction (swelling, pain, redness)
  - DPT, Pentavalent : Local reaction (swelling ,pain, redness), fever
  - Hepatitis B: Local reaction (swelling, pain, redness), fever
  - OPV: None
  - IPV: None
  - Tetanus: local reaction (swelling, pain, redness), malaise and non-specific symptoms
- Rare serious adverse events mentioned in **Table 2.5**.

Table 2.5: Rare serious adverse events.

Vaccine	Reaction
BCG	Suppurative lymphadenitis, BCG osteitis, disseminated BCG infection
Hepatitis B	Guillain-Barre syndrome (plasma derived), Anaphylaxis
Measles	Febrile seizures, anaphylaxis, thrombocytopenia
OPV	Vaccine-associated paralytic polio, vaccine derived polio virus
Tetanus	Brachial neuritis, thrombocytopenia
DPT	Persistent (>3 hours) inconsolable screaming, seizures Hypotonic hyporesponsive episode (HHE), Anaphylaxis/shock Encephalopathy

Contraindication of Vaccine

- Live vaccine: Pregnancy, radiation therapy
- BCG: Symptomatic HIV infection
- Pertussis: Neurological disease, anaphylactic reaction to previous dose
- All other vaccines: Any current serious illness, anaphylactic reaction to previous dose.

Responsibilities of ANM for routine immunization session: ANM can take help from ASHA and AWW.

- Map of area under SC with names of villages, urban areas including all hamlets (tola), sub-villages, sub-wards, sector, mohalla, hard to reach areas, etc.).
- Demarcation map—allocate areas for each ANM if more than 2 ANMs are present in a SC. It can also show the exact boundaries and areas for ASHAs and AWWs.
- Master list of the area–this list includes all villages/tolas/HRAs/wards/mohalls
  - An estimation of beneficiaries.
  - An estimation of vaccines and logistics.
  - ANM work plan including mobilization plan.

Types of Routine Immunization Session

- **Fixed:** These sessions are held where vaccine storage is possible because of availability of ILR and deep freezer (DF), i.e., the sessions conducted at PHC/CHC.
- **Outreach:** All sessions conducted where vaccine has to be taken by vaccine carrier.
- **Mobile:** Sessions conducted using a vehicle which moves from site to site along with the immunization team and vaccine.
- **Tagged:** Site/area which does not have a session but is linked to the nearest session site.

Give These Four Key Messages to the Caregiver after Vaccination

1. What vaccine was given and what disease it prevents (e.g. BCG for preventing TB).
2. When to come for the next visit.
3. What are the minor side-effects and how to deal with them.
4. To keep the vaccination card safe and to bring it along for the next visit.

BIBLIOGRAPHY

1. https://nhm.gov.in/New_Updates_2018/NHM_Components/Immunization/Guildelines_for_immunization/Immunization_Handbook_for_Medical_Officers%202017.pdf
2. https://main.mohfw.gov.in/sites/default/files/Universal.pdf

CHAPTER 3

Demography, Surveillance, and Data

CHAPTER OUTLINE

- 3.1 Demography: Background, scope and definition
- 3.2 Demography cycle
- 3.3 population pyramid, dependency ratio and other important definitions
- 3.4 Sex ratio
- 3.5 Important vital statistics indicators
- 3.6 Sources of vital statistics
- 3.7 Summary of common sampling methods
- 3.8 Data: Source, methods of collection, analysis, and interpretation
- 3.9 National population policy
- 3.10 Basics of surveillance including IDSP and IHIP

3.1 DEMOGRAPHY: BACKGROUND, SCOPE AND DEFINITION

DEMOGRAPHY

- It is defined as scientific study of population size, composition and distribution of human population.
- Demo means people and graphy means recording.
- India's area is 2.4% of total world while 17.4% of total world population.
- Demography includes marriage, fertility, migration, social mobility and mortality.
- Study of demography is useful to measure the change in population and it will help to control population growth and also study the social, economical and political problem.
- John Graunt is known as father of demography.
- Population dynamics is a study and measurement of population changes and components of change overtime.
- Birth, death and migration affect the size, composition and distribution of population.

DEMOGRAPHIC TRANSITION IN INDIA

- Definition of **"demographic transition"** the transition from a largely rural agrarian society with high fertility and mortality rates to a predominantly urban industrial society with low fertility and mortality rates.
- It denotes change in population size from a condition in which both the birth and death rates are high, to another condition in which both rates are low.
- Before and after transition the population size is relatively stable.

Phases of Demographic Transition (Fig. 3.1)

Phase I: Pretransition phase (1990–1921)
- Also known as "big divide" because up to 1921, population of India was stable but then after it is steadily increasing that's why 1921 is known as "big divide" **(Fig. 3.2)**.
- Before 1921 the BR was almost equal to DR. So, negligible increase in population.
- High death rate was due to large scale famine and epidemics.

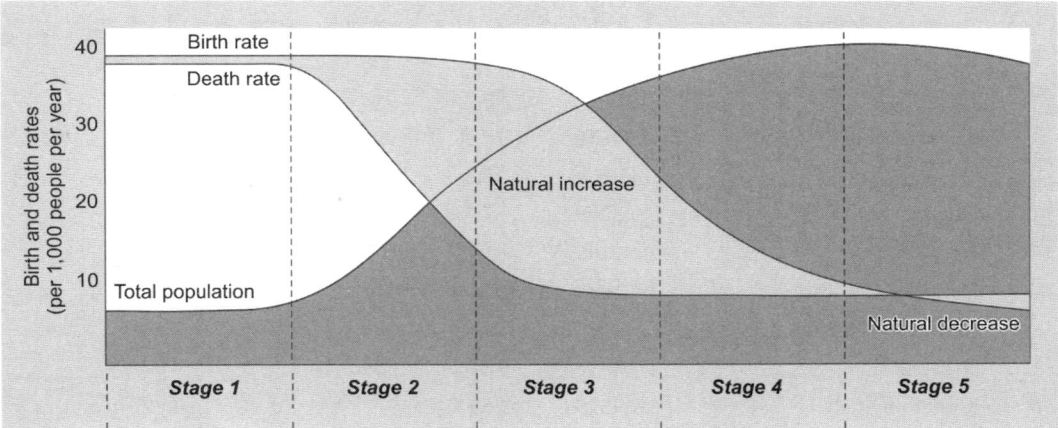

Fig. 3.1: Phases of demographic transition.

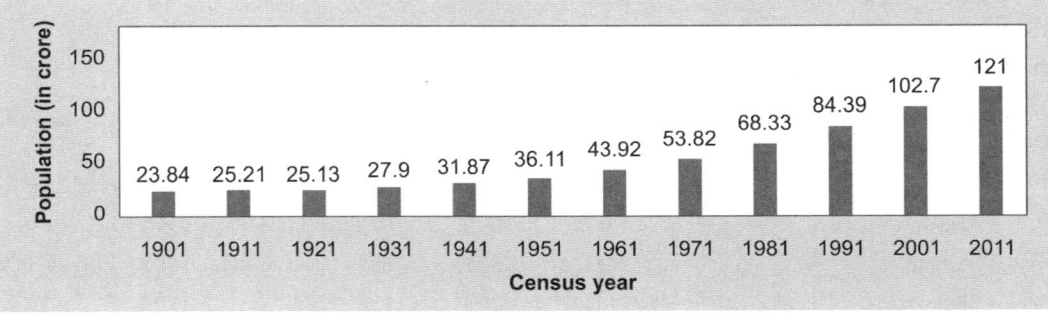

Fig. 3.2: Decadal growth of Indian population (1901–2011).

Phase II: Early transition stage (1921–1951)—slow but steady growth.

Phase III: Mid transition stage (1951–2001)—population explosion phase.

Phase IV: Late transition stage (2001–2010)—birth rate and death rate both have come down due to achievement of TFR.

Phase V: Post transition phase—Population becomes stable. India will achieve this stage by 2045.

Phase VI: Declining stage—Death rate is more than birth rate, e.g., Germany.

1921 known as a big divide because population has been steadily increasing since 1921.

Table 3.1: Census 2011: Statewise data of population, sex ratio, and population density.

Sl. No.	India/state/union territory	Population	Rural %	Sex ratio	Population density (per sq. km)
	INDIA	1210854977	68.9	943	382
1.	Andhra Pradesh**	49386799	70.4	993	308
2.	Arunachal Pradesh	1383727	77.1	938	17
3.	Assam	31205576	85.9	958	398
4.	Bihar	104099452	88.7	918	1106
5.	Chhattisgarh	25545198	76.8	991	189
6.	Goa	1458545	37.8	973	394
7.	Gujarat	60439692	57.4	919	308
8.	Haryana	25351462	65.1	879	573
9.	Himachal Pradesh	6864602	90.0	972	123
10.	Jammu and Kashmir	12541302	72.6	889	56
11.	Jharkhand	32988134	76.0	949	414
12.	Karnataka	61095297	61.3	973	319
13.	Kerala	33406061	52.3	1084	860
14.	Madhya Pradesh	72626809	72.4	931	236
15.	Maharashtra	112374333	54.8	929	365
16.	Manipur*	2855794	70.8	992	128
17.	Meghalaya	2966889	79.9	989	132
18.	Mizoram	1097206	47.9	976	52
19.	Nagaland	1978502	71.1	931	119
20.	Odisha	41974218	83.3	979	270
21.	Punjab	27743338	62.5	895	551
22.	Rajasthan	68548437	75.1	928	200
23.	Sikkim	610577	74.8	890	86

Sl. No.	India/state/union territory	Population	Rural %	Sex ratio	Population density (per sq. km)
24.	Tamil Nadu	72147030	51.6	996	555
25.	Telangana**	35193978	61.3	—	306
26.	Tripura	3673917	73.8	960	350
27.	Uttarakhand	10086292	69.8	963	189
28.	Uttar Pradesh	199812341	77.7	912	829
29.	West Bengal	91276115	68.1	950	1028
30.	Andaman and Nicobar Island	380581	62.3	876	46
31.	Chandigarh	1055450	2.7	818	9258
32.	Dadra and Nagar Haveli	343709	53.3	774	700
33.	Daman and Diu	243247	24.8	618	2191
34.	Delhi	16787941	2.5	868	11320
35.	Lakshadweep	64473	21.9	947	2149
36.	Puducherry	1247953	31.7	1037	2547

3.2 DEMOGRAPHY CYCLE

- **Demographic cycle:** A demographic cycle has 5 stages through which a nation passes.
- **Demographic cycle stage:**

Stage	Population status	DR	BR
First stage	High stationary	High	High
Second stage	Early expanding Ex. Africa	Starts to decline	Unchanged
Third stage	Late expanding Ex. India	Declines still further	Starts to fall
Fourth stage	Low stationary	Low BR	Low DR
Fifth stage	Declining E.g., Germany and Hungary	BR is lower than DR	

3.3 POPULATION PYRAMID, DEPENDENCY RATIO AND OTHER IMPORTANT DEFINITIONS

- **Concept of population pyramid with examples:** Population pyramid is a graphical representation of the age and sex composition of a given population in the form of two histograms, one for each gender where the numbers are shown horizontally and the ages vertically.

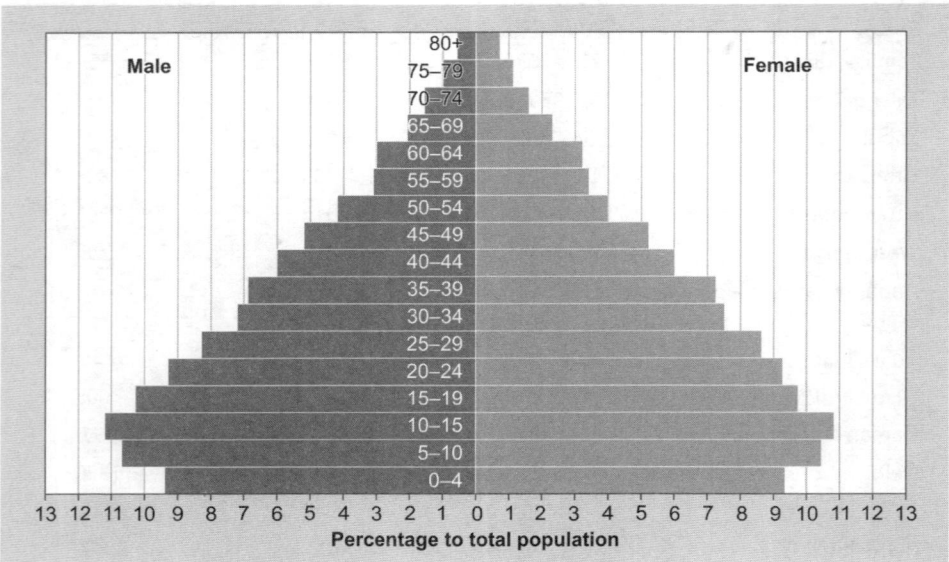

Fig. 3.3: Actual population pyramid of India as per census 2011.

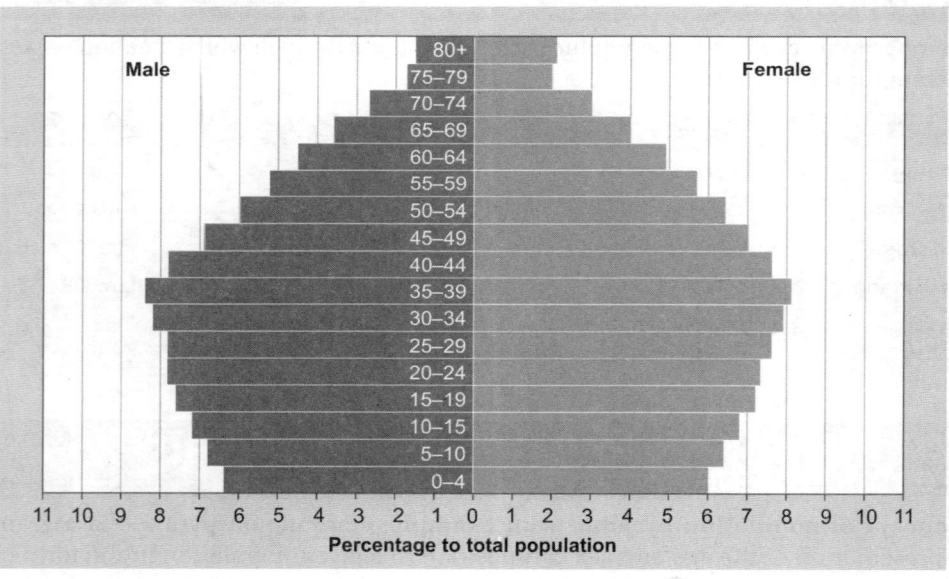

Fig. 3.4: Projected population pyramid of India for the year 2036.

By comparing population pyramid of 2011 and 2036 **(Figs. 3.3 and 3.4)**, it is clearly understandable that the old age people cohort would be smaller than younger population cohort while due to expected decline in fertility, the base of pyramid would be narrow down and middle of the pyramid would be broadened in 2036.

Demography, Surveillance, and Data

- **Demographic dividend:** According to United Nations Population Fund (UNFPA), demographic dividend means, "the economic growth potential that can result from shifts in a population's age structure, mainly when the share of the working-age population (15 to 64) is larger than the non-working-age share of the population (14 and younger, and 65 and older)".
- **Demographic burden:** Demographic burden is represented by dependency ratios.
- **Dependency ratio:** The dependency ratio, which is the ratio of economically active to economically inactive persons, is dependent on age composition.
  Formula:
  $$\frac{\text{No. of children 0–14 years + 65 years or more}}{\text{No. of person between 15 to 64 years}}$$
  - It is the ratio of the financially dependent population over economically productive population. Current (census 2011) dependency ratio is 652 it means 1000 productive age group need to earn for 1652 persons (1000 themselves and 652 dependents).
  - As we know there are two types of dependency ratio: young dependency and old dependency ratio.
  - India's young dependency ratio is declining as currently it is 510 (census 2011) as compared to 621 (census 2001). It means our programs related to family planning are working and this also been seen in terms of reduction in TFR.
  - India's old dependency ratio is increasing from 131(census 2001) to 142 (census 2011) and this is because of rising in life expectancy.
  - As fertility levels decline, the dependency ratio falls initially because the proportion of children decreases while the proportion of the population of working age increases. The period when the dependency ratio declines is known as the "window of opportunity" when a "demographic dividend" may be reaped because society has a growing number of potential producers relative to the number of consumers.
  - However, as fertility levels continue to decline, dependency ratios eventually increase because of the proportion of working age starts declining and the proportion of older persons continues to increase.
  - As populations grow older, increases in old-age dependency ratios are indicators of the added pressures that social security and public health systems have to withstand.
- **Natural growth rate:** It is a difference between Birth rate and Death rate.
- **Population density:** Number of the people living in per square kilometer of area.
- **Poverty:** It is an inability to gratify the physiological needs that is need for survival, safety and security.
- **Definition of BPL family:** If person is earning money that is not enough to manage 2400 Kcal per day per person in rural area and 2100 Kcal in Urban area then he/she is considered as below poverty line. Currently 22% of the Indian population is BPL.
- **Tendulkar committee poverty definition:**
  27 ₹ per capita per day: Rural
  33 ₹ per capita per day: Urban
- **Income based definition (according to C. Rangarajan committee) (2014)**
  32 ₹ per capita per day: Rural
  47 ₹ per capita per day: Urban

- **World bank definition:** Person earns <1.90 $ per day then he/she is below poverty line. (updated in October 2015, from 1.25 $ to 1.90 $)
- **Literacy:** Person aged 7 years or more who can read and write with understanding in any national language will be considered as literate. About 74.04% of the Indian population is literate (census 2011).

3.4 SEX RATIO

- It is defined as the number of females per 1000 males.
- It is affected by sex ratio at birth, sex selective abortion, sex selective migration and mortality pattern.
- Male child preference leads to lower sex ratio.
- Sex determination test and sex selective abortion need to be strictly stopped with the help of PCPNDT Act.
- **Beti Bachao Beti Padhao** scheme aims to address declining child sex ratio and related issue of empowerment of girl. The scheme is being implemented in all districts of the country through multisectoral intervention. The Scheme has stirred up collective consciousness towards changing the mind-set of the Nation towards valuing the girl child. This is reflected in the improvement of **Sex Ratio at Birth** (SRB) by **16 points** at National level, from **918** in 2014–15 to **934 in 2021-22** (HMIS).
- Child sex ratio include 0-6 years of age group.
- Sex ratio = $\frac{\text{No. of females}}{\text{Number of males}} \times 1000$
- As per NFHS-5, Sex ratio of the total population is 1037 per 1000 males while as per census 2011, it is 943 per 1000 males.

3.5 IMPORTANT VITAL STATISTICS INDICATORS

Rate

- **Crude rate**

$$= \frac{\text{No. of events that occurring in a given geographic area during the year}}{\text{Estimated mid-year population of that year}} \times 1000$$

- **Specific rate**

$$= \frac{\text{No. of events that occurring in a specific group of the population given geographic area during the year}}{\text{Mid-year population of the specific group of the population in the same geographic area during the same year}} \times 1000$$

Measures of Fertility

- **Crude birth rate**

$$= \frac{\text{No. of live births during the year}}{\text{Estimated mid-year population of that year}} \times 1000$$

- **General fertility rate (GFR)**

$$= \frac{\text{No. of live births in defined area in a year}}{\text{Mid-year population of women aged 15–49 years}} \times 1000$$

Demography, Surveillance, and Data

- **General marital fertility rate (GMFR)**

$$= \frac{\text{No. of live births in defined area in a year}}{\text{Mid-year population of married women aged 15–49 years}} \times 1000$$

- **Age specific fertility rate (ASFR)**

$$= \frac{\text{No. of live births to mother of a specific age group}}{\text{Mid-year population of women of same age group}} \times 1000$$

Note: It is useful to identifying the age group with highest reproductive potential, so family planning measures are targeted to these age groups.

- **Age specific marital fertility rate (ASMFR)**

$$= \frac{\text{No. of live births to mother of a specific age group}}{\text{Mid year population of married women of same age group}} \times 1000$$

Total Fertility Rate (TFR)

- It is defined as the average number of children a woman would be bear during her whole reproductive years.
- It is useful to identify how many children a woman would have on an average and it gives approximate Completed Family Size.
- **Formula:**

$$\text{TFR} = \frac{5 \times \sum_{15-19}^{45-49} \text{ASFR}}{1000}$$

- **Total marital fertility rate (TMFR):** Average number of children that would be born to a married woman if she experiences the current fertility pattern throughout her reproductive life years.

$$\text{TMFR} = \frac{5 \times \sum_{15-19}^{45-49} \text{ASMFR}}{1000}$$

- **Gross reproduction rate (GRR):** It is the average number of girl child that would be born to a woman if she experiences current fertility rate throughout her reproductive span with **assumption of no mortality**.

$$= \frac{\text{No. of female children born to women in cohort sample}}{\text{Total no. of women in the same cohort sample}} \times 1000$$

$$\text{GRR} = \frac{5 \times \sum_{15-19}^{45-49} \text{ASFR for female live birth}}{1000}$$

Net reproduction rate (NRR): NRR is different from GRR as NRR takes into consideration current mortality rate also.

- NRR is defined as the number of daughters, a newborn girl will bear during her lifetime assuming fixed age-specific fertility and mortality rates.

- It is average no. of female live birth that occur to female newborn as she grow up and passes through her entire reproductive age group provided she were subject to current rate of fertility as well as mortality.
- It is sensitive indicator of population growth.
- Goal is to achieve NRR = 1 (Which is equivalent to attaining approximately 2 child norm)

$$NRR = \frac{\text{No. of girls survived after the mortality experience}}{\text{No. of cohort women survived at end of reproductive period as per mortality experiences}} \times 1000$$

Crude Marriage Rate

$$= \frac{\text{Marriage registered in a year}}{\text{Estimated mid-year population of that year}} \times 1000$$

General Marriage Rate

$$= \frac{\text{Marriage registered in a year}}{\text{No of unmarried person age 15-49 years}} \times 1000$$

Pregnancy Rate

$$= \frac{\text{Total pregnancies in married women in 15-44 years}}{\text{Number of married women in same age group}} \times 1000$$

Abortion Ratio

$$= \frac{\text{No. of all type of abortion}}{\text{Number of live births}} \times 1000$$

Child Woman Ratio

$$= \frac{\text{No. of children in age group 0-4 years}}{\text{Number of women in 15-44 years}} \times 1000$$

Important Mortality Indicators

- **Maternal mortality ratio (MMR):**

$$= \frac{\text{Total no. of female deaths due to complications of pregnancy, childbirth or within 42 days of delivery from "puerperal causes" in an area in a given year}}{\text{Total no. of live births in the same area and year}} \times 100{,}000$$

- **Stillbirth rate**

$$= \frac{\text{Fetal deaths weighing over 1000 gm at birth during the year}}{\text{Total live births + stillbirth weighing over 1000 gm at birth during the year}} \times 1000$$

- **Perinatal mortality rate**

$$= \frac{\text{Late fetal deaths (28 weeks gestation and more) + early neonatal death (within 1 week)}}{\text{Total births in a year (live + stillbirth)}} \times 1000$$

- **Neonatal mortality rate**

$$= \frac{\text{Number of deaths of children under 28 days of age in a year}}{\text{Total live births in the same year}} \times 1000$$

Demography, Surveillance, and Data

- **Early neonatal mortality rate**

$$= \frac{\text{Number of deaths in children under 7 days of age in a year}}{\text{Total live births in the same year}} \times 1000$$

- **Postneonatal mortality rate**

$$= \frac{\text{No. of death of children after 28 days and before one year of age in given year}}{\text{Live birth in a year}} \times 1000$$

- **Infant mortality rate** (IMR)

$$= \frac{\text{Number of deaths of children less than 1 year of age in a year}}{\text{Number of live births in the same year}} \times 1000$$

- **Fetal death ratio**

$$= \frac{\text{Fetal death}}{\text{Live birth}} \times 1000$$

- **1-4 year mortality rate/Child death rate**

$$= \frac{\text{No. of deaths of children aged 1-4 years during a year}}{\text{Total no. of children aged 1-4 years at given year}} \times 1000$$

- **Under 5 mortality rate**

$$= \frac{\text{Number of deaths of children less than 5 years of age in a given year}}{\text{Number of live births in the same year}} \times 1000$$

- **Crude death rate**

$$= \frac{\text{No. of death during the year}}{\text{Estimated mid-year population of that year}} \times 1000$$

- **Case fatality rate**

$$= \frac{\text{No. of death due to specific disease}}{\text{Total no of cases}} \times 100$$

- **Proportional mortality rate**

$$= \frac{\text{No. of death due to specific disease}}{\text{Total no of deaths}} \times 100$$

Expectation of Life

- Life expectancy at birth is "the average number of years that will be lived by those born alive into a population if the current age-specific mortality rates persist".
- It is estimated for both gender separately.
- It is a good indicator of socioeconomic development in general and also improvement of overall health status.
- It can be considered as a positive health indicator.

Years of Potential Life Lost (YPLL)

It is defined as one that occurs before the age to which a dying person could have expected to survive (before an arbitrary determined age, usually taken age 75 years).

Specific Death Rates

- **Age specific death rate**

$$= \frac{\text{No. of death in particular age group during the year}}{\text{Estimated mid-year population of that age group}} \times 1000$$

- **Gender specific death rate**

$$= \frac{\text{No. of death in particular gender during the year}}{\text{Estimated mid-year population of particular gender}} \times 1000$$

- **Cause specific death rate**

$$= \frac{\text{No. of death due to specific disease}}{\text{Estimated mid-year population of that year}} \times 1000$$

Morbidity Indicators

- Incidence and prevalence
- Notification rates
- Admission, readmission and discharge rates
- Duration of stay in hospital
- Attendance rates at out-patient departments, health centers, etc.
- Spells of sickness or absence from work or school.

3.6 SOURCES OF VITAL STATISTICS

Sources of Demographic Data

- Census
- Sample Registration System (SRS)
- Civil Registration System (CRS)
- National Family Health Survey (NFHS)
- Periodic Publications:
  - World Health Organization (WHO)
  - Registrar General, India
  - Directorate General Health Services (DGHS), New Delhi
  - State Health Directorates

Census	• According to United Nations, the census of population is defined as "the total process of collecting, compiling and publishing demographic, economic and social data pertaining, at a specified time or times to all persons in a country or delimited territory." • The Indian Census is largest administrative and statistical exercise in the world. • A "de jure" census tallies people according to their regular or legal residence, whereas a "de facto" census allocates them to the place where enumerated normally where they spend the night of the day enumerated. Currently census being conducted as per 'De jure' method. • Census is the purview of ministry of home affairs. It is conducted under the guidance of the census commissioner of India. • First census conducted on 1881. • The Census Operations in India have been carried out in two phases: (i) House Listing and Housing Census and (ii) Population Enumeration. • It takes places every 10 years in India and last one was conducted in 2011 and latest one to be conducted in 2022–2023. This one will be the 16th census overall and 8th post-independence. • Census 2022–2023 will be the digital census. The theme slogan of the ongoing census is "**Janganana se Jan Kalyan**".

Demography, Surveillance, and Data

- Census is the biggest source of primary data at village, town and ward level providing micro level data on various parameters including Housing Condition; Amenities and Assets, Demography, Religion, caste related data, Language, Literacy and Education, Economic Activity, Migration and Fertility.
- The population census is the primary source of basic national population data required for administrative purposes and for many aspects of economic and social research and planning.
- Census stops on 1st March.

SRS
- Sample registration system (SRS) is a large-scale demographic survey which provides data annually for infant mortality rate, birth rate, death rate and other fertility and mortality related indicators.
- Started as pilot project by the OFFICE OF THE REGISTRAR GENERAL, INDIA in a few selected states in 1964-65 and it became fully operational during 1969-70.
- Base-line survey of the sample units is done to collect demographic details of the usual resident population of the sample areas.
- Continuous (longitudinal) enumeration of vital events pertaining to usual resident population is done by the enumerator.
- It is dual recording system as continuous enumeration of births and deaths in selected sample units is carried out by part time enumerators who is generally anganwadi workers and teachers, and an independent survey is done every six months by full time SRS supervisors.
- The data obtained by these two independent enumerators (part time and full time) are matched and the unmatched or partially matched data are re-verified in the field and thereafter an unduplicated data about births and deaths is obtained.
- In rural areas the sample is a village or a part of it when the population of village is 2000 or more. In urban areas, the sampling unit is a census enumeration block with population ranging from 750 to 1000.
- Useful to provide information on fertility and mortality indicator like CBR, CDR, TFR, IMR, MMR, etc.

CRS
- Registration of birth and death (Birth and Death Registration Act, 1969) is compulsory at their place of occurrence.
- By knowing birth and death scenario it helps in better understanding of demography, health and other needs of the people.
- The Registrar General of India is overall authority.
- In rural area local registrars are from Panchayat while in urban area, health officers of the municipalities are the registrars.
- Every registrar sends periodical reports to the chief registrar and in turn who sends those reports to the registrar general of India.
- On the basis of these reports, the registrar general of India brings a comprehensive reports titled as "vital statistics of India".
- Civil Registration System (CRS) useful to provide information on various important indicator.
- Private practitioner is bound to give the death certificate free of cost.

  Time limit for registration:
  - Births must be registered within: 21 days
  - Deaths must be registered within: 21 days
  - Marriages must be registered within: Variable limits within India

  If registration is delayed, Penalty provision as follow:
- After 21 days till 30 days: Late fee Rs 2
- After 30 days till 1 year: Late fee Rs 5 + affidavit
- After 1 year: Late fee Rs 10 + magistrate order

NFHS

- The National Family Health Survey (NFHS) is a large-scale, multi-round survey conducted in a representative sample of households throughout India.
- Each of these households have been visited and information obtained about the household using household questionnaire.
- The survey provides state and national information for India on fertility, infant and child mortality, the practice of family planning, maternal and child health, reproductive health, nutrition, anemia, utilization and quality of health and family planning services.
- Each successive round of the NFHS has had two specific goals:
  - To provide essential data on health and family welfare needed by the Ministry of Health and Family Welfare and other agencies for policy and program purposes, and
  - To provide information on important emerging health and family welfare issues.
- The Ministry of Health and Family Welfare (MOHFW), Government of India, designated the International Institute for Population Sciences (IIPS) Mumbai, as the nodal agency, responsible for providing coordination and technical guidance for the survey.
- So far 5 rounds of NFHS have been completed.
  - NFHS 1: 1992-1993
  - NFHS 2: 1998-1999
  - NFHS 3: 2005-2006
  - NFHS 4: 2015-2016
  - NFHS 5: 2019-2021
  - NFHS 6: 2023-2024 (ongoing)

3.7 SUMMARY OF COMMON SAMPLING METHODS

It is very important that sample should be representative of study population because we conduct studies on samples but making the inferences about the study population. That's why the study participants should be recruited and interviewed with caution.

Sampling Techniques

There are mainly two types of sampling.
1. **Probability sampling:** In this technique, each participant has an equal and known chance of being selected in a study. This technique ensures that the sample is true representative of a population.
2. **Non-probability sampling:** In this technique, each participant does not have an equal and known chance of being selected in a study.

Classification of sampling techniques:

Probability sampling	Non-probability sampling
Simple random sampling	Consecutive/sequential sampling
Systematic random sampling	Convenience/accidental/opportunity sampling
Stratified random sampling	Purposive/judgmental sampling
Multistage sampling	Quota sampling
Multiphase sampling	Snowball sampling
Cluster sampling	

Probability Sampling

Simple Random Sampling

Characteristics
- Simplest method: Each participant within study frame has an equal chance of inclusion in a study.
- More representative
- It is a method of choice when population is small, homogenous and list of the population available.
- This method is also known as an unrestricted random sampling.

Methods: There are two methods for simple random sampling.
1. Lottery method
2. Table of random number method (recommended method).

Systematic Sampling

Characteristics
- This method is used in case when complete list of population is available.
- It is used when population is large, scattered and non homogeneous.
- Each participant is selected by using sample interval (K).
- **K = Total population/Desired Sample size.**
- This sampling interval will be added in previously selected participant's assigned number and the number which we get that numbered participant will be our next study participant.
- Thus, same process will be followed until our desired sample size is achieved.

Example: If in study there are 500 individuals and required or desired sample size is 100 then, K = 500/100 = 5. So K is 5.

Now we need to select the first participants randomly from 1 to K^{th} element means from 1 to 5, after that, we will add 5 in the number of this randomly selected participant. For example that number is 4 then 4 + 5 = 9. So our second study participant is 9th numbered individual. Third participant will be 9 + 5 =14, so 14th numbered individual will be our third participant.

Stratified Random Sampling

Characteristics
- This method is used when population is non-homogeneous.
- In this sampling method that divides the population into the homogenous subgroup based on gender, age or socioeconomic condition which is known as strata and sample is selected from each stratum.
- After making strata any of the random sampling method can be used to select participants from each stratum.
- Main purpose of stratified sampling is to make different strata comparable.
- More accurate and representative sample of the population.

Example: We want to know the relationship between religion and low birth weight among children born in particular village in particular year. Now we will make line list of all births of that year according to religion. For our current study let's say for example, decided sample size is 80. To ensure that equal number of children would have selected from each religion community to have better representation, we need to select randomly 20 children from Hindu, 20 from Muslim, 20 from Sikh, and 20 from Christian community.

Multistage Sampling
Characteristics
- It is used when sample is to be drawn from a huge population like world, country or state. It is commonly used in large scale survey.
- Flexibility is the key feature of this sampling technique.
- It is one of the less time consuming and less expensive methods.

Example: We want to do the survey to know the vitamin B12 deficiency in Indian population.
- **Stage 1:** Out of total 640 districts we will randomly select 100 districts.
- **Stage 2:** Out of selected 100 districts, we will select randomly 100 talukas (tehsils).
- **Stage 3:** Out of selected 100 tehsils we will select randomly 100 villages.
- **Stage 4:** Out of 100 villages we will select every 10th family of each village to have study participants for this large scale survey.

Multiphase Sampling
Characteristics
- Some of the information is obtained from the whole sample and additional information is obtained at the same time or later from the subgroup or subsamples of that entire sample.
- Most commonly used method is two phase sampling but it could be three or four phase sampling as well.
- More purposeful type of sampling as we are getting closer to our aim at the end of each phase of sampling.
- More useful when some screening tests are too costly.

Example: Let's assume that we want to screen all the final MBBS students of the particular medical college for having TB.
- **Phase 1:** All the final year MBBS students will be asked for having cough for more than 2 weeks.
- **Phase 2:** All symptomatic students will be asked to go for sputum smear microscopy.

Cluster Sampling
Characteristics
- Population divided into clusters of homogeneous units which is usually based on geographical contiguity.
- Sampling units are groups rather than individuals.
- Fewer resources are required. It reduces travel and other administrative costs.
- Less time consuming.
- Requires only list of all clusters, and detailed information is required only about those individuals who are from the chosen clusters.
- We can estimate characteristics of both cluster and population.
- Simple as complete list of sampling units within population not required.
- Often used to evaluate vaccination coverage.

Two types of cluster sampling:
- One-stage sampling: All the members or elements within selected clusters are included in the sample.
- Two-stage sampling: In the First stage a sample of areas is selected; and in Second stage a sample of respondents within those areas is selected.

Methodology
- First make a List of all cities, towns, villages and wards of cities with their population.
- Calculate total cumulative population.
- Generally 30 clusters are selected as WHO often do the survey for immunization coverage evaluation with 30*7 methods. But it is not necessary to have 30 clusters only; it could be any number of clusters.
- Divide cumulative population by 30 and that will give sampling interval.
- Select a random number less than or equal to sampling interval having same number of digits. (this random number can be selected by using currency note method or by using random number table method)
- Look at the list of cluster with their respective population and try to match this random number with the population.
- Where the random number falls in the list of cluster population that will be our 1st cluster.
- Now 2nd cluster = Random number + sampling interval
- 3rd cluster = Second cluster population + sampling interval
- Last or 30th cluster = 29th cluster population + sampling interval
- All units from the selected clusters are studied.

Nonprobability Sampling

Consecutive/Sequential Sampling

Characteristics
- It is selection of all the accessible individuals who are meeting the selection criteria.
- It is the best method among nonprobability sampling techniques as it minimizes selection bias.
- We keep enrolling all the coming patients or participants sequentially until our desired sample size is achieved.

Example:
- We want to know the HIV infection prevalence of pregnant women. Let's assume our estimated sample size is 100.
- Then we will seat in gynecology OPD from 8 to 12 am and will enroll first 100 women who makes visit on that day and meeting the selection criteria.

Convenience/Accidental/Opportunity Sampling

Characteristics
- It is nonprobability sampling which takes the sample from that part of the population which is close to reach.
- It means from the population which is readily available, accessible and convenient.
- It is also known as accessibility or haphazard sampling.
- Easy, fast and less costly method but with selection bias.
- The researcher cannot make generalizations of the results of the study because this sample would not be representative enough for the whole population.
- This type of sampling is most useful for pilot testing as purpose of pilot study is to either to make correction in the proforma or to have idea about the sample size.
- It is one of the commonly used methods in clinical research.

Example:
- Suppose we want to know the extent of stress among postgraduate medical students. Our desired sample size is 40.
- Researcher is having more than 50 colleagues in his department.
- He interviewed 40 out of these 50 PG students who were readily accessible and available to him.
- Result about among PG students will be biased due to improper selection of study population.

Purposive/Judgmental Sampling

Characteristics
- The researcher chooses the sample based on who they think would be appropriate for the study.
- It is deliberate subjective choice of participants for ease of access.
- This is used primarily when there is a limited number of people that have expertise in the area being researched.

Example:
Agency X wants to show low immunization coverage in particular city so they will recruit children living in slum area only so the coverage of immunization will be less.

Quota Sampling

Characteristics
- It is basically similar to stratified random sampling method but nonrandom or non-probabilistic in nature.
- In this method we first divide the population into mutually exclusive subgroups or strata like in stratified sampling.
- Thus, Subsets are chosen and then either convenience or judgmental sampling is used to choose people from each subset. The researcher decides how many of each category is selected.
- Non-randomization is the key difference between stratified sampling and quota sampling.
- So first step of quota sampling is random sampling and second step is non-random sampling in the form of either accidental sampling or judgmental sampling.
- Quota sampling is useful when time is limited, when sampling frame is not available or the budget is very low or when detailed accuracy is not important.

Example:
- In the given college, 44% of the students are male and 56% are female.
- Let's assume that desired sample size is 100.
- That's why researcher knows that 44 males and 56 females will need to be interviewed from that population.

Snowball Sampling

Characteristics
- It is method of choice when study participants are difficult to identify, access.
- This sampling technique is often used in hidden populations.
- It is generally used when research subject is more sensitive or involved subjects are hard to reach like homosexuals, commercial sex workers or IV drug users.
- It works on the principle of snowball which keep on increasing as you roll it.

- It is based on chain of referrals of subjects.
- That's why it is also called as chain sampling, chain-referral sampling, referral sampling.

Example
- We want to know the prevalence of IV drug user among college students of a particular city.
- Then we should begin by identifying one student who meets our selection criteria.
- Then now we can ask him to recommend other students name.

3.8 DATA: SOURCE, METHODS OF COLLECTION, ANALYSIS, AND INTERPRETATION

Use of Health Information
- To measure the health status of the people and to quantify their health problems
- For comparisons of health status at local, national and international level
- For assessment of health service delivery and their effectiveness and efficiency
- For planning, administration and effective management of health services and programs
- For assessing degree of satisfaction of the beneficiaries with the health system; and
- For research in health problem and disease.

Methods of Demographic Data
- There are three main methods of data collection: Surveys, Records and Experiments.
- Data could be primary data or secondary data.
- If investigator him/herself collected the data then it will be called as primary data while if we are using already published data then it will be called as secondary data.

Types of Data
- **Data:** A merely observation made on the subjects is called raw data. Raw data becomes useful only when they are arranged and organized in a manner that can extract information from the data and communicate it to others.
- **Types of data:** There are mainly two types of data.

Qualitative Data
- It is usually referred as enumeration or counting type of data.
- It represents a particular quality or attribute.
- It cannot be measured in the units of measurement (for example in kg, cm)
- It is generally of discrete type of data.

Measurement Scales of Qualitative Data
Nominal
- It can be arranged in any order.
- Binary or dichotomous—for example, gender (male or female), vaccination status (vaccinated or unvaccinated).
- Polychotomous—for example, marital status (married, unmarried, remarried, divorced), country of origin (India, America, Japan, South Africa)

Ordinal
- Its classification is based on an order or rank
- It must be in some meaningful ascending or descending order.
- For example—pain scale (mild, moderate, severe, very severe), or Likert scale (strongly agree, agree, neutral, disagree, strongly disagree).

Quantitative Data
- It is also called as measurement data
- Measurement can be fractional
- Implies amount or quantity
- It may be discrete or continuous type of data.

Measurement Scales Quantitative Data
Interval
- Interval tells about order and exact values between two units but it does not have absolute zero.
- For example, temperature

Ratio
- Ratio is the ultimate scale of measurement of data as it tells exact order, distance (between two values) and also have absolute zero point which indicates the absence of the quantity being measure.
- For example, weight

Methods of Data Presentation
- **Presentation of data:** There are two main methods:
  1. Tabulation (classwise or groupwise tabulation)
  2. Drawing:
     - Drawings are of two types namely **graphs** as presentation of quantitative data and **diagram** as presentation of qualitative data which is given below.

Quantitative data	Qualitative data
• Histograms • Frequency polygon • Frequency curve • Line chart or graph • Cumulative frequency curve • Scatter or dot diagram	• Bar diagram • Pie or sector diagram • Pictogram or picture diagram • Map diagram or spot map

- **Tabulation:**
  - Some definitions:
    - **Frequency:** Count or number of observations within an interval or group
    - **Cumulative frequency:** Count within the current interval and all preceding intervals
    - **Relative frequency:** Count within an interval divided by the total number of observations
    - **Cumulative relative frequency:** Count within the current interval and all preceding intervals divided by the total number of observations

From the same above example we can have understanding about these definitions in the following table:

Frequency Distribution table:

Interval	Frequency	Cumulative frequency	Relative frequency	Cumulative relative frequency
20–29	2	2	0.2 (2/10)	0.2
30–39	3	5	0.3	0.5 (0.2 + 0.3)
40–49	3	8 (5 + 3)	0.3	0.8
50–59	2	10	0.2	1.0
Total	10		1.0	

Drawing

Graphs

Histogram

- A frequency histogram is very useful display graph applicable to frequency distribution of the quantitative (measured or counted) data.
- A histogram contains no scale breaks (gaps) along the x axis. (bar chart have scale gaps)
- The independent variable is divided into class intervals which are plotted on the x axis (**Fig. 3.5**).

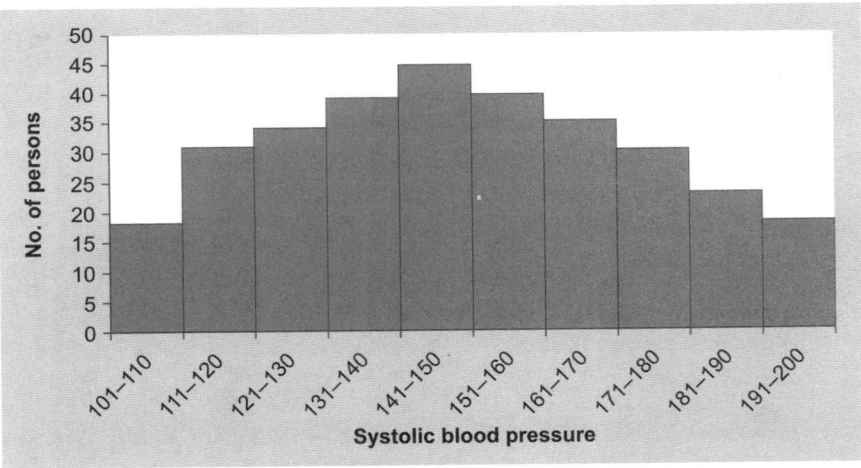

Fig. 3.5: Histogram.

- Usually we take class intervals between 5 and 20 but it depends on the range of the data and the total number of observations.
- The width of class intervals is always same.
- The number of observations or frequency is plotted on y- axis.
- "Area Under the Curve" is the area of the histogram calculated by multiplying the height with the width of each class interval.
- Shape of a frequency histogram helps to decide the type of distribution (**Fig. 3.6**):
  - Normal Distribution: mean = median = mode
  - Positive (right) Skewed distribution: mean > median > mode
  - Negative (left) Skewed distribution: mean < median < mode

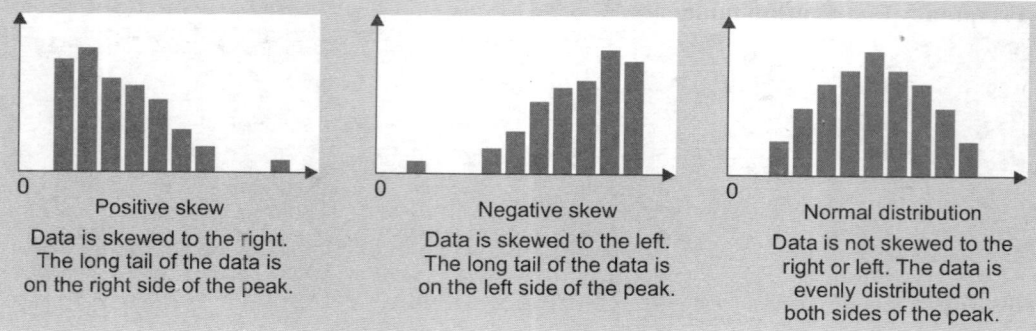

Fig. 3.6: Types of distribution.

- **Frequency polygon (polygon means figure with angles):**
  - It is area graph drawn over a histogram by joining the mid points of the top of each column for each class interval **(Fig. 3.7)**.
  - A frequency polygon is used when more than one frequency distribution to be shown on one graph.
  - The area under the curve represents the total number of observations.

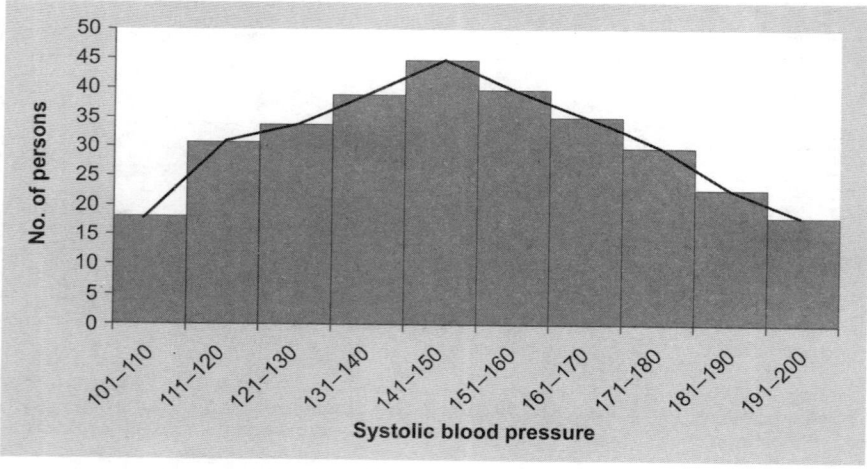

Fig. 3.7: Frequency polygon.

- **Frequency curve:**
  - When numbers of observations are large and group interval is reduced the frequency polygon tends to lose its angulation and gives a smooth curve known as frequency curve.
- **Line chart or graph:**
  - It is used to show the trend of an event that occurring over period of time **(Fig. 3.8)**.
  - The class interval can be a month, a year, or even decade.
  - Deteriorating or improving of any disease status after implementing any public health measure can be assessed with help of line chart.

Demography, Surveillance, and Data

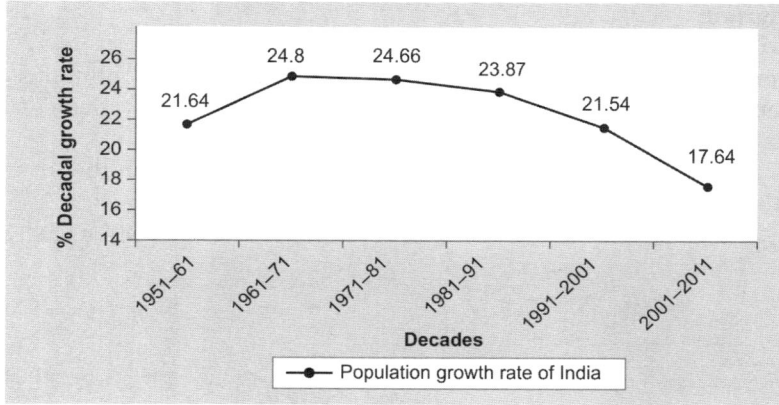

Fig. 3.8: Line chart or graph.

- **Cumulative frequency diagram or "ogive":**
  - Ogive is a graph of the cumulative relative frequency distribution.
  - As we already talked how to convert the frequency into cumulative frequency, in that way we will convert the frequency distribution into the cumulative frequency distribution and then will get the histogram **(Fig. 3.9)**.
  - Then with smooth hand we will join the point to get the curve which is called as ogive.

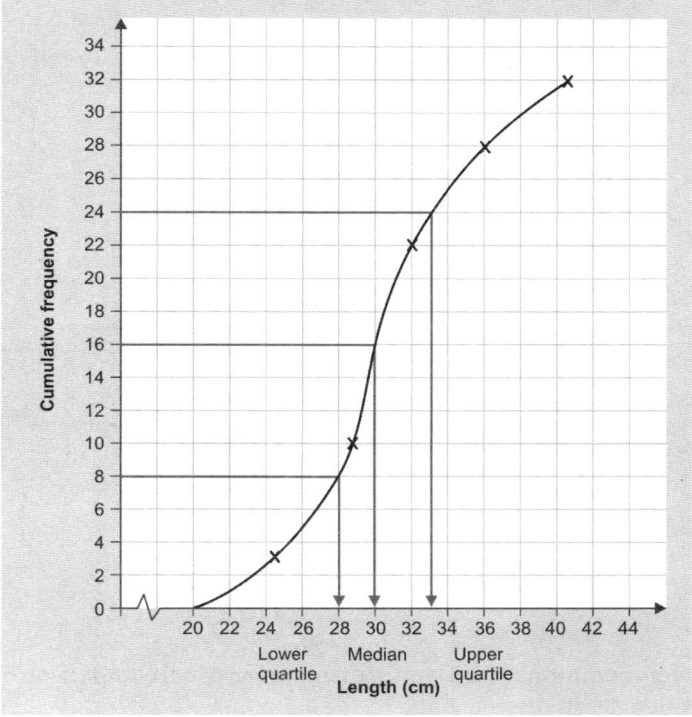

Fig. 3.9: Cumulative frequency diagram or ogive.

Demography, Surveillance, and Data

- **Scatter diagram:**
  - It is also called as **correlation diagram**.
  - It is useful to show the relationship or association between two continuous variables.
  - It is a graphical presentation to show the correlation between two variables such as height and weight.
  - Depending on the clustering of scatter points of paired data on the diagram, we can decide that it is positive, negative or no correlation.
  - The scatter diagram given below is an example of positive correlation **(Fig. 3.10)**.

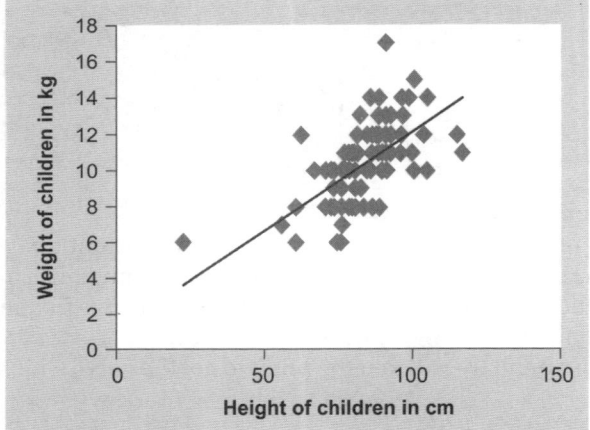

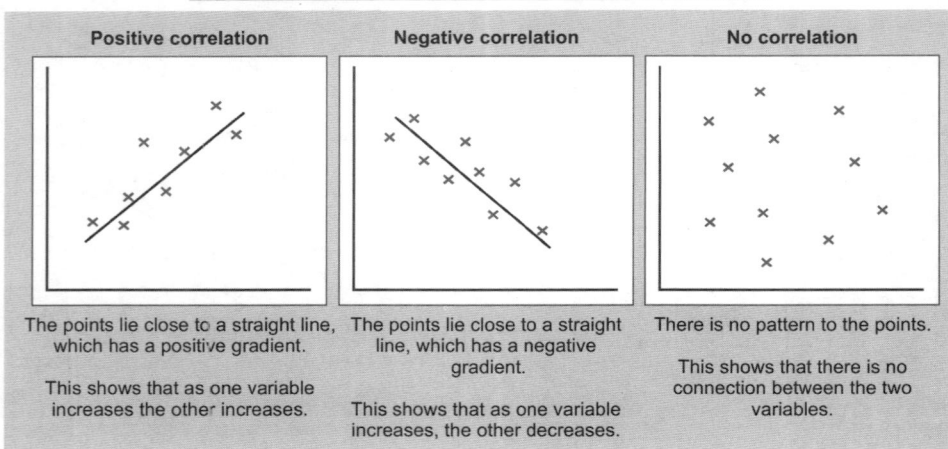

Fig. 3.10: Scatter diagram.

Diagrams

Bar Diagram

- Bar diagram is very commonly used type of diagram for visual comparison of the magnitude of different frequencies in discrete data.
- Bar may be drawn vertically or horizontally and in ascending or descending order.
- Spacing between two bars must be equal and it should be half of the width of the bar.

- In bar chart there will be presence of scale breaks or gaps between its columns or bars.
- Example: There are three types of bar diagram.
    1. Simple bar diagram
    2. Multiple bar diagram
    3. Proportional bar diagram

Simple Bar Diagram

- In this figure we can see that there is single bar showing the distribution of study participants according to blood group **(Fig. 3.11)**.

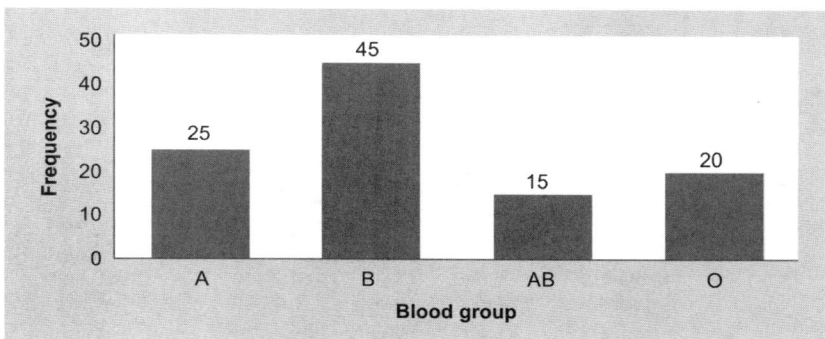

Fig. 3.11: Simple bar diagram.

Multiple Bar Diagram

- In this type of bar diagram it shows frequencies of two or more type discrete data.
- Genderwise distribution of children according to grade of undernutrition **(Fig. 3.12)**:

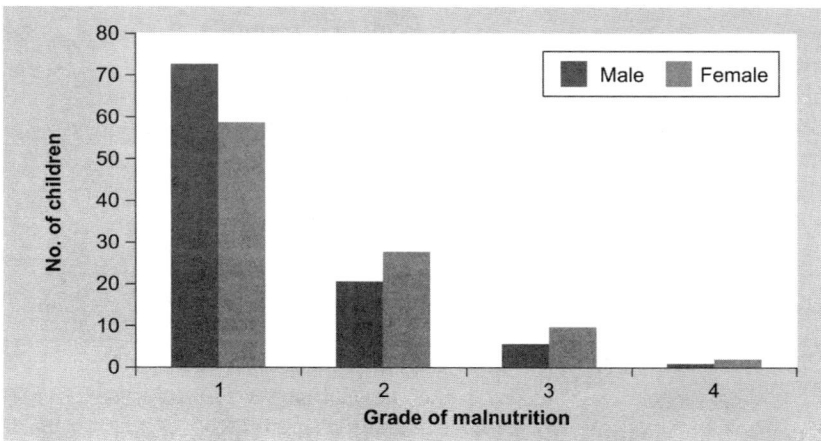

Fig. 3.12: Multiple bar diagram.

Proportional Bar Diagram

❑ The bars are divided into two or more parts; each part represents proportional to the magnitude of that item.
❑ Figure shows distribution of metabolic risk factors according to gender **(Fig. 3.13)**.

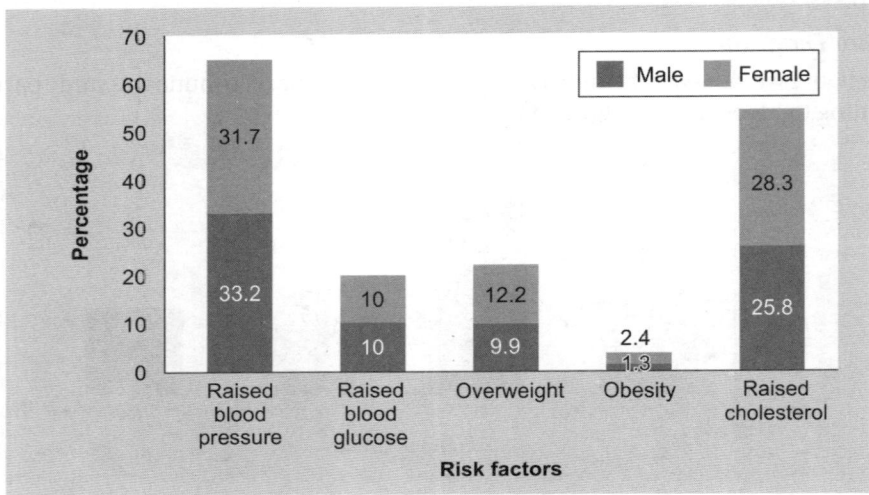

Fig. 3.13: Proportional bar diagram.

Pie or Sector Diagram

This is also commonly used diagram for the presentation of discrete type of qualitative data.
❑ Degree of angle shows the frequency.
❑ It is very easy to make comparison between different attributes.
❑ **size of angle = {class frequency/total observations} × 360**
❑ **size of angle = class percentage × 3.6**
  • Distribution of children according to place of delivery **(Fig. 3.14)**

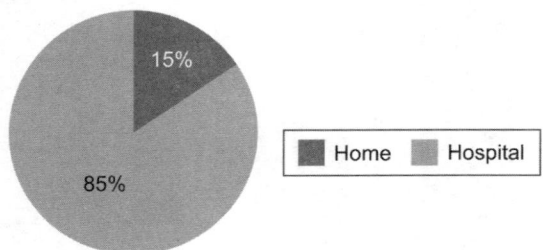

Fig. 3.14: Pie or sector diagram.

Pictogram

❑ It is a very useful method of presenting data to the layman person to understand easily.
❑ To represent certain number of units of variable, we need to choose suitable symbol first.
❑ Each value in the given series of data is represented either by taking similar symbol, its size being proportional to the value or by taking number of symbols of same size **(Fig. 3.15)**.

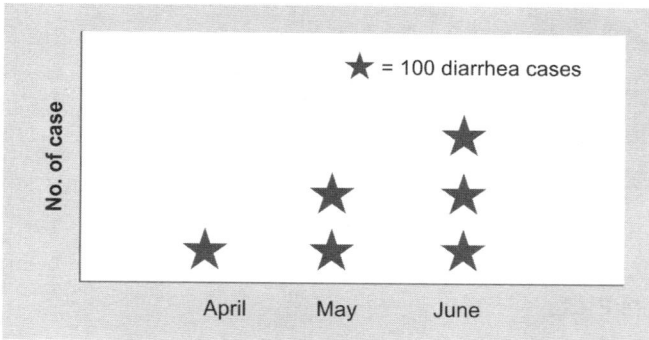

Fig. 3.15: Pictogram.

Map Diagram

- It is useful to show geographical distribution of frequencies of characteristics.
- The map given below shows the state wise PLHIV on ART as on March 2022 **(Fig. 3.16)**.

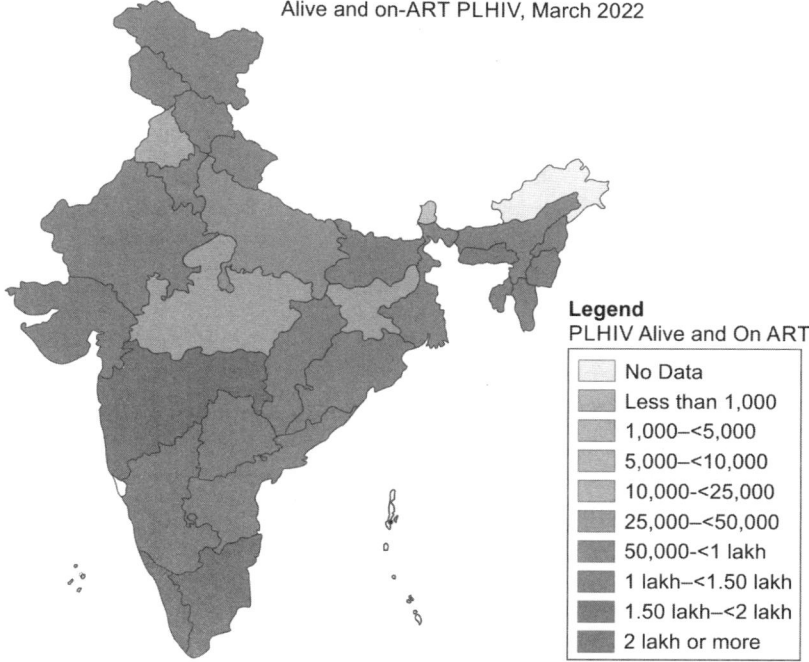

Fig. 3.16: Map diagram.

Venn Diagram

- It is useful to show the degree of overlap and exclusivity for two or more characteristics within a sample.
- In the following Venn diagram we have shown the distribution of the factors helping in deaddiction **(Fig. 3.17)**.

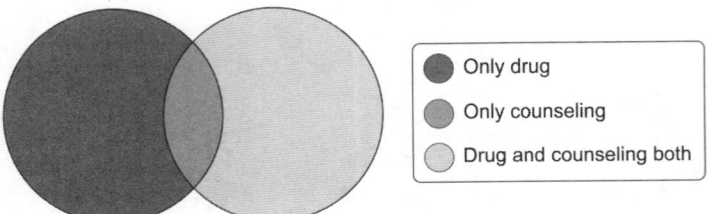

Fig. 3.17: Venn diagram.

Box-and-whiskers Plots
- It is useful in comparing the distribution of two or more groups.
- It is also known as five number summary which includes median, the lower quartile, upper quartile, and the smallest and greatest values in the distribution **(Fig. 3.18)**.
- It displays the center, the spread, and the overall range of distribution.

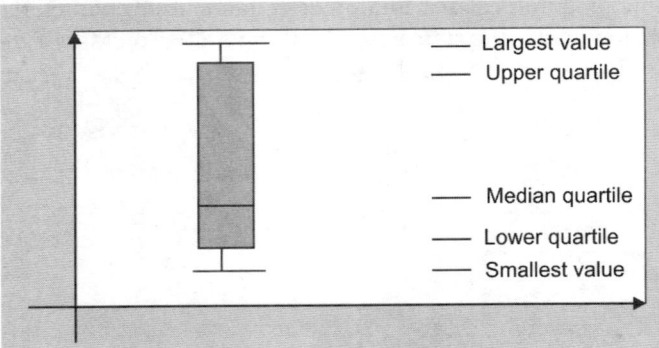

Fig. 3.18: Box and whisker plots.

Measure of Central Tendency
- Generally biological data are not equal but they have tendency to cluster around a particular level and this tendency is called as central tendency.
- All data generally cluster around common central value which is also called as an 'average.'
- There are various types of measurement of central tendency.
- For example:
  - Mean
  - Median
  - Mode
  - Quartiles

Mean
- It is the simplest form of measurement of central tendency.
- It is calculated by dividing the sums of all the observations by the number of observation.

Arithmetic Mean
For Ungrouped Data
Formula: $\bar{x} = \Sigma x/n$

$$= \frac{x_1 + x_2 + \ldots x_n}{n}$$

Example: Hb of 10 ANC women is as follows: 9.5, 11.5, 12.5, 10, 11.7, 13.0, 10.8, 12.7, 13.2 and 14.2 mg/dL.

Mean Hb,

$(\bar{x}) = \Sigma x/n$

$$= \frac{9.5 + 11.5 + 12.5 + 10 + 11.7 + 13.0 + 10.8 + 12.7 + 13.2 + 14.2}{10}$$

Mean Hb = 11.91 mg/dL.

For Grouped Data
- **Arithmetic mean for grouped data of discrete type:**
  Formula: $\bar{x} = \Sigma fx / \Sigma(f)$
  Example: Calculate the average period duration of menstrual cycle.

Days of periods (x)	No. of women (f)	fx
3	22	22 × 3 = 66
4	34	34 × 4 = 136
5	25	25 × 5 = 125
6	18	18 × 6 = 108
7	12	12 × 7 = 84
	=111	Σfx = 519

$\bar{x} = \Sigma fx / \Sigma(f)$
  = 519/111
  = 4.67 days of periods

Arithmetic Mean of Grouped Data of Continuous Type
Calculation of Mean
Example: Calculate average daily protein intake of adult male from the following data of 200 male.

On the basis of their protein intake we can summarize data in frequency distribution table as follows.

Class interval (on the basis of daily protein intake)	No. of male (f)	Midpoint of class interval	fx
15–25	15	20	300
25–35	20	30	600
35–45	50	40	2000
45–55	55	50	2750
55–65	40	60	2400

Class interval (on the basis of daily protein intake)	No. of male (f)	Midpoint of class interval	fx
65–75	15	70	1050
75–85	05	80	400
	$\Sigma(f) = 200$		$\Sigma fx = 9500$

$\bar{x} = \Sigma fx / \Sigma(f)$
  $= 9500/200$
  $= 47.5$

- **Merits of arithmetic mean:**
  - It is easy to calculate and to understand.
  - It can be treated further mathematically to know the dispersion and to apply other statistical tests.
  - It is based on all observation and least affected by sampling fluctuations.
- **Demerits of arithmetic mean:**
  - It is not possible to calculate mean for qualitative data.
  - It is very sensitive to extreme observation.
  - It cannot be determined graphically
  - It cannot be calculated in open end series.

Median

- **Ungrouped data**
  - First arrange the observations in the ascending or descending order.
  - The central value gives us the median.
  - Formula for median for ungrouped data are of two types depends on number of observations:

For odd number of observation

$$\text{Median} = \frac{(n+1)^{th}}{2} \text{ observation}$$

For even Number of observation:

$$\text{Median} = \frac{(n/2)^{th} + (n/2+1)^{th}}{2}$$

Example

- **For odd** observation: 640, 230, 686, 400, 520.
  - Here N is 5 (odd)
  - Ascending order = 220, 400, 520, 640, 680
  - Median $= \frac{(n+1)}{2}$
      $= \frac{5+1}{2}$
      $= 3$ rd observation is median.

  So, Median = 520
- **For even** observation: 640, 220, 330, 680, 440, 520
  - N = 6 (even)
  - Ascending order = 220, 330, 400, 520, 640, 680

Demography, Surveillance, and Data

- Median $= \dfrac{(n/2)^{th} + (n/2+1)^{th}}{2}$

  $= \dfrac{3rd + 4th}{2}$

  $= \dfrac{400 + 520}{2}$

  $= \dfrac{920}{2}$

  Median $= 460$

Median for General Grouped Data

We will use the same data which we used for calculation of mean for grouped data.

Daily protein intake by adult male	No. of Male	Cumulative frequency
15–25	15	15
15–35	20	35
35–45	50	85
45–55	55	140
55–65	40	180
65–75	15	195
75–85	5	200
	(Σf) = 200	

Formula for median $= L + \dfrac{(n/2 - cf)}{F} \times c$

Where, L = Lower limit of median class
N = total number of observation
Cf = cumulative frequency upto the median class
F = frequency of median class
C = class interval

Steps

1. Median class $= n/2$
   $= 200/2$
   $= 100$
2. Find the class interval of median class
   Here in this example it is 45–55 as 100 falls in cumulative frequency of 140.
3. Find the L = it is the lower limit of median class
   So, L is 45
4. CF = cumulative frequency is taken just above the median class
   So, CF = 85
5. F = it is the frequency of median class.
   So, F is 55
6. Class interval (c) in the example is 10. (45 – 55 = 10)

Formula: $= L + \dfrac{(n/2 - cf)}{F} \times c$

$= 45 + \dfrac{(100 - 85)}{55} \times 10$

$= 45 + 150/55$

$= 45 + 2.72$

$= 47.72$

Note: Median also can be obtained graphically with the help of cumulative frequency polygon called a as ogive.

Merits and Demerits of Median
- Just like mean it is also easy to calculate and easy to understand.
- It is very important to note that median can be found for distribution with open end classes also.
- It can be obtained graphically too.
- Two main important features which makes median very important measure of central tendency and they are as follows:
  - It is not affected due to extreme observation.
  - It is applicable to both quantitative and qualitative data.

Mode

- It is the most frequently occurring event or observation.
  - **For ungrouped data**
    80, 86, 82, 80, 78, 80, 84, 85,
    Mode is 80
    Mode may be more than one.
  - **For grouped data**

    $\text{Mode} = L + \dfrac{fm - f1}{2fm - f1 - f2} \times C$

    Where
    L = lower boundary of modal class
    Fm = frequency of modal class, Modal class is class with highest frequency
    F1 = frequency of premodal class
    F2 = frequency of postmodal class
    C = class interval

Now we will extract all required information from previous example.

L = 45, fm = 55, f1 = 50, f2 = 40, c = 10

$\text{Mode} = 45 + \dfrac{(55 - 50)}{110 - 55 - 40} \times 10$

$= 45 + (5/15) \times 10$

$= 45 + 50/15$

Mode = 48.33

Merits and Demerits of Mode

Merits
- It is just like median applicable to both qualitative and quantitative type of data.
- It is not affected by extreme value.
- It also works with open end classes type of distribution also.

Demerits
- It is not true representative of all observation as it is not based on all the observations.
- It is not possible to have further mathematical calculation with mode.

Formula to find out mode, when median and mean are known as:
  Mode = 3 Median − 2 Mean

3.9 NATIONAL POPULATION POLICY

- **The immediate objective** of the NPP 2000 is to address the unmet needs for contraception, healthcare infrastructure, and health personnel, and to provide integrated service delivery for basic reproductive and child healthcare.
- **The medium-term objective** is to bring the TFR to replacement levels by 2010, through vigorous implementation of intersectoral operational strategies.
- **The long-term objective** is to achieve a stable population by 2045, at a level consistent with the requirements of sustainable economic growth, social development, and environmental protection.

National Sociodemographic Goals for 2010

- Address the unmet needs for basic reproductive and child health services, supplies and infrastructure.
- Make school education up to age 14 free and compulsory, and reduce drop outs at primary and secondary school levels to below 20% for both boys and girls.
- Reduce infant mortality rate to below 30 per 1,000 live births.
- Reduce maternal mortality ratio to below 100 per 100,000 live births.
- Achieve universal immunization of children against all vaccine preventable diseases.
- Promote delayed marriage for girls, not earlier than age 18 and preferably after 20 years of age. Achieve 80% institutional deliveries and 100% deliveries by trained persons.
- Achieve universal access to information/counseling, and services for fertility regulation and contraception with a wide basket of choices.
- Achieve 100% registration of births, deaths, marriage and pregnancy.
- Contain the spread of Acquired Immunodeficiency Syndrome (AIDS), and promote greater integration between the management of reproductive tract infections (RTI) and sexually transmitted infections (STI) and the National AIDS Control Organization.
- Prevent and control communicable diseases.
- Integrate Indian Systems of Medicine (ISM) in the provision of reproductive and child health services, and in reaching out to households.

- Promote vigorously the small family norm to achieve replacement levels of TFR.
- Bring about convergence in implementation of related social sector programs so that family welfare becomes a people centered program.

3.10 BASICS OF SURVEILLANCE INCLUDING IDSP AND IHIP

Introduction

- Launched in 2004 as Project with world bank assistance in selected states and later on with NHM fund it is now pan India implemented.
- **Integrated disease surveillance program:** Here integration means sharing of surveillance information of various disease control programs, developing effective partnership with health and non-health sectors in surveillance, including communicable and non-communicable diseases in the surveillance system, working with the private sector and non-governmental organization and bringing academic institutions and medical colleges into disease surveillance.

Objectives

- Integration and decentralization of surveillance activities through establishment of surveillance units at Centre, State and District level, so:
  - Districts would be able to detect **early warning signals** of impending outbreaks and timely, effective public health actions can be initiated
  - Disease **trends** can be traced over a period of time
  - Districts can provide essential data to **monitor progress of ongoing disease Control Programs** and Control strategies can be periodically evaluated and suitably tailored
  - **Health resources can be allocated more efficiently**
- Human resource development—Training of state surveillance officers, District Surveillance Officers, rapid response team and other medical and paramedical staff on principles of disease surveillance.
- Information communication technology—for collection, collation, compilation, analysis and dissemination of data.
- Strengthening of public health laboratories.
- To **involve all stakeholders** including private sectors and communities in surveillance activities.
- Program components and reporting mechanism of IDSP is explained in **Figures 3.19 and 3.20.**

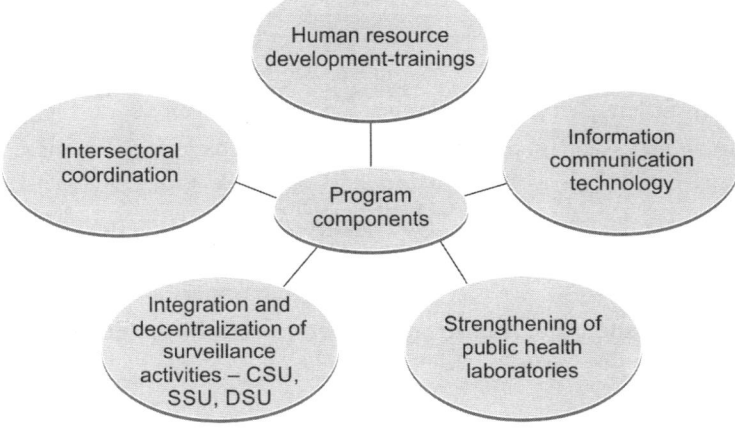

Fig. 3.19: Program components.

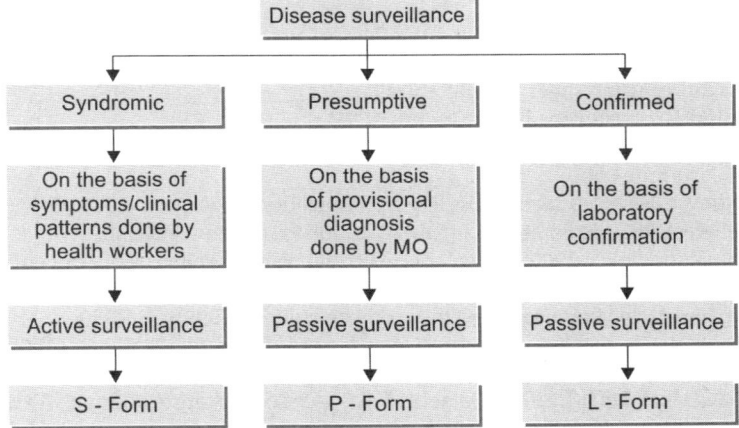

Fig. 3.20: Reporting mechanism.

Organizational Structure of IDSP

Central Surveillance Unit (CSU): Integrated administratively and financially with National Centre for Disease Control (NCDC), Delhi.

State Surveillance Unit (SSU): One in each State/UT with a regular officer identified as State Surveillance Officer (SSO). Supported by 7 contractual staff.

District Surveillance Unit (DSU): One in each district with a regular officer as District Surveillance Officer (DSO). Supported by 3 contractual staff.

Differences between IDSP and IHIP

IDSP portal	IHIP portal
Capture aggregate data only	Capture disaggregate data of persons at all levels
Paper-based data collection	Web based Data Collection
Manually links data from S, P and L forms	Electronically linked data of S, P, L forms
Weekly surveillance	Capture real-time or daily surveillance data
Monitoring 22 health conditions	Monitor more than 33+ health conditions
Not being done	Integrate with ongoing surveillance programs Provide analysis on mobile and electronic devices

Current demographic and other important indicators of India are given in the Annexure 2.

BIBLIOGRAPHY

1. Arun Bhandra Khanal, Mahajan's methods in Biostatistics for medical students and research workers, eighth edition, New Delhi, Jaypee Brothers Medical Publication. 2016. p.10.
2. Basics of Statistics; Jarkko Isotalo
3. Bogue, D.N. (1969). Principles of Demography John Wiley.
4. Correlation, available at; https://www.simplypsychology.org/correlation.html, accessed on 24-7-2017
5. http://rchiips.org/nfhs/factsheet_NFHS-5.shtml
6. https://censusindia.gov.in/census.website/node/294
7. https://censusindia.gov.in/vital_statistics/SRS_Reports_2019.html
8. https://idsp.nic.in/index.php
9. https://nhm.gov.in/New_Updates_2018/Report_Population_Projection_2019.pdf
10. Marie Diener-West, PhD, Exploratory Data Analysis, Johns Hopkins University.
11. National population policy 2000, Ministry of Health and Family Welfare, Government of India
12. PSS Sundar Rao, J. Richard. An Introduction to Biostatistics: A manual for students in health sciences, third edition, New Delhi, Prentice hall of India private limited, (1999), pp.16-30.
13. Quota Sampling, available at: http://www.fao.org/docrep/W3241E/w3241e08.htm#quota%20sampling.
14. Sky Graph, available at; https://d203algebra.wikispaces.com/Statistics-Target+A-Shape+It-Guided+Learning, accessed on 24 September, 2017.

CHAPTER 4

Population and Family Welfare

CHAPTER OUTLINE

- 4.1 Population explosion: Reasons, impact and population control
- 4.2 Basics of family planning and different family planning measures
- 4.3 Emergency contraception
- 4.4 The Medical Termination of Pregnancy (MTP) Act, 1971
- 4.5 National Family Welfare Program
- 4.6 Population Stabilization Fund/Jansankhya Sthirata Kosh
- 4.7 Mission Parivar Vikas
- 4.8 National Family Planning Indemnity Scheme (NFPIS)
- 4.9 Counseling in reproductive and sexual health problems of adolescents
- 4.10 Family Planning 2020 and 2030
- 4.11 Miscellaneous

4.1 POPULATION EXPLOSION: REASONS, IMPACT AND POPULATION CONTROL

Population explosion: Population explosion is the sudden increase in the size of the population. This term was coined by the American Sociologist, Kingsley Davis.

Doubling time of population has declined gradually from 64 to 34 years, this faster growth of population is known as population explosion.

Population Doubling Cycle

Rating	Annual GR (%)	Population doubling time
Stationary population	None	–
Slow growth	<0.5	>139 years
Moderate growth	0.5–1.0	139–70 years

Population and Family Welfare

Rating	Annual GR (%)	Population doubling time
Rapid growth	1–1.5	70–47 years
Very rapid growth	**1.5–2.0**	**47–35 years (INDIA)**
Explosive growth	2.0–2.5	35–28 years
Explosive growth	2.5–3.0	28–23 years
Explosive growth	3.0–3.5	23–20 years
Explosive growth	3.5–4.0	20–18 years

Reason for Population Explosion in India

- Widening gap between birth and death rates due to high birth rate and declining death rate:
  - Reasons for high birth rate: poverty, illiteracy, attitude towards male child preference, early marriage
  - Death rate has been declined due to control of epidemics and availability of medical facilities.
- Low age at marriage (including child marriage)
- High illiteracy
- Religious attitude towards family planning
- Other causes. Example: hot climatic condition (early maturity), migration, lack of social security scheme, preference of male child, arrival of refugees.

Impact of Population Explosion

- Unemployment
- Poverty
- Poor living condition
- Increase economic burden
- A high inequality lesser resources
- Greater exploitation of natural resources (e.g., Deforestation)
- High prices
- Burden of dependents
- Reduce growth of agriculture and industry, etc.

Population Control

- Marriages should be encouraged as per legal age for girl and boy, to reduce the period of reproduction among the females, bringing down the birth rate. Minimum age at marriage: 21 for boys and 18 for girls which also to make 21 as government is already made draft.
- Literacy as it helps both male and female in adopting small family norms
- By addressing the unmet need of family planning by encouragement of women to use birth control measures, providing birth control measures free or at very low cost.
- Spread of awareness and education regarding benefits of small family size.
- Due to fear of child death, people produce more children. To prevent this, we should have brought down infant mortality rate.
- Women empowerment and education
- Strengthening and expansion of social security schemes which will reduce the desire for having children as a support of old age life.

Population and Family Welfare

- Economic growth increases standard of living which in turn helps to accept small family norms.
- Urbanization has been proven in reducing TFR.
- Awareness related to marriage practice, gender bias and acceptance of family planning.

4.2 BASICS OF FAMILY PLANNING AND DIFFERENT FAMILY PLANNING MEASURES

- WHO defined **family planning** as "a way of thinking and living that is adopted voluntarily, upon the basis of knowledge, attitudes and responsible decisions by individuals and couples, in order to promote the health and welfare of the family group and thus contribute effectively to the social development of a country".
- **Small family norm**: It is an objective of family welfare program. In 1970 campaign slogan was "*do ya teen bas.* In 1980 campaign was on "2—child norm". The current themes are: "Sons or Daughters—two will do"; "Second child after 3 years", and "Universal Immunization".
- **Eligible couple** refers to a currently married couple wherein the wife is in the reproductive age, which is generally assumed to lie between the ages of 15 and 45.
- **Target couple**: It includes families with one child or even newly married couple.
- To avoid unwanted pregnancies, preventive methods to help women are known as fertility regulating methods or contraceptive methods.

Details about Different Family Planning Measures (Fig. 4.1)

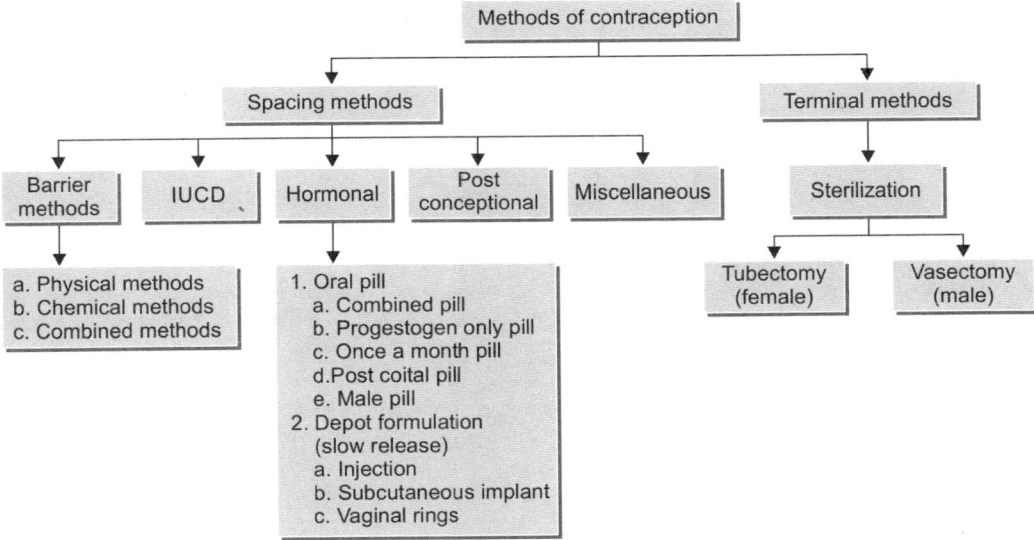

Fig. 4.1: Classification of different method.

Characteristics of Ideal Contraceptive

Safe, effective, acceptable, inexpensive, reversible, simple to administer, independent of coitus, long-lasting enough to obviate frequent administration and requiring little or no medical supervision.

Family Planning Methods

Barrier Methods

I. PHYSICAL METHODS

Condom (NIRODH)	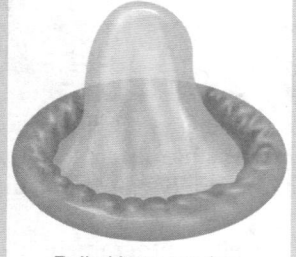 Rolled latex condom
Methods	Barrier methods, (Physical methods)
M/A	Prevent semen being deposited in vagina and thus prevent the meeting of the sperm with ovum.
Instruction	Fitted on erect penis, air must be removed from teat, Held carefully at a time of withdrawal
Failure rate	2–3 to 14 per 100 women years due to incorrect use
Remarks	May contain spermicidal (Nonoxynol, octoxynol) that immobilize and kill sperm **Advantage:** Readily available, protect against STD, cheap, simple without side effect, light, compact and disposable **Disadvantage:** Tear or slip off during coitus due to incorrect use, interfere with sex sensation **Side effect:** Allergy due to latex material
Female condom	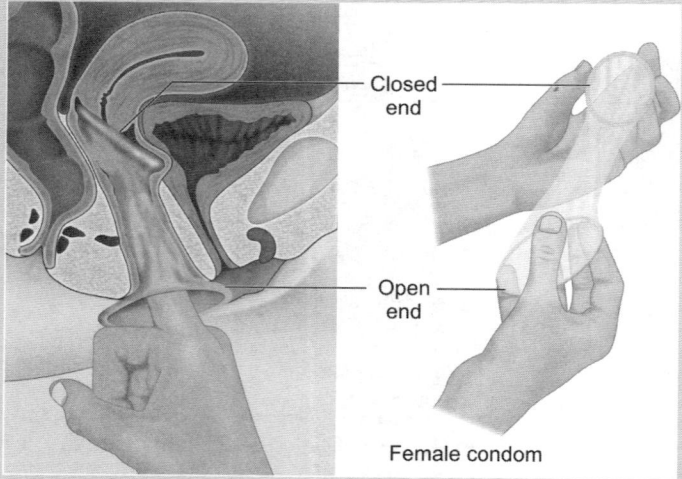 Female condom
Methods	Barrier methods (Physical methods)
M/A	Prevent semen being deposited in vagina

Instruction	The smaller closed end ring fits on cervix and the large outer ring remain outside the vagina
Failure rate	5–21/100 women years
Remarks	There is no need of spermicide. Because it is prelubricated with silicon. Also prevent STD infection **Limitation:** High cost, acceptability
Diaphragm/cervical cap/dutch cap	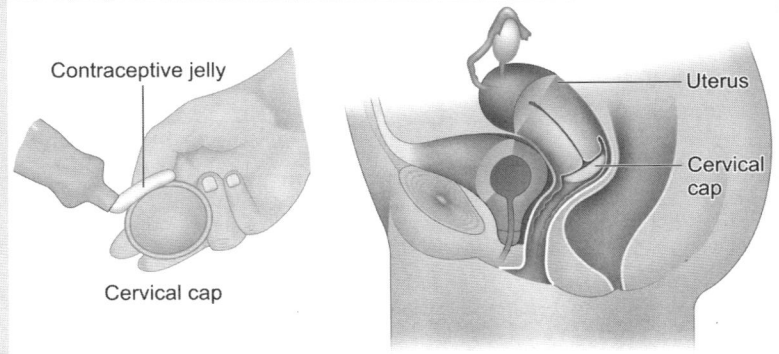
Methods	Barrier methods, (Physical methods)
M/A	Prevent semen being deposited in vagina
Instruction	It should be inserted before sexual intercourse. Spermicidal jelly is to be filled into it before insertion. It must remain in place for more than 6 hours after course
Failure Rate	6–12/100 women years
Remarks	There is a chance of toxic shock syndrome if diaphragm is left in vagina for a long period. Practice for insertion is also required
Vaginal Sponge	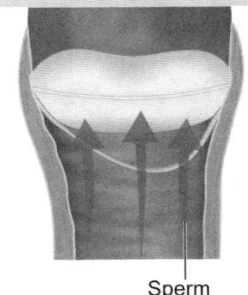
Methods	Barrier methods (Physical methods)
M/A	It releases spermicide during coitus, it absorbs ejaculate, it blocks the entrance to the cervical canal
Instruction	The sponge is moistened with water, squeezed and inserted high in vagina
Failure Rate	9–20/100 women years in nulliparous and 20–40 in parous women
Remarks	Trade name '**TODAY**'. Used with spermicidal nonoxynol 9

II. CHEMICAL METHODS

Chemical Methods	Foams: foam tablets, foam aerosols Creams, jellies and pastes—squeezed from a tube Suppositories—inserted manually, and Soluble films—C-film inserted manually

INTRAUTERINE DEVICES

IUCD	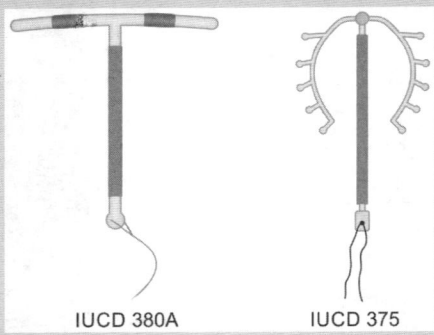 IUCD 380A IUCD 375
Methods	Intrauterine devices may have all types of mechanism like mechanical and hormonal
M/A	Impair viability of gamete and thus reduce the chances of fertilization. Cu ion alter the biochemical composition of cervical mucus, affect sperm motility, capacitation and survival. Increase the viscosity of mucus. IUCDs exhibit foreign body like reaction.
Instruction	Ideal timing: Within 10 days of menstruation period or immediately after delivery of placenta within 48 hours or after 6 weeks of delivery (PPIUCD: Postpartum IUCD) **Follow-up schedule:** After first menstrual period and then after the third menstrual period and then after six-month or one-year intervals
Failure Rate	Cu T 200: 1-5/100 women years, Cu T 380-A: 0.6-0.8/100 women years
Remarks	**1st generation:** Lippes loop, **2nd generation:** Cu T 380 A (effective for 10 years), Cu T 375 (effective for 5 years) **3rd generation:** Progestasert, Mirena (LNG 20) **Ideal candidate for IUCD:** • Having at least one child, • No history of pelvic disease, • Willingness to check the IUCD thread, • Monogamous relationship • Ready for follow up visit and treatment if any problems starts **Advantages of copper devices** • Less side effects • Decrease expulsion rate • Improve the effectiveness • Easier to insert in nulliparous women • Better tolerated by nullipara

Advantages of the IUCD:
- Simple insertion procedures required only few minutes and no requirement of hospitalization
- Highly effective and reversible method
- Once inserted IUD stays in place as long as required
- Reversible contraceptive effect
- Inexpensive
- No any systemic metabolic side-effects
- Highest continuation rate

Common Side effects:
Bleeding (mc), Pain (mc reason for removal), Pelvic infection

Rare Side Effects
Uterine perforation, pregnancy, ectopic pregnancy, fertility after removal, expulsion, cancer and teratogenesis, mortality

Contraindications:
- **Absolute:** Pregnancy, unexplained vaginal bleeding, suspected cancer of genital tract, PID, previous history of ectopic pregnancy
- **Relative:** Anemia, History of PID, Menorrhagia, Anatomical deformity due to fibroid, congenital malformation, purulent cervical discharge

Cu T 380 A:
Cu: copper, T for T shape. 380 is a surface area in sq.mm over the device where copper wire is present, A denotes arm which is horizontal and having copper sleeves. This extra copper increases effectiveness of copper T

LNG-20/Mirena: IUD releasing 20 mcg of levonorgestrel it has a low pregnancy rate (0.2 per 100 women) and a smaller number of ectopic pregnancies.

HORMONAL CONTRACEPTIVES

Combined oral contraceptive pills	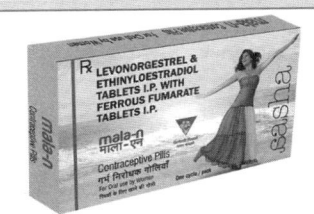 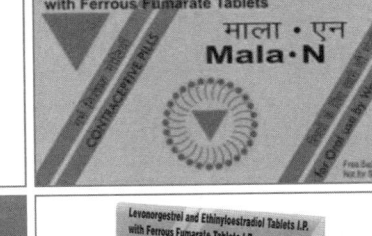 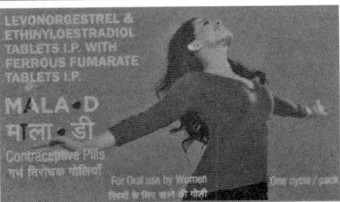 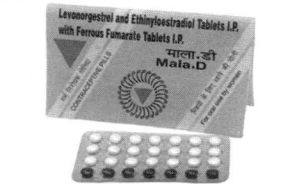
Methods	Hormonal contraception
M/A	Prevent the release of ovum from ovary, Inhibit sperm penetration and tubal motility, Delayed transport of sperm
Instruction	Start within 5 days of menstruation, every day take one pill on fixed time when packets of 28 pills over new packet should start from next day. (21 hormonal pills (white) and 7 non-hormonal pills (red) total 28 pills per packet).

Failure rate	0.1/100 women years
Remarks	**MALA-D** Estrogen (Ethinyl estradiol) **30** mcg and Levonorgestrel **0.15** mg. **MALA-N** MALA-N free in government supply. **Indication:** • Women with anemia, • Women with heavy or irregular menstrual cycle • Women who are on ART • Adolescent • Newly married couple • Women with family history of ovarian cancer **Absolute contraindication:** Breast cancer, genital cancer, thromboembolism history, abnormal uterine bleeding, liver disorder, congenital hyperlipidemia **Relative contraindication:** Women with hypertension, diabetes, smokers (>15 cigarettes per day), lactation **Adverse effect:** Metabolic, cardiovascular, carcinogenesis, liver disease **Common adverse effect:** Weight gain, breast tenderness, migraine, headache, bleeding **Noncontraceptive benefits:** Protection against benign breast disorders including fibrocystic disease and fibroadenoma, iron deficiency anemia, ectopic pregnancy, pelvic inflammatory disease, ovarian cysts, PCOD, and ovarian cancer
Progestogen only pill (POP)/Minipill/Micro pill	**Contain:** norethisterone and levonorgestrel. **Indication:** women having cardiovascular risk or tumor **Limitation:** high failure rate
Male pill	It is a derivative of cotton seed oil.
Methods	Hormonal contraception
M/A	Prevent the spermatogenesis, Prevent the sperm transport, Interfering with sperm storage and maturation, Affecting the constitute of seminal fluid
Instruction	One pill daily
Remarks	**Gossypol** is the trade name of the pill.
Injectable contraceptives	**Progestogen-only injectables** Depot-medroxyprogesterone acetate (DMPA) NET-EN (Norethisterone enanthate) DMPA-SC
DMPA (Depot medroxy progesterone acetate) *150 mg*	Medroxyprogesterone Injection IP — Contraceptive Injection — Antara Programme — Sterile Aqueous Suspension 1ml For deep intramuscular use only. Single Use Only — अंतरा
Methods	Hormonal contraception

M/A	Suppression of ovulation
Instruction	Intramuscular injection of 150 mg every 3 months.
Failure rate	0.1/100 women years
Remarks	DMPA/Depo-provera as "**Antara**" trade name included in the National Family Planning Program It is effective for 3 months Most common side effect unpredictable bleeding

NET-EN (Norethisterone enanthate) *200* mg

Methods	Hormonal contraception
M/A	suppression of ovulation
Instruction	Intramuscular injection of 200 mg every 2 months.
Failure rate	0.4/100 women years
Remarks	It is effective for 2 months Most common side effect unpredictable bleeding

DMPA-SC *104* mg

Methods	Hormonal contraception
M/A	Suppression of ovulation
Instruction	Subcutaneous injection of (Depo sub Q provera) 104 mg
Failure rate	0.3/100 women years
Remarks	Effective for 3 months Most common side effect unpredictable bleeding

Combined *Injectable* Contraceptives

Methods	Hormonal contraception
M/A	suppression of ovulation+ effects due to progesterone
Instruction	Effective for 1 month
Failure rate	0.2/100 women years
Remarks	Contains estrogens and progesterone Given at monthly interval

Sustained release system

Subdermal implant

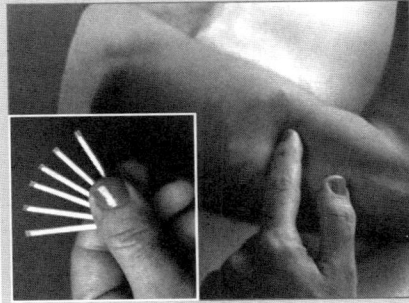

Population and Family Welfare

Methods	Hormonal contraception
M/A	Prevent the release of ovum from ovary, Thicken cervical mucus
Instruction	Silastic capsule of rod implanted beneath the skin of forearm of upper arm
Remarks	**Norplant**: 6 silastic capsule having 35 mg levonorgestrel **Norplant (R) 2:** only two small rods Protect for 5 years **Vaginal ring:** levonorgestrel absorbed through vaginal mucosa. Ring use up to 3 weeks of cycle then need to change.

Nonhormonal contraception

Nonhormonal contraception chhaya/saheli	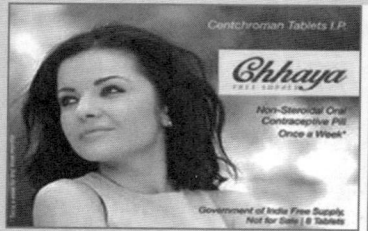 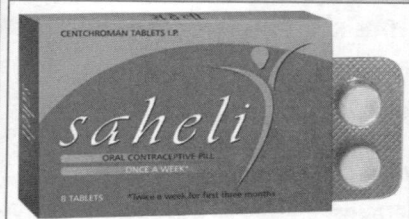
Methods	Nonhormonal contraception
M/A	Defective implantation of blastocyst Due to abnormal decidualization or blastocyst abnormality
Instruction	It is started on the first day of menstruation, given twice a week for the first 3 months and then once weekly.
Failure rate	1.6/100 women years
Remarks	Active ingredient is ormeloxifene also known as **centchroman** The only Nonsteroidal Nonhormonal Birth control pill **"Chhaya"** trade name included in the National Family Planning Program and as a **Saheli** trade name which is available in private sector. Indicated for women who cannot tolerate hormonal methods

TERMINAL METHODS

Female sterilization	**Laparoscopic tubal occlusion:** • Short operating time, shorter stay in hospital and a small scar • Through abdominal approach with a specialized instrument called "laparoscope" • The abdomen is inflated with gas (carbon dioxide, nitrous oxide or air) and the instrument is introduced into the abdominal cavity to visualize the tubes. Once the tubes are accessible, the Falope rings (or clips) are applied to occlude the tubes • Condition: Not history of heart disease, respiratory disease, diabetes and hypertension. Not within 6 weeks of postpartum **Minilap operation:** • Much simpler procedure requiring a smaller abdominal incision of only 2.5 to 3 cm conducted under local anesthesia. The minilap/Pomeroy technique is considered a revolutionary procedure for female sterilization. Advantage is a safe and easy method. • Also suitable for postpartum tubal sterilization

Male sterilization vasectomy	• Simple procedure performed under local anesthesia • It can be done by NSV method or conventional. • Vas deferens is cut at least 1 cm after clamping and tied so it prevents the sperm entering into seminal stream. **Advantage:** Less bleeding, highly effective **Instruction:** At least 30 ejaculations are necessary before seminal examination, wear scrotal support or T bandage for 15 days. And for next 3 months use another contraceptive method. **Complication:** Sperm granule, autoimmune response, spontaneous recanalization ▪ Failure rate is only 0.15 per 100 person year due to mistake during identification of vas.

- **Miscellaneous methods**
  - **Abstinence:** This is an effective method but practically not advisable and possible.
  - **Rhythm method:** Also known as calendar method or safe period. Last day is calculated by longest cycle minus 10 days and first day is calculated by shortest cycle minus 18 days. Then we get safe period. Sometimes cycle is not regular, illiterate couple who unable to calculate, they have to avoid intercourse from 8th to 22nd days of cycle. Failure rate high (9%).
  - **Natural method:** It includes cervical mucus method, basal body temperature and Symptothermic method.
  - **Coitus interruptus:** In this method male withdraws before ejaculation so, prevent deposition of semen in vagina. Failure rate is high (25%) reason behind this is unable to timely withdrawn.
  - **Lactation amenorrhea method:** LAM is only effective if mother exclusively breastfeed her child, child less than 6 month and till menstruation not started after childbirth.
  - **Birth control vaccine:** It is under research about use of human chorionic gonadotropin (hCG).
- **Postpartum and post-abortion family planning:** Women is very receptive at this time. Method of choice in this periods are IUCD (PPIUCD), Condom and sterilization. If women are breastfeeding, then only lactational amenorrhea method is also effective.

Types of Contraceptive Method for Different Needs

Needs for	Contraceptive option
Delaying the first child	Condoms Oral contraceptive pills Intrauterine contraceptive devices (IUCD 380 A and 375) Injectable contraceptive MPA Emergency contraceptive pills (not to be used routinely)
Healthy spacing between two pregnancies	Condoms Intrauterine contraceptive devices (IUCD 380 A and 375) OCPs (not given till breastfeeding) Injectable contraceptive MPA
Limiting methods	Female sterilization Male sterilization/ Vasectomy Long acting reversible methods (ex. IUCD 380 A and 375, injectable contraceptive)

Family Planning Methods According to Service Provider

Family planning method	Service provider service	Location
Spacing methods		
IUD 380 A/IUCD 375	Trained and certified ANMs, LHVs, SNs and doctors	Subcenter and higher levels
Oral Contraceptive Pills (OCPs)	Trained ASHAs, ANMs, LHVs, SNs and doctors	Village level
Condoms	Trained ASHAs, ANMs, LHVs, SNs and doctors	Village level
Limiting methods		
Minilap	Trained and certified MBBS doctors and specialist doctors	PHC and higher levels
Laparoscopic sterilization	Trained and certified MBBS doctors and specialist doctors	Usually CHC and higher levels
NSV: No scalpel vasectomy	Trained and certified MBBS doctors and specialist doctors	PHC and higher levels
Emergency contraception		
Emergency contraceptive pills (ECP)	Trained ASHAs, ANMs, LHVs, SNs and doctors	Village level, subcenter and higher levels

4.3 EMERGENCY CONTRACEPTION

- Emergency contraception refers to back-up methods for contraceptive emergencies which women can use within the first few days after unprotected intercourse to prevent an unwanted pregnancy.
- It is also known as **postcoital contraception, back-up with birth control, the morning after pill.**

Use of Emergency Contraception

- After voluntary sexual act without contraceptive protection
- Incorrect or inconsistent use of regular contraceptive methods: failure to take oral contraceptives for more than 3 days, being late for contraceptive injection
- In case of contraceptive failure or mishaps: miscalculation of infertile period, failed coitus interruptus, expulsion of an intrauterine device and, or in case of slippage/leakage/breakage of condom
- In the event of sexual assault.

Emergency contraception

Emergency oral contraception (ECP)	Ezy pill
Methods	Hormonal contraception
Instruction	Used within 72 hours of unprotected sexual intercourse
Failure rate	Less than 1%
Remarks	**Brief about** methods used as emergency contraception: • **Levonorgestrel:** *0.75* mg within *72* hour of unprotected sex and 2nd *12* hour of 1st dose • **Yuzpe's regimen** 4 OCP pills followed by 4 more after 12 hours. • Two pills of *50* mcg estrogen within *72* hours and same dose after *12* hours • **Mifepristone *10*** mg once within *72* hours • IUD within 5 days (nonhormonal method)

4.4 THE MEDICAL TERMINATION OF PREGNANCY (MTP) ACT, 1971

- It is based on the recommendations of the Shah committee.
- It was formulated on 10th August 1971 but came into force in 1st April 1972.
- It is amended in 1975, 2002 and 2021.
- It is intended to prevent illegal abortion and thus prevent sex selective abortion and also to reduce the maternal mortality ratio.
- It guides when, where and by whom the pregnancy should be terminated.
- It was also enacted to control the population of India.
- **Conditions when termination of pregnancy is permitted under this Act:**
  - **Therapeutic condition:** The life of woman is at risk if pregnancy is continued.
  - **Eugenic condition:** Substantially high risk of having physically or mentally abnormal child will be born if pregnancy is continued.
  - **Humanitarian condition:** For example, if pregnancy is resulted due to rape.
  - **Social condition:** For example, when pregnancy is due to contraceptive failure or social condition is not suitable for the continuation of the pregnancy.
  - Age of unmarried women is less than 18 years.
- **Duration of pregnancy:**
  - Up to 12 weeks opinion of one registered medical practitioner will be suffice.
  - From 12 weeks to 20 weeks duration of pregnancy opinion of two registered practitioners will be required in the favor of termination of pregnancy.
  - Beyond 20 weeks termination of pregnancy is not permitted under this act.

Population and Family Welfare

- But as per the latest medical termination of pregnancy (MTP) (Amendment) Bill, 2020, termination of pregnancy period has extended from 20 weeks to 24 weeks to make easier for women to safely and legally terminate an unwanted pregnancy. This enhanced the gestation limit for **'special categories' of women** which includes: survivors of rape, victims of incest, differently-abled women and **minors**.
- As per this The Bill, there will be requirement of the opinion of **one** registered medical practitioner (instead of two or more) for termination of pregnancy up to 20 weeks of gestation (fetal development period from the time of conception until birth) while opinion of **two** registered medical practitioners **for termination of pregnancy** of **20–24 weeks of gestation.**
- For pregnancies diagnosed with substantial fetal abnormalities, it has been proposed, that no upper gestation limit would apply for termination but opinion of the state-level medical board is essential for a pregnancy to be terminated after 24 weeks.
- If woman is less than 18 years than consent of guardian is compulsory.
- And though she is more than 18 years but mentally ill (earlier lunatic word was used) then also the consent of guardian is mandatory.
- To increase the legal abortion service providers medical practitioners of other stream like ayurvedic or homeopathic will be trained for medical termination of pregnancy.
- Confidentiality and privacy will be ensured for the unmarried women.

❑ **By whom the pregnancy can be terminated**:
  - MD in obstetrics and gynecology.
  - A medical practitioner who has assisted at least 25 terminations of pregnancy including 5 MTP performed independently.
  - Doctor who did 6 months of housemanship in obstetrics and gynecology department before this act implementation.

❑ **Provision of penalty**:
  - Medical practitioner is not registered—2 to 7 years of imprisonment
  - Place or hospital is not registered—2 to 7 years of imprisonment

4.5 NATIONAL FAMILY WELFARE PROGRAM

❑ **History and approach (Fig. 4.2)**

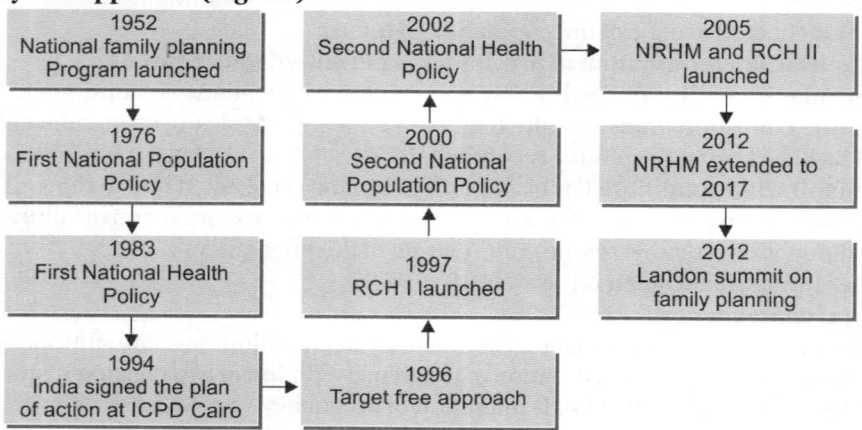

Fig. 4.2: Evolution of family planning program in India.

Population and Family Welfare

- India was the first country in the world to have launched a National Program for Family Planning in 1952.
- Over the decades, the program has undergone transformation in terms of policy and actual program implementation and currently being repositioned to not only achieve **population stabilization** goals but also promote **reproductive health** and reduce **maternal, infant and child mortality and morbidity.**

Key strategies include:
- Providing more choices through newly introduced contraceptives: Injectable Contraceptive, MPA (Medroxyprogesterone acetate) under Antara program and Chaya (earlier marketed as Saheli) will be made freely available to all government hospitals.
- Emphasis on Spacing methods like IUCD
- Revitalizing Postpartum Family Planning including PPIUCD in order to capitalize on the opportunity provided by increased institutional deliveries. Appointment of counselors at high institutional delivery facilities is a key activity.
- Strengthening community-based distribution of contraceptives by involving ASHAs and Focused IEC/ BCC efforts for enhancing demand and creating awareness on family planning
- Availability of fixed day static services at all facilities.
- Emphasis on minilap tubectomy services because of its logistical simplicity and requirement of only MBBS doctors and not postgraduate gynecologists/surgeons.
- A rational human resource development plan for IUCD, minilap and NSV be chalked up to empower the facilities (DH, CHC, PHC, SHC) with at least one provider each for each of the services and Subcenter's with ANMs trained in IUD insertion
- Ensuring quality care in Family Planning services by establishing Quality Assurance Committees at state and district levels Plan for accreditation of more private/NGO facilities to increase the provider base for family planning services under PPP.
- Increasing male participation and promoting non-scalpel vasectomy.
- Demand generation activities in the form of display of posters, billboards and other audio and video materials in the various facilities be planned and budgeted.
- Strong political will and advocacy at the highest level, especially in states with high fertility rates.

JANSANKHYA STHIRATA KOSH

4.6 POPULATION STABILIZATION FUND/JANSANKHYA STHIRATA KOSH

Strategy	Beneficiary	Condition	Financial award
Prerna	Under this strategy, awards are given to the couples who have broken the tradition of early marriage and early childbirth.	• Couple from below poverty line (BPL) family. • Age of woman should be <30 years of age. • The girl's age should be ≥19 years at the time of marriage. • There should be gap of at least 2 years between the first child birth and marriage.	If four condition fulfilled, then: Award of 10000/- in the case of boy child or 12000/- in the case of girl child If above all six conditions are fulfilled, then payment of award:

Population and Family Welfare

Strategy	Beneficiary	Condition	Financial award
		• There should be gap of at least 3 years between the first child birth and second child birth. • Either parent voluntarily accepts permanent method of family planning within 1 year of second child birth	15,000/- if both boy child 17,000/- if one boy and one girl child 19,000/- if both girl child.
Santushti	High populated states, such as Bihar, Uttar Pradesh, Madhya Pradesh, Rajasthan, Jharkhand, Chhattisgarh and Odisha	Invites private sector gynecologists and vasectomy surgeons to do tubectomy/vasectomy	Incentive for conducting 10 or more tubectomy/vasectomy cases in a month
Call center	For adolescents, newly married and about to be married couples	The information on reproductive health and family planning is given in both languages English and Hindi.	–
Private practitioner for IUCD 380 A	For private sector Promotion of IUCD 380A	–	–
Virtual resource center (VRC)	Anyone can receive the material on CD free of cost	Gives access to films, posters, photos related to gender discrimination, maternal and infant mortality, the declining sex ratio, adolescent health, spacing of birth, etc.	–
IEC activities like poster	All eligible population	–	–

Note: The JSK has been discontinued on 08/02/2019 vide the cabinet decision on 07.02.2018 and various schemes for population control are being supported under National Health Mission.

4.7 MISSION PARIVAR VIKAS

- "**Mission Parivar Vikas**" has been launched in 145 high focus districts with highest total fertility rate (TFR) more than/equal to 3.0, to reach the replacement level fertility goals of 2.1 by 2025".
- The key strategies are as follows:

Population and Family Welfare

1. Delivering Assured Services

- Roll out of injectable contraceptive DMPA (Antara) up to Sub-center level and Incentivizing ASHAs @ ₹ 100/dose while Incentivizing beneficiary @ ₹ 100/dose received.
- PPIUCD Services to be made available at all delivery points. ₹ 300 will be given to the acceptors of PPIUCD to cover their incidental cost and the travel cost for two follow-up visits.
- Augmentation of Sterilization services through compensation scheme in government facilities:

States	Type of operation	Acceptor	ASHA/ Health worker	others	Total (amount in ₹)
11 High focus states (Uttar Pradesh, Bihar, Madhya Pradesh, Rajasthan, Chhattisgarh, Jharkhand, Odisha, Uttarakhand, Assam, Haryana, Gujarat)	Vasectomy	2000	300	400	2700
	Tubectomy	1400	200	400	2000
Mission Parivar Vikas district	Vasectomy	3000	400	600	4000
	Tubectomy	2000	300	500	2800
	Tubectomy (PPS)	3000	400	600	4000
	Vasectomy (COT)	3000	400	1600	5000
	Tubectomy (COT)	2000	300	2200	4500
Other High focus states (North-East States, J & K, Himachal Pradesh)	Vasectomy	1100	200	200	1500
	Tubectomy	600	150	250	1000
Non-high focus states	Vasectomy	1100	200	200	1500
	Tubectomy (BPL + SC/ST only)	600	150	250	1000
	Tubectomy (APL)	250	150	250	650

- Condom boxes to be established at strategic locations like heath facilities, Gram Panchayat Bhavan etc.
- Social marketing of condoms and pills will be strengthened.
- There will be four round 'Mission Parivar Vikas' Campaigns per year in HFD districts during month of April, July, October and January (11th to 25th of the designated months). In July and October the activity will be clubbed with WPD and Vasectomy Fortnight.

2. Promotional Schemes

- **"NAYI PAHEL"**: It is an FP KIT for "Newly Weds" that would be given to the newly-wed couple by the ASHA. ASHA will receive @ ₹ 100/ASHA/Nayi Pahel kit distributed. This Kit includes jute bag, marriage registration form, pamphlet, 3 packet of condoms, oral contraceptive pills (Mala N) cycles, emergency contraceptive pill (E pill), Grooming/hygiene bag, pregnancy testing kit, information card.

- **Saas Bahu Sammelan:** Saas Bahu Sammelan is aimed to facilitate improved communication between mothers-in-law and daughters-in-law through interactive games and exercises. ₹ 1600 can be spent per meeting (₹ 1500-for organizing sammelan and token gifts (maximum permissible limit); ₹ 100 for ASHA incentive).
- **SAARTHI:** "SAARTHI" is a smartly designed bus/van equipped with interactive communication devices, IEC material and FP commodities which will help during "mission parivar vikas" campaign".
- Local radio spots with messages from local actors.

3. Ensuring Commodity Security

A management information system will track the supplies and consumption to different facilities and designated FP logistic manager would look after smooth functioning of this system.

4. Capacity Building/HRD for Enhanced Service Delivery

These districts are having shortage of trained providers and the high demand generated, so that need to be satisfied with by giving training to Approx. 47,600 providers for injectables (Antara Program) and PPIUCD/IUCD.

5. Creating Enabling Environment

Advocacy and intersectoral convergence to reduce TFR for a healthy mother and child will be done at all level including national, state, district and block level.

4.8 NATIONAL FAMILY PLANNING INDEMNITY SCHEME (NFPIS)

Under this scheme, any event of death/failures/complications/indemnity cover to doctors/health facilities during sterilization process accepters can claim payment.

Section	Coverage	Limits
Section I (A-D) For beneficiaries		
IA	Death following sterilization in hospital or within 7 days from the date of discharge	₹ 2 lakh
IB	Death following sterilization within 8-30 days from the date of discharge from the hospital	₹ 50,000/-
IC	Failure of sterilization	₹ 30,000/-
ID	Cost of treatment in hospital if complication due to sterilization within 60 days	Actual not exceeding ₹ 25,000/-
Section II: Empanelled Doctors under Public and Accredited Private/NGO Sector and Health Facilities under Public and Accredited Private/NGO Sector		
II	Indemnity coverage up to 4 cases of litigations per doctor and per health facility in a year	Up to ₹ 2 Lakh per cases of litigation

4.9 COUNSELING IN REPRODUCTIVE AND SEXUAL HEALTH PROBLEMS OF ADOLESCENTS

Counseling is a two-way communication between a healthcare worker (counselor) and a client, where the counselor builds rapport with the client for the purpose of facilitating decision making by the client regarding adoption of healthy behavior/s or availing health service/s and reducing health risks.

Tasks Involved in Counseling

- Creating appropriate and supportive counseling environment with privacy
- Actively and empathetically listening to clients' problems and work with them to find solutions that fits into their context in order to build trust and confidence. Because it is a sensitive matter to discuss with any age groups.
- Providing information appropriate to clients' problems and needs
- Assisting the clients in making voluntary and informed decisions
- **Voluntarism:** Family planning services are voluntary. Unlike other services couples are given information about methods relevant for them and it is the couples' right to choose a method.
- **Couple counseling:** Acceptance and continuation of the method is higher when couples are counseled together.
- **Culturally sensitive:** The counsellor should understand and be sensitive to cultural and psychological factors that may affect couple's need and decision for adopting contraceptive method.
- **Informed choice**: The purpose of informed choice is to ensure that all clients choose the best option/s for their healthcare needs after receiving full information about all available options. Informed choice is a pre-condition for informed consent.
- **Informed consent** means that a client understands the procedure (medical or surgical) and then decides to receive the care. Informed consent can be verbal or written. However, informed consent alone does not constitute informed choice.

Counseling Adolescents

- During adolescence, boys and girls undergo many physical, emotional/psychological as well as social changes due to sudden spurt in the hormones.
- Most adolescents get confused due to these sudden changes and find it challenging to cope with them.
- Role of counselor is to reassure them that these changes are normal during adolescence and occur due to the rapid development in the brain and production of hormones. Their misconceptions/myths/fears related to these changes need to be clarified.
- Married adolescents want contraception to delay the child and unmarried adolescents may not seek contraceptive services due to lack of privacy and fear of being judged.
- Counsel and discuss about various risks with the teenage pregnancy
- If pregnancy occur then counsel and educate about all the pregnancy care

- Refer the adolescents at risk of STIs/HIV/AIDS to Integrated counseling and testing centers, if needed. Counsel on safer sex including use condoms for protection against STIs/HIV
- Counselor should discuss the preventive measures for RTIs/STIs with adolescents:
  - Maintain proper genital and menstrual hygiene
  - Avoiding sex with unknown or multiple partners or an infected partner of STI/RTI

Six Essential Steps for Counseling Adolescents

- **Connect:** with the adolescents
- **Reassure:** the adolescents
- **Stabilize:** provide support
- Address their needs and concerns
- **Provide support:** emotional, psychosocial, physiological
- Facilitate coping.

Basic Principles of Adolescent Centered Counseling

- Respect and accept their norms and concerns
- Listen carefully and avoid any discrimination
- Be nonjudgmental and ensure confidentiality of information shared
- Be empathetic and offer nondirective suggestions
- Provide resources with problem-solving skills.

Communication Skills for Counseling

Verbal Communication

- Clear diction
- Positive tone of voice
- Use of simple language and culturally appropriate words and phrases
- Emphasizing main points
- Active listening.

Nonverbal Cues

- Smiling and maintaining eye-contact
- Facial expressions showing interest and concern
- Leaning towards the client and nodding.

Tips for Interacting with Adolescents

- Start the conversation with non-threatening issues in a friendly and non-judgmental tone and assure confidentiality to build rapport and trust.
- After listening, reassure them of an appropriate solution, e.g., when adolescents come with signs/symptoms of STI, do not scare them but tell them about the treatment, discuss the preventive measures and encourage them to make informed decisions on their own.

GATHER approach: It is the counseling approach commonly used in family planning while dealing with the choice of methods of contraception:
- G: Greet (show respect and trust)
- A: Ask (encourage them to tell the problem)
- T: Tell (provide accurate and specific needed information)
- H: Help (help them to make correct decisions)
- E: Explain (clear the doubts or any misunderstanding)
- R: Return (follow-up visit).

4.10 FAMILY PLANNING 2020 AND 2030

- Family Planning (FP) program in India was the first national program in the world which helping it emerge as a global leader to provide learning platforms to the world **(Fig. 4.3)**.

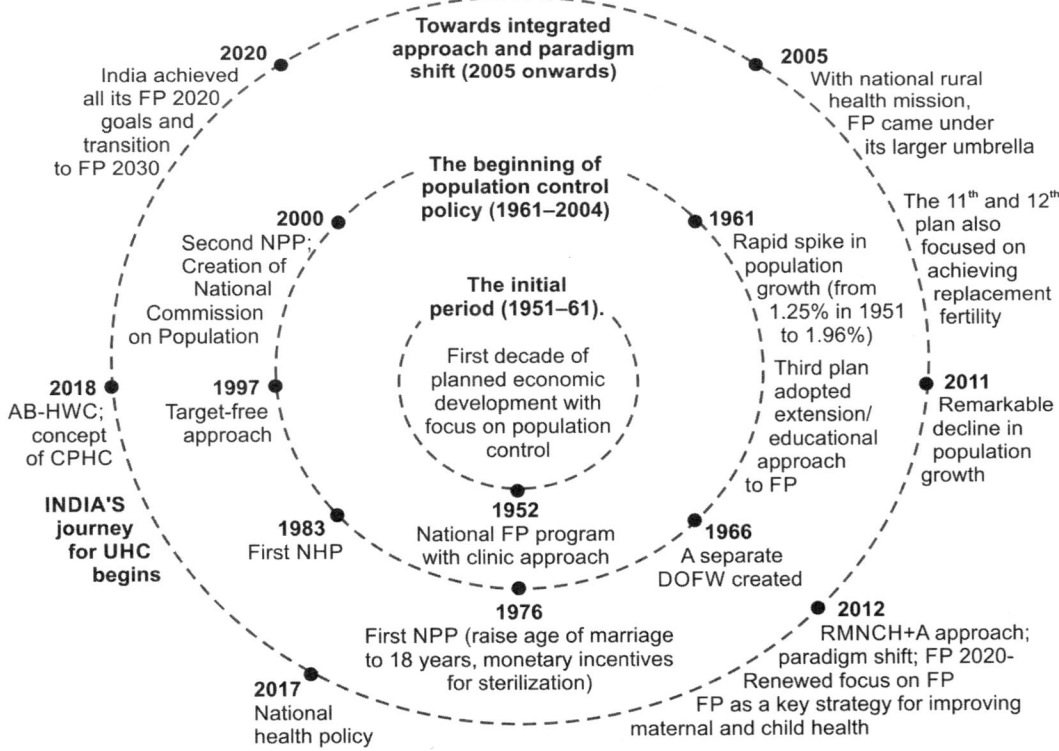

Fig. 4.3: Advent of family planning program in India.

Different Strategic Approaches under FP Program (Fig. 4.4)

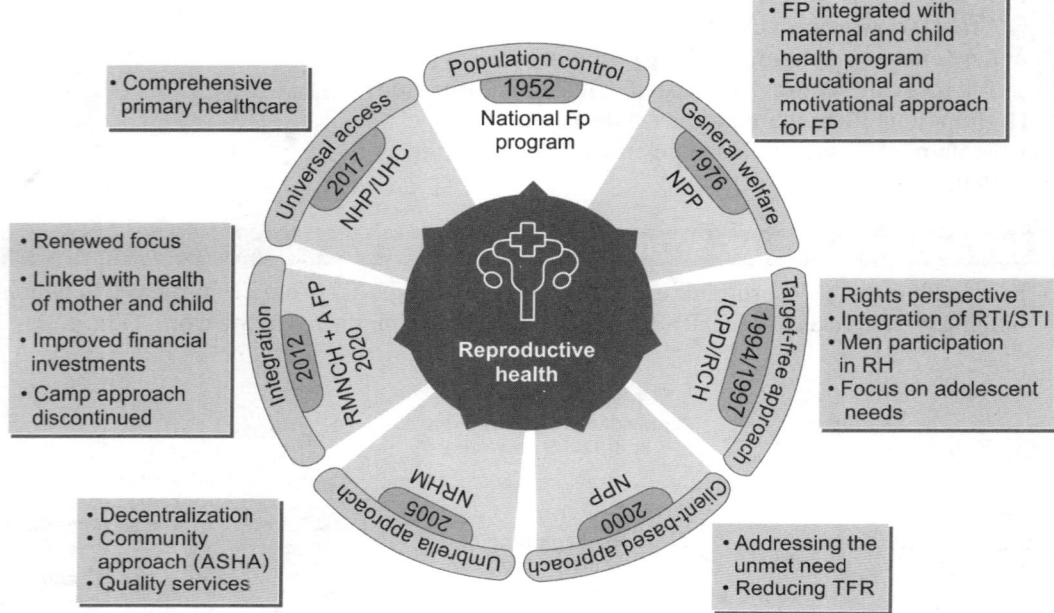

Fig. 4.4: Strategic approach under FP program.

Key Supply Side Strategies for FP 2020

Year	Strategies
2012	• Paradigm shift • Expansion of contraceptive basket–Introduction of IUCD 375
2013	• HR strengthening–task sharing • Dedicated counselors • PPIUCD service strengthening
2014	• Focus on quality–technical guidelines • Drop back scheme • HR development–onsite training model (EAISI)
2015	• Focus on quality–camps discontinuation, replaced by FDS • Improved packaging • Statewise annual review and capacity building
2016	• Introduction of injectable MPA–antara program • Introduction of centchroman • Revival of PAFP
2017	• Supply chain strengthening–FP logistics management information system • Improving access to FP–Mission Parivar Vikas. • Clinical outreach teams (COT).
2018	• HR development–extensive trainings for pan India roll out of MPA, centchroman pills and FPLMIS. • Institutionalizing monitoring–ongoing state-specific reviews.
2019	• Improving quality–state specific reviews and capacity building for quality compliances.
2020	• Pandemic response–guidelines and reviews for continuation of essential services.

Key Demand Side Strategies for FP 2020

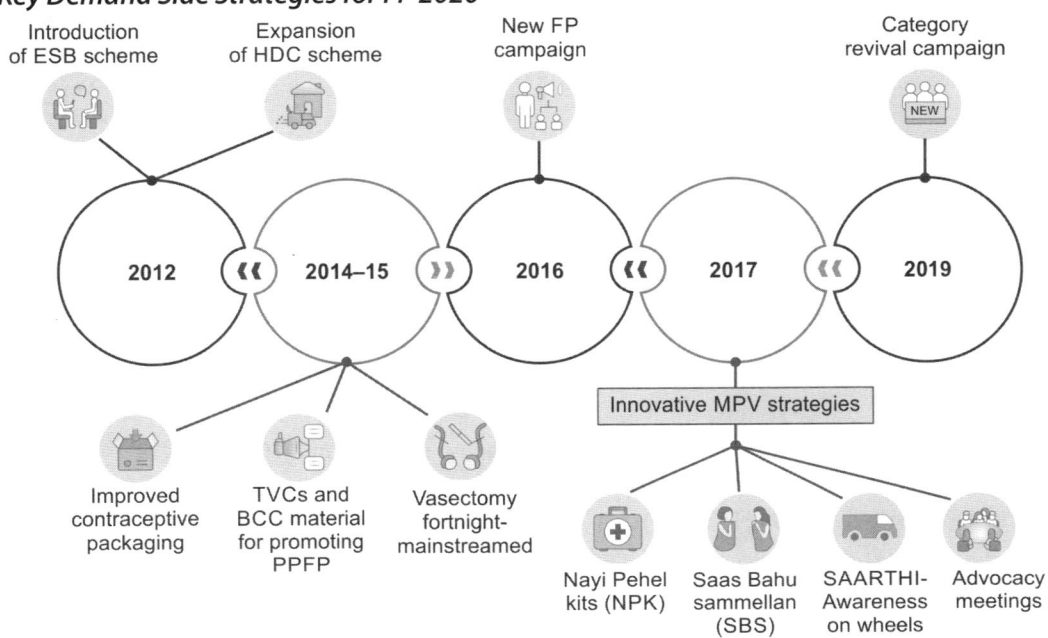

Fig. 4.5: Evolution strategies of family planning program.

- The modern contraceptive use shows an increasing trend with a substantial gain during FP 2020 era. The rate of increase is almost 55% in 28 years—from 36.5% in 1992–93 to 56.5% in 2019–21—almost one-third of this increase happened during the FP 2020 period (from 47.8% in 2015–16 to 56.5% in 2019–21) **(Fig. 4.5)**.
- In NFHS-5, unmet need for FP shows a significant decline from 12.9% (NFHS-4) to 9.4%.
- The share of spacing doubled from 16.2% in 1992–93 to 32.3% in 2019–21 (NFHS). This shift is a testimony of success of GoI schemes like MPV, PPIUCD, Condom boxes, HDC, ESB, etc.
- India has achieved the replacement fertility level. The current TFR for the country is 2.0 (NFHS-5). While fertility has declined across 31 States/UTs of India, 5 States still have high TFR (Bihar-3, Meghalaya-2.9, UP-2.3, Jharkhand-2.3 and Manipur-2.2). There is also urban-rural variation in the country. In terms of rural India, 7 States (out of 36) are yet to achieve replacement TFR.
- Trends in Prevalence of Modern Contraceptive Methods and TFR, India, 1992–2021 **(Fig. 4.6)**.
- India's Achievements towards FP 2020 Commitments Under FP 2020, India committed:
  - Ensuring total allocation of US $3 billion for Family Planning from 2012-2020.
  - Increasing annual modern Contraceptive Prevalence Rate by 0.4% so as to attain 54.3%
  - Increasing demand satisfied by modern contraceptives to 74% by 2020. **All the three goals were successfully achieved by the country.**

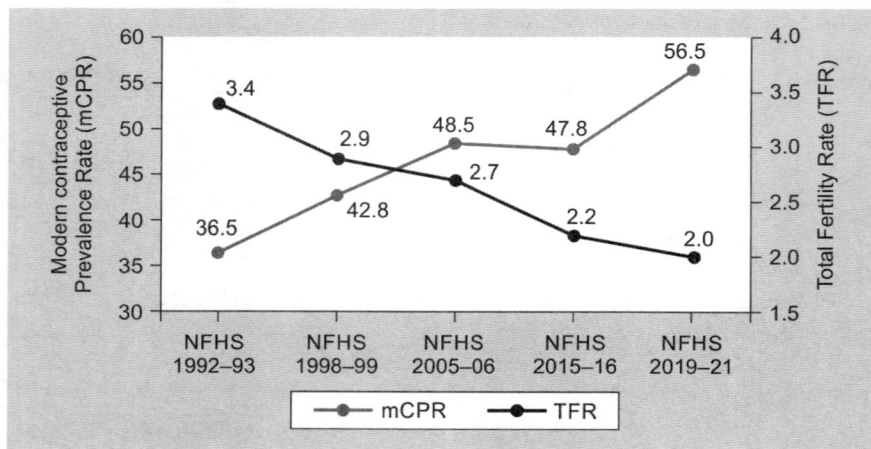

Fig. 4.6: Trends in prevalence of modern contraceptive methods and TFR, India, 1992–2021.

Family Planning 2030 (FP 2030)
- India successfully achieved its FP 2020 country goals well before the stipulated time frame. This is reflective of the success of various strategies, initiatives and collaborative efforts undertaken in the country.
- The road to FP 2030 will run on the guiding principles for UHC.

India's Vision for FP 2030
By the end of 2030, India's Family Planning vision is to provide access to high quality comprehensive Family Planning services to all people of reproductive age group including those from marginalized groups by ensuring equitable, affordable and appropriate contraceptive choices and information till last mile through improved health systems and community engagement within the country's UHC framework.

FP 2030–India's Commitments
- Expanding range and reach of contraceptive options by 2030 by exploring the introduction of new contraceptives.
- Ensuring healthy timing and spacing of pregnancies by improving the demand, uptake, and quality for post-pregnancy contraception services.
- Scaling up of Mission Parivar Vikas (MPV) for delivering assured quality of services in the hardest-to-reach rural and urban areas by providing a full-service package at all levels in all MPV Districts.
- Intensifying social and behavior change activities (SBC) for Family Planning and strengthening access to information and services for all girls and women and couples with specific focus on young people.
- Civil society commitments for creating awareness on family planning commodities and services and mobilizing community for increasing uptake as well as providing services through civil society organizations.

Strategic Priorities

- Addressing the FP needs of vulnerable population (ensuring universal, equitable, non-discriminatory and comprehensive services)
- Ensuring male participation (ensuring equitable and comprehensive services)
- Improving access and availability of contraceptive services (ensuring universal, comprehensive, choice based and quality services)
- Engaging community and other stakeholders (ensuring community participation and accountability).

4.11 MISCELLANEOUS

Example 1. There are 220 eligible couple living in village A with population of 1200. In this village couple are using different types of contraceptive methods and details about that given in following table. On the basis of this data calculate couple protection rate.

Method of contraception	No. of couple using particular method
Condom	42
OC pill	19
IUCD	16
Tubectomy	13
Vasectomy	6

Total eligible couple in village A = 220
Total couple using contraceptive methods = 96

Method of contraception	Effectiveness of contraception method	No. of couple using particular method	Effectively protected couple
Condom	50%	42	21#
IUCD	95%	16	15
OC pill	100%	19	19
Tubectomy	100%	13	13
Vasectomy	100%	6	6
Total		96	74

#Effective protected couple calculation example = (42 × 50/100) = 21. In this way we can calculate for other methods.

Couple Protection Rate

$$\text{CPR} = \frac{\text{Total number of couple protected by contraceptive methods}}{\text{Total number of couple in village}} \times 100$$

$$= \frac{96 \times 100}{220} = 43.64\%$$

Effective Couple Protection Rate

$$\text{ECPR} = \frac{\text{Total number of couple effectively protected by contraceptive methods}}{\text{Total number of couple in village}} \times 100$$

$$= \frac{74 \times 100}{220} = 33.64\%$$

Example 2

In village X, 150 women were using contraceptive method "A" for 2 years. Among them, during 2-year period, 60 women conceived pregnancy. Calculate Pearl index of contraceptive method "A".

Total months of exposure = no. of women × no. of months of contraceptive use
$$= 150 \times 24 = 3600$$

Accidental pregnancy (contraception failure) occurred in 60 women in village X.

Pearl index

$$= \frac{\text{Number of accidental pregnancy}}{\text{Total months of exposure}} \times 1200$$

$$= \frac{60 \times 1200}{3600} = 20 \text{ per hundred women year}$$

BIBLIOGRAPHY

1. http://www.rncollegehajipur.in/rn/uploads/products/Measures%20to%20Control%20Population%20Growth%20in%20India.pdf
2. https://fp2030.org/sites/default/files/India_FP2030_Vision_Document.pdf
3. https://nhm.gov.in/images/pdf/programmes/familyplaning/guidelines/MPV/MPV_guidelines.pdf
4. https://pib.gov.in/newsite/mbErel.aspx?relid=151049
5. https://pib.gov.in/PressReleasePage.aspx?PRID=1600916
6. Jansankhya Sthirata Kosh, pib, govt. of India, MOHFW, Available at: http://pib.nic.in/newsite/PrintRelease.aspx?relid = 101231.
7. JSK strategies, Jansankhya Sthirata Kosh, MOHFW, govt. of India. available at: http://www.jsk.gov.in/jsk_strategies.asp.
8. K Park. Park's Textbook of Preventive and Social Medicine, 26th edn., Bhanot Publishers, Jabalpur; 2021.
9. Lal S, Adarsh, Pankaj. Textbook of Community Medicine, 2nd edn. CBS Publishers and Distributors, New Delhi; 2010.
10. Reference manual for integrated Reproductive, Maternal, Neonatal, Child, Adolescent Health and Nutrition (RMNCAH+N) Counseling, Family Planning Division, Ministry of Health and Family Welfare, Government of India,2021
11. The gazette of India. The medical termination of pregnancy act, 1971 and Draft of medical termination of pregnancy (amendment) bill 2014.

CHAPTER 5

Occupational Health

CHAPTER OUTLINE

- 5.1 Occupational health hazards
- 5.2 Occupational diseases
- 5.3 The Factory Act, 1948
- 5.4 The Employees State Insurance (ESI) Act, 1948
- 5.5 National Program for Control and Treatment of Occupational Diseases
- 5.6 Role of a nurse in occupational health services

5.1 OCCUPATIONAL HEALTH HAZARDS

OCCUPATIONAL HEALTH

Definition of **Occupational Health** (by joint ILO and WHO Committee): Occupational health should aim at the promotion and maintenance of the highest degree of physical, mental and social well-being of workers in all occupations; the prevention among workers of departures from health caused by their working conditions; the protection of workers in their employment from risks resulting from factors adverse to health; the placing and maintenance of the worker in an occupational environment adapted to his physiological and psychological equipment, and, to summarize, the adaptation of work to man and of each man to his job.

ERGONOMICS

- The word "ergonomics" is derived from the Greek word ergon, meaning work and nomos, meaning law
- It means "fitting the job to the worker"
- Aim is to achieve the best mutual adjustment of man and his work, for the improvement of human efficiency and well-being

❑ Training in ergonomics includes working method and environment, appropriate designing of machines, tools, equipment and manufacturing processes, lay-out of the places of work in order to achieve greater efficiency of both man and machine. It is indirectly helpful to reduce industrial accidents.

Occupational Environment

Three types of interaction in a working occupational environment: these all factors affect the health and efficiency of worker. Equilibrium between all these factors is necessary for better outcome.

1. **Man and physical, chemical and biological agents**
   - *Physical agents:* Heat, cold, air movement, vibrations, heat radiation, humidity light, noise and ionizing radiation.
   - *Chemical agents:* Number of chemicals, gases and toxic dusts which are potential hazards to the health of the workers.
   - *Biological agents:* Bacterial, viral, rickettsial and parasitic agents
2. **Man and machine:** For mass production, use of machines is increased in industry. Lack of safety measures and wrong technique sometimes are causes accidents. During long working hours in unphysiological postures is the causes of backache, fatigue, muscle ache, and joint pain.
3. **Man and man:** The psychosocial factors are the human relationships amongst workers themselves on the one hand, and those in authority over them on the other. Examples are type of work, service conditions, job satisfaction, work stability, leadership style, security, workers participation, communication, payment system, incentives, welfare conditions, trade union activities, etc.

Occupational hazards: Depending upon type of occupation, an industrial worker may be exposed to major five types of hazards.
❑ Physical hazards
❑ Chemical hazards
❑ Biological hazards
❑ Mechanical hazards
❑ Psychosocial hazards

Hazards and its effect mentioned below.

Hazards	Effects
Physical hazards	
Heat and cold	Burns, heat exhaustion, heat stroke and heat cramps
Noise	**Auditory effects:** Temporary or permanent hearing loss **Non-auditory effects:** Fatigue, nervousness, decreased efficiency
Light	**The acute effects** of poor illumination effect: headache, eye strain, eye pain, lachrymation, eye fatigue **The chronic effects:** Miner's nystagmus **Exposure to excessive brightness or glare:** Discomfort, visual fatigue

Hazards	Effects
Vibration	Work with pneumatic tools such as drills and hammers. Vibration usually affects the hands and arms After some months or years of exposure, spasm of fine blood vessels of the hand cause white fingers Exposure to vibration may also produce injuries of the joints of the hands, elbows and shoulders
Ionizing radiation	X-rays and radioactive isotopes damage certain tissues such as bone marrow. Effects like malformation, genetic changes, cancer, leukemia, ulceration, sterility and in extreme cases of death.
Ultraviolet radiation	Arc welding worker may develop intense conjunctivitis and keratitis (welder's flash)
Chemical hazards: Local action of chemical produce ulcer, eczema, dermatitis and due to pneumoconiosis develop due to inhalation and some hazards develop after ingestion of substances	
Mechanical hazards: Accident	
Biological hazards: Brucellosis, fungal infections, leptospirosis, tetanus, anthrax, psittacosis, encephalitis, schistosomiasis	
Psychosocial hazards: Lack of job satisfaction, insecurity, frustration, anxiety, depression, poor human relationships	

BIBLIOGRAPHY

1. https://www.who.int/tools/occupational-hazards-in-health-sector.

5.2 OCCUPATIONAL DISEASES

Major occupational diseases can be divided into following categories:
- Occupational injuries
- Occupational lung diseases
- Occupational cancers
- Occupational infections
- Occupational dermatitis
- Others.

Occupational Lung Diseases

Lung disease occurs due to long exposure of dust which size range of 0.5 to 3 micron is known as a pneumoconiosis. The important dust diseases are given in **Table 5.1**.

Table 5.1: Pneumoconiosis.

Name	Exposure	Industry	Clinical features	X-ray findings	Remarks
Silicosis (Miner's Phthisis, Grinder's disease)	Free silica (silicon dioxide)	Mining of mica, coal, gold, silver, lead and zinc etc., ceramic industry, pottery industry, sand blasting and construction work	Irritating cough, pain in the chest, and dyspnea on exertion. Pathologically it causes **"Nodular fibrosis"**	**"Snow storm appearance"** Apical part involvement is common.	1. **"Silicotuber-culosis"** 2. Silicosis is notifiable under factories and mines Act
Anthracosis	Coal dust	Mining of coal, carbon electrode manufacturer	There are two phases: 1. Simple Pneumoconiosis 2. Progressive massive fibrosis (results in severe respiratory insufficiency)		Once pneumoconiosis due to coal dust has set in then massive fibrosis will develop even without having further exposure. Notifiable under mines Act and compensable under Workmen's Compensation Act
Byssinosis	Cotton fiber dust	Textile industry	Chronic cough, progressive dyspnea		It is called **"Monday fever"** while metal fume fever is called as **"Monday Morning fever"**
Bagassosis	Bagasse or sugarcane dust (due to growth of thermoactinomyces sacchari)	Cardboard manufacturing industry, paper and rayon industry	It is fungal infection results in acute bronchitis and Bronchospasm. Breathlessness, cough, hemoptysis, and fever. It is reversible condition if treated.	**"Mottling in lung shadow"**	It was reported for the first time in India by Ganguli and Pal. Moisture content more than 20% and spraying of 2% propionic acid can keep bagasse safe for use
Asbestosis	Serpentine type (chrysolite) and amphibole type. There are varieties of amphibole, Amosite, Crocidolite and anthophyllite	Fireproof textiles, roof tiling, brake lining, and gaskets and asbestos cement industry		**"Ground glass appearance"** in lower two thirds of the lung fields (basal fibrosis)	Once the disease is developed then it is progressive even after removal of exposure. Mesothelioma occurs due to crocidolite type of asbestos. Chrysolite and amosite are safer types of asbestosis
Farmers' lung	Mouldy hay or grain dust (Micropolyspora faeni)	Agriculture work	It is fungal infection results in acute bronchitis and bronchopneumonia		30% or more moisture content and temperature between 40 and 50 deg. Enhance growth of actinomycetes particularly of Micropolyspora faeni in the grain dust
Siderosis	Iron dust	Foundry workers, welders	No tissue reaction so not lung impairment		

Occupational Cancer

The characteristics are:
- History of prolonged exposure
- The long period between exposure and development of the disease
- The average age incidence is earlier than that for cancer in general
- The disease may develop even after the cessation of exposure.

Type	Details
Skin cancer	• 75% of occupational cancers • Carcinogens: UV rays, coal tar, soot, oils and dyes, X-rays • At risk group: Gas workers, oil refiners, coke oven workers, dyestuff workers, road makers
Lung cancer	• Carcinogens: arsenic, asbestos, beryllium, chromium, tobacco, coal tar, nickel • At risk group: Asbestos factory, gas industry, uranium mines, nickel, cigarette smoking
Cancer bladder	• Carcinogens: aromatic amines, β-naphthylamine, para amino diphenyl, benzidine, auramine, and magenta • At risk group: dyestuffs and dyeing industry, rubber industry, gas industry, electric cable industry
Leukemia	• Carcinogen: benzol, roentgen rays, radioactive substances • At risk group: atomic energy research department and radiology department

Occupational Dermatitis

- These are the diseases of the skin arising out of the occupation or during the course of employment.
- Agents causing dermatitis: Primary irritants and sensitizing substances
- Causes:
    - Physical: Heat, cold, moisture, friction, pressure, X-rays
    - Chemical: Acids, alkalis, grease, oils, phenols, dyes, solvents, tar
    - Biological: Viruses, bacteria, fungi, parasites
    - Plant products: Leaves, fruits, flowers, vegetables, plants

Lead Poisoning

- Most toxic metal poisoning
- Toxic lead compound: Lead carbonate, lead arsenate, lead oxide

Sources:
- **Occupational:** Mines of lead ores, manufacture of storage batteries, glass manufacture, printing and potteries, rubber industry, ship building, plumbing works
- **Nonoccupational:** Gasoline (leaded petrol), drinking water, insecticides, children—chewing lead paint on windows and toys
- **Clinical features:** Anemia, blue lines on the gums (burton's lines/burtonian lines), colicky abdomen, encephalopathy, fatigue, growth failure among children, headache, irritability, mental confusion, delirium, nausea, oliguria, wrist drop and foot drop.

Occupational Hazards in the Health Sector

- **Occupational infections:** Most common occupational infections of concern in the health sector are tuberculosis, hepatitis B and C, HIV/AIDS and respiratory infections (coronaviruses, influenza)
- **Exposure to hazardous chemicals:** It includes cleaning and disinfecting agents, mercury, sterilants, toxic drugs, anesthetic gases and laboratory chemicals and reagents
- **Unsafe patient handling:** Lifting, transferring, repositioning and moving patients without using proper techniques or handing equipment can cause musculoskeletal injury (e.g., back injury and chronic back pain)
- **Exposure to radiation:** Ionizing (X-rays, radionuclides) and non-ionizing radiation (UV, lasers) exposure may occur in healthcare settings. It may cause skin and blood damage, cataract, infertility, birth defects, cancer, etc.
- **Occupational stress and fatigue:** Time pressure, lack of control over work tasks, long working hours, shift work, lack of support and moral injury are important risk factors for stress.

Prevention of Occupational Diseases

It includes medical, engineering and statutory or legislative.

Medical Measures

- **Preplacement examination:** It is done at the time of employment and it includes the worker's medical, family, and occupational history. Physical examination, biological and radiological examinations like, e.g., chest X-ray, vision testing, electrocardiogram, urine and blood examination are included.
- **Periodical examination:**
  - The frequency and content of periodical medical examinations will depend upon the type of occupational exposure.
  - Routinely ordinarily workers are examined once a year. Occupational exposures like lead, toxic dyes, radium monthly examinations are indicated.
- **Medical services:**
  - First aid services should be made available within the factory.
  - Employees State Insurance Scheme provides medical care to the worker and his family.
- **Supervision:**
  - It is helpful to prevent occupational disabilities.
  - During periodic visit the physician gets the information of occupational environment like temperature, noise, ventilation, etc., types of raw material and product, working duration. On the basis of that effective preventive measure of occupational diseases can be taken.
- **Notification:** The main aim of notification is to initiate measures for prevention and protection of occupational disease. List of disease included under the different laws like Factories Act and Mines Act.
- **Maintenance of records:** It is necessary for future follow-up and proper planning.
- **Health education and counseling:** At the time of work placement, health education is compulsory to the worker for how to use personal protective equipment, nature of chemical and risk of hazards.

Engineering Measures

- **Building design:** It includes type of walls, floor, roof, ceiling etc.
- **Ventilation:** As per the Indian Factories Act, a minimum of 500 cu. ft. of air space require for each worker. It is helpful to decrease airborne hazard.
- **Good house-keeping**
- **Isolation:** Hazardous in industry should be isolated in separate building or room.
- **Protective devices:** It includes ear plug, helmets, safety shoes, respirators, aprons, gloves, goggles, boots, etc.
- **Local exhaust ventilation:** It is required to remove dusts, gases, fumes and other injurious substances.
- **Substitution:** It means replacement of a harmful material by a harmless one. For example, acetone in place of benzene, zinc and iron in place of lead.
- **Mechanization:** Contact hazard is decreased by mechanical devices, pipelines, etc.
- **Dusts:** It is controlled by water spray.
- **Enclosure:** Enclosure of harmful material process prevent escape in environment.
- **Statistical and environmental monitoring:** It is helpful to decide the role of PPE to prevent the hazard and effect of environmental measure.
- **Research:** It is helpful to decide permissible limit of toxic material.

Legislative Measures

Important measures are like Factory Act,1948, ESI Act,1948, Mines Act,1952, The Workman's Compensation Act, 1923, The Maternity Benefit Act, 1961.

BIBLIOGRAPHY

1. https://www.hopkinsmedicine.org/healthlibrary/conditions/respiratory_disorders/pneumoconiosis_134,162
2. https://www.who.int/tools/occupational-hazards-in-health-sector
3. Vinaya S. Karkhanis and J.M. Joshi, Pneumoconiosis, The Indian Journal of Chest Diseases and Allied Sciences, 2013; Vol.55, p.25-34.

5.3 THE FACTORY ACT, 1948

The Act was revised and amended several times, the latest being the factories (Amendment) Act, 1987.

- **Scope:** The Act defines factory as an establishment employing 10 or more workers where power is used, and 20 or more workers where power is not used. There is no distinction between perennial and seasonal factories.
- **Health, safety and welfare** (Chapter III, IV, IVA, and V):
  - Elaborate provisions have been made for the
    - Health, safety and welfare of the workers
    - Cleanliness, lighting and ventilation
    - Treatment of wastes and effluents so as to render them innocuous, and for their disposal
    - The elimination of dusts and fumes
    - The provision of spittoons, control of temperature
    - Supply of cool drinking water during summer

- A minimum of **500 Cu.ft** of space for each worker has been prescribed and for factories installed before the 1948 Act, a minimum of 350 Cu.ft of space has been prescribed.
- The Act contains a separate Chapter (Chapter V) relating to specific welfare measures, e.g., washing facilities, facilities for storing and drying clothes, facilities for sitting, first-aid appliances, shelters, rest-rooms and lunch rooms, canteens and creches.
- When more than 250 workers are employed, a **canteen** shall be provided.
- The 1976 amendment provides for **creches** in every factory wherein more than 30 women workers are ordinarily employed.
- In every factory, wherein 500 or more workers are ordinarily employed, a **Welfare Officer** should be appointed.
- The 1976 amendment (Section 40 B) states that a **'Safety Officers'** in every factory wherein 1,000 or more workers are ordinarily employed.

☐ **Employment of young persons:**
- The Act prohibits employment of children below the age of 14 years and declares persons between the ages 15 and 18 to be adolescents.
- Child who has not completed his fourteenth year of age has been restricted from employment in any factory.
- Adolescents should be duly certified by the "Certifying Surgeons" regarding their fitness for work. Adolescent employee is allowed to work only between 6 AM and 7 PM

☐ **Hours of work:**
- The Act has prescribed a maximum of 48 working hours per week, not exceeding 9 hours per day with rest for at least ½ hour after 5 hours of continuous work.
- For adolescents, the hours of work have been reduced from 5 to 4½ hr per day.
- The total number of hours of work in a week including overtime shall not exceed 60.

☐ **Leave with wages:**
- The Act lays down that besides weekly holidays, every worker will be entitled to leave with wages after 12 month's continuous service at the following rate:
- Adult: One day for every 20 days of work, children: one day for every 15 days of work.
- The leave can be accumulated up to 30 days in case of adults and 40 days in case of children.

☐ **Occupational diseases:**
- It is obligatory on the part of the factory management to give information regarding specified accidents which cause death, serious bodily injury or regarding occupational diseases contracted by employees.
- The Act gives a schedule of notifiable diseases. The 1976 amendment includes Byssinosis, Asbestosis, occupational dermatitis and noise-induced hearing loss among the list of notifiable diseases and provides for enquiry in every case of a fatal accident.

☐ **Employment in hazardous processes:**
- The Central Government has incorporated a new Chapter IV-A by the Factories (Amendment) Act, 1987, relating to hazardous processes.
- Site Appraisal Committee consisting of Chief Inspector and other members, not more than 14 in number, for examination of service conditions of employees in a factory, involving hazardous processes, is to be constituted for recommendations.

Note: **The Occupational Safety, Health and Working Conditions Code, 2020** is a code to consolidate and amend the laws regulating the occupational safety and health and working conditions of the persons employed in an establishment. The Act will replace 13 old central labor laws including factory Act. As of now this code is being considered and it is under revision.

BIBLIOGRAPHY

1. The gazette of India. The factory act, 1948.

5.4 THE EMPLOYEES STATE INSURANCE (ESI) ACT, 1948

ESI Act is designed to accomplish the task of protecting the employees against the impact of incidences of sickness, maternity, disablement and death due to employment injury and to provide medical care to insured persons and their families.

- It is applicable to factories and other establishments like road transport, hotels, restaurants, cinemas, newspaper industry, shops and educational institutions.
- It is applicable above mentioned institutions wherein 10 or more persons are employed irrespective of aid of power. (**amended from 20 to 10 persons**)
- Since 1st August 2015, ESI Act has been extended to construction sites workers.
- World Economic Forum (WEF) 1st October 2016, employee's wage up to ₹ **21,000 per month** (amended from ₹ 15,000 per month to ₹ 21,000 per month) are entitled to social security under the ESI Act.
- Contribution for the premium will be 3.25% of daily wages from the employer side and 0.75% of daily wages from the employee side.
- Employees earning less than ₹ **176 per day** are exempted of their share of contribution.
- Summary of different benefits discussed in **Table 5.2**.

Table 5.2: Summary of different benefits under ESI Act.

Benefit	Contributory condition	Duration	Rate
Medical benefit	From day one	All reasonable medical care till he remains employed.	
Sickness benefit			
Sickness benefit	At least 78 days in corresponding contribution period	Up to 91 days in two consecutive benefit periods	70% of the average daily wages
Enhanced Sickness benefit	Same as above	14 days for tubectomy 7 days for vasectomy	100% of the average daily wages
Extended Sickness benefit (it is given for 34 specified long term diseases)	Continuous insurable employment for two years with minimum 156 days contribution in four consecutive contribution periods.	124 days and can be extended to two years.	80% of the average daily wages

Disablement benefit			
Temporary disablement	From day one for the disablement due to employment injury	As long as temporary disablement lasts	90% of the average daily wages
Permanent disablement	From day one for the disablement due to employment injury	For whole life	90% of the average daily wages
Dependents benefit	From day one for the disablement due to employment injury	It will be given whole life for widows and for dependent children it will be given for 25 years of age.	90% of the average daily wages sharable in fixed proportions among all dependents
Maternity benefit	For 70 days in two preceding contribution periods	• It will be given for 12 weeks in case of confinement(pregnancy) and extendable for one more month on medical advice. • Under maternity benefit act it has been increased up to 26 weeks. • For case of miscarriage it, will be leave for 6 weeks. • If ESI medical services are not available then ₹ 5,000 per confinement for maximum two confinement are given.	100% of the average daily wages

Funeral expenses: ₹ 10,000

For vocational training: For case of physical disablement ₹ 123 per day or actual expense for training whichever is higher is given.

Unemployment allowance: Under RGSKY in case of involuntary loss of job, 50% of the daily wages is given for 12 months. (earlier it was 6 months)

- **Benefits for the employer:**
  - Exemption from the applicability of Maternity Benefit Act and Workmen's Employee's Compensation Act.
  - Income tax benefit
  - No any other medical allowances to be paid to employees.

Brief introduction of "2nd Generation Reforms Agenda" named as **'ESIC-2.0'**:

"ESIC-2.0"

- Online availability of electronic health record of ESI beneficiaries (insured persons and their family members).
- **Abhiyan Indradhanush:** Ensuring the change of bed sheet according to VIBGYOR pattern during the week, i.e., to be changed everyday.

Occupational Health

- Medical Helpline No. 1800 11 3839 for emergency and seeking guidance from casualty/emergency of ESIC Hospitals.
- Special OPD for senior citizens and differently-abled persons in ESIC hospitals.
- Under the project 'Panchdeep', the ESI Corporation has undertaken the computerization of its core activities and its records. Now, these health records will be made available online. The records will also include laboratory reports in digital form.
- As an extension of the National Drive of Swachh Bharat Abhiyan, all the ESIC Hospitals have been directed to complete white washing, painting of the building along with minor repair. To ensure the change of bed sheets, different following color-bed sheets will be used on different days in all the hospitals of ESIC using **VIBGYOR pattern (Table 5.3).**

Table 5.3: VIBGYOR pattern used by hospitals of ESIC.

Day	Color of bed sheet
Sunday	Violet
Monday	Indigo
Tuesday	Blue
Wednesday	Green
Thursday	Yellow
Friday	Orange
Saturday	Red

New Provisions of the ESI Act

- ESIC launched a scheme named '**Atal Bimit Vyakti Kalyan Yojana**' (ABVKY) on 1st July 2018 which, in case the insured person (IP) is rendered unemployed, provides relief to the extent of 25% of the average per day earning during the previous four contribution periods to be paid for up to maximum three months (90 days) of unemployment once in lifetime.
- If an employer does not to deposit the employee's ESI contribution after 42 days, then there will be the penalty of ₹ 10,000/.
- ESIC-2.0 mobile app is also launched.
- Now it is mandatory for employees of the organized sector to obtain ESIC registration online within 10 days from the date of their appointment.
- Now it is compulsory for employees to collect their biometric scanned ESI registration Permanent Card from the nearest ESIC branch office as soon as they get their online ESIC registration.

BIBLIOGRAPHY

1. http://www.esicgoa.org.in/en/benefit-at-a-glance
2. https://www.esic.nic.in/finance
3. http://esic.nic.in/backend/images/launch_esic/fba167f69bc82aa6f57e14ec2d96c99d.pdf

5.5 NATIONAL PROGRAM FOR CONTROL AND TREATMENT OF OCCUPATIONAL DISEASES

Ministry of Health and Family Welfare, Government of India has launched this scheme in 1998–99. The National Institute of Occupational Health, Ahmedabad (ICMR) is the nodal agency.

Following research projects has been proposed by the Government:
- Prevention, control and treatment of silicosis and silico-tuberculosis in agate industry.
- Occupational health problems of tobacco harvesters and their prevention.
- Hazardous process and chemicals, database generation, documentation, and information dissemination
- Capacity building to promote research, education, training at national institute of occupational disease.
- Health risk assessment and development of intervention programs in cottage industries with high-risk of silicosis.
- Prevention and control of occupational health hazards among salt workers in the remote desert areas of Gujarat and Western Rajasthan.

GLOBAL STRATEGY FOR OCCUPATIONAL HEALTH

The global strategy given by WHO-SEARO includes the following major areas for action:
- Strengthening of international and national policies for health at work and development of policy tools.
- Developing healthy work environments.
- Developing healthy work practices and promoting health at work.
- Strengthening occupational health services.
- Establishing support services for occupational health.
- Developing occupational health standards based on scientific risk assessment.
- Developing human resources for occupational health.
- Establishing registration and data system including development of information services for experts, effective transmission of data, and raising public awareness through strengthened public information system.
- Strengthening research.
- Developing collaboration in occupational health services and organizations.

BIBLIOGRAPHY

1. http://www.nihfw.org/NationalHealthProgramme/NATIONALPROGRAMMEFORCONTROL.html

5.6 ROLE OF NURSE IN OCCUPATIONAL HEALTH SERVICES

Role of occupational health nurse are as follows:
- Assistance in general administration, maintenance and arrangement of health facilities in the workplace
- Provides emergency and primary treatment of accidents and illness based on standing orders from physicians
- Assistance with replacement and other medical examinations
- Assistance in general preventive health measures of the work force
- Cooperation with and referral of workers to general community agencies for help as and when necessary.
- Maintenance of the physical and psychosocial environment, and conductive to recovery and health
- Arranging follow-up treatment wherever indicated including health supervision of employees returning to work after illness
- Assistance in supervision of workplace hygiene and accident prevention
- Advice for protective equipment
- Identify and correct the working factors
- Health education and counseling
- Maintenance of records
- Assist health assessment at the time of preplacement examination, periodic examination, routine surveillance, fitness to work, rehabilitation activity.

BIBLIOGRAPHY

1. https://www.who.int/publications/i/item/the-role-of-the-occupational-health-nurse-in-workplace-health-management

CHAPTER 6

Geriatric Health

CHAPTER OUTLINE
6.1 Health problems of older adults
6.2 National Program for Health Care of Elderly (NPHCE)
6.3 Schemes for welfare of older adults
6.4 Role of frontline healthcare workers in geriatric health

6.1 HEALTH PROBLEMS OF OLDER ADULTS

- As per Ministry of Health and Family Welfare, citizens above the age of 60 years are considered to be elderly.
- India recorded a significant improvement in life expectancy at birth, which was 47 years in 1969, growing to 60 years in 1994 and 69 years in 2019.
- The share of population of elderly was 8% in 2015, i.e., 106 million (10 crores plus) across the nation, making India the second largest global population of elderly citizens.
- Further, it has been projected that by 2050 the elderly population will increase to 19%.
- Therefore, to identify the health needs of the elderly, it is necessary to understand aging and age-related changes.
- The special features of the elderly population in India are:
  - Majority (80%) of them are in the rural areas, thus making service delivery a challenge
  - Feminization of the elderly population
  - Increase in the number of the older-old (persons above 80 years)
  - Large percentage (30%) of the elderly are below poverty line.
- With increased access and advancement in healthcare combined with several other factors, people all over the world are now living longer than before.
- It is natural, therefore, that healthcare workers are likely to encounter older patients frequently in their practice and service.
- Old age is a sensitive phase—elderly people need care and comfort to lead a healthy life without worries and anxiety.

Age-related Changes in Human Body System

- Vision impairment
- Hearing impairment
- Disturbed sleep
- Loss of teeth
- Change in taste
- Decline in functions of lungs
- Decline in functions of heart
- Decline in functions of kidney
- Wrinkling of skin
- Decrease in muscle strength
- Decrease in bone strength
- Loss of bladder control
- Loss of appetite
- Decrease in sexual function
- Decrease in memory
- Increase in tiredness.

Problems of Geriatric Population

- Lack of awareness regarding the changing behavioral patterns in elderly people at home leads to abuse of them by their kin.
- Various issues affect the lives of senior citizens and further complicate into major physiological and psychological problems.
- The elderly population have various complex needs (physical, emotional, nutritional, financial) and the inability of the younger family members to understand these needs lead to them regarding the elderly individuals as a burden.
- The elderly suffers from multiple and chronic diseases.
- They need long-term and constant care.
- Their health problems also need care from various disciplines, e.g., ophthalmology, orthopedics, psychiatry, cardiovascular, dental, urology, etc.

The problems of geriatric population can be classified broadly into four following groups:

1. Health Problems

- Hypertension
- Atherosclerosis
- Coronary artery disease (CAD)
- **Nutritional excess or deficiencies**: Obesity, anemia, avitaminosis, etc.
- **Eyes:** Senile cataract, glaucoma
- **Ears:** Nerve deafness, vertigo, tinnitus
- **Skin:** Loss of elasticity of skin leading to wrinkling and dryness.
- **Articular disorders:** Osteoarthritis, spondylosis of spine—lumbar and cervical, gout
- **Fractures due to falls:** Fracture neck of femur and hip, fires, traffic collisions are extremely common among elderly
- **Respiratory system:** Chronic bronchitis, emphysema, asthma

- **Central nervous system:** Cerebrovascular accidents, peripheral neuritis, Alzheimer's disease, Parkinson's disease
- **Endocrine system:** Diabetes mellitus, hypothyroidism
- **Malignancies—Females:** Ca cervix, ca ovary; **Males:** lung ca, prostate ca
- **Dental:** Dental caries and loss of teeth.
- **GI system:** Indigestion due to reduced metabolism and malabsorption, constipation.
- **Genitourinary system—Males:** BPH; **Females:** Uterine prolapse, nonspecific vaginitis, cervicitis.

2. Psychological Problems
- Emotional disturbance
- Feel lonely
- Neglected and unwanted
- Anxiety
- Sexual problems
- Depression and suicidal tendencies
- Impaired memory
- Rigid outlook.

3. Social Problems
- Loneliness and social isolation.
- Rapid disintegration of joint family.
- Change in social contacts due to retirement.
- Death of spouse/siblings, close relatives, friends, or separation of their children after marriage.
- Diminished participation in social and cultural activities like marriages, ceremonies, visiting temples, etc.
- Diminished role in the family and community, even if they participate their role is not much appreciated.
- Problems of leisure
- Absence of job.

4. Economic Problems
- More common in women than men.
- Retirement of people employed in government services, local bodies, public sector and private organizations.
- Self-employee like agriculturists, businessmen, daily wage earners who cannot earn their livelihood due to disease and disability, etc.

Findings of LASI Study
- The Longitudinal Ageing Study in India (LASI) Wave 1, 2017–18, launched under the aegis of Ministry of Health and Family Welfare.
- The self-reported prevalence of cardiovascular disease was 34% among those in age 60–74 which increases to 37% among those age 75 and above.

- 32% of the elderly reported hypertension, 14.2% reported diabetes, 4.7% reported anemia, 8.3% reported chronic lung disease, 5.9% reported asthma, 2.6% reported neurological and psychiatric problems.
- 55.3% reported vision-related problems, 9.6% reported ear-related problems.
- A higher proportion of elderly age 60 and above experienced difficulty in stooping, kneeling, or crouching (58%), followed by difficulty in climbing upstairs without resting (57%) and pulling/pushing large objects (53%).
- 11% of the elderly age 60 and above reported having at least one form of impairment (locomotor, mental, visual and hearing impairment).
- A quarter (24%) of the elderly age 60 and above reported having at least one Activity of Daily Living (ADL) limitation; difficulty in using the toilet facility is the most common ADL limitation faced.
- Although 43.3% of elderly people use some kind of supportive device. However, 37.5% uses spectacles/contact lens due to presbyopia, 3.1% uses dentures, 8.3% uses walker/walker sticks and 0.7% uses hearing aids.
- More than a third (36%) are widowed. The proportion of widowed is higher among older adult women (30%) than older adult men (10%).

BIBLIOGRAPHY

1. https://nhsrcindia.org/sites/default/files/202106/Operational%20Guidelines%20for%20Elderly%20Care%20at%20HWC.pdf

6.2 NATIONAL PROGRAM FOR HEALTH CARE OF ELDERLY (NPHCE)

Vision of the NPHCE
- To provide accessible, affordable, and high-quality long-term, comprehensive and dedicated care services to an aging population.
- Creating a new "architecture" for aging.
- To build a framework to create an enabling environment for "a society for all ages".
- To promote the concept of active and healthy ageing.

Specific Objectives of NPHCE
- To provide an easy access to promotional, preventive, curative and rehabilitative services to the elderly through community-based primary health care approach.
- To identify health problems in the elderly and provide appropriate health interventions in the community with a strong referral backup support.
- To build capacity of the medical and paramedical professionals as well as the caretakers within the family for providing health care to the elderly.
- To provide referral services to the elderly patients through district hospitals, regional medical institutions.

- Convergence with National Rural Health Mission, AYUSH and other line departments like Ministry of Social Justice and Empowerment.

Core Strategies
- Community-based primary health care approach including domiciliary visits by trained healthcare workers.
- Dedicated services at PHC/CHC level including provision of machinery, equipment, training, additional human resources (CHC), Information, Education and Communication (IEC), etc.
- Dedicated facilities at District Hospital with 10 bedded wards, additional human resources, machinery and equipment, consumables and drugs, training and IEC.
- Strengthening of 8 Regional Medical Institutes to provide dedicated tertiary level medical facilities for the Elderly, introducing PG courses in Geriatric Medicine, and in-service training of health personnel at all levels.
- Information, Education and Communication (IEC) using mass media, folk media and other communication channels to reach out to the target community.
- Continuous monitoring and independent evaluation of the Programme and research in Geriatrics and implementation of NPHCE.

Supplementary Strategies
- Promotion of public private partnerships in geriatric health care.
- Mainstreaming AYUSH—revitalizing local health traditions, and convergence with programs of Ministry of Social Justice and Empowerment in the field of geriatrics.
- Reorienting medical education to support geriatric issues.

Organization of Geriatric Health Services
- NPHCE has component for primary and secondary care service delivery through district hospital, CHC, PHC, subcenter/health and wellness centers. Tertiary care services through Regional Geriatric Centers and National Centers of Aging **(Fig. 6.1)**.
- The State Non Communicable Diseases (NCD) Cells constituted under NPCDCS implements and monitors NPHCE.

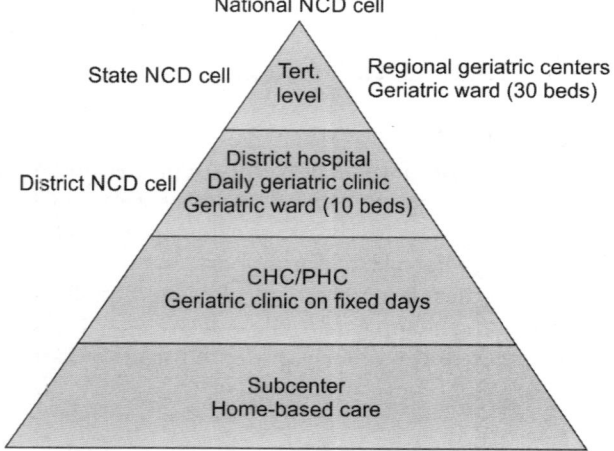

Fig. 6.1: Organization of geriatric health services.

ACTIVITIES UNDER NPHCE AT VARIOUS LEVELS

Subcenter
- The ANM/Male Health Workers will do domiciliary visits to the elderly persons in their areas and also give training to the family healthcare providers about care of bedridden elderly persons.
- The ANM/Male Health Worker will provide information about:
  - Health education related to healthy aging
  - Environmental modifications
  - Nutritional requirements,
  - Lifestyles and behavioral changes.
- They will arrange calipers and supportive devices for the elderly disabled persons.
- They arrange annual check-up of all the elderly at village level.

Primary Health Center
- **A weekly geriatric clinic** will be arranged at PHC level
- Simple clinical examination is carried out to assess vision, hearing, BP, blood sugar, etc. and all the information will be recorded as baseline data.
- Proper advice on chronic diseases like chronic obstructive lung disease, diabetes, hypertension, etc. will be given.
- Provision of medicines to the elderly people.
- Referral for further investigations and treatment to higher level facility as per need.
- Public awareness on promotional, preventive and rehabilitative aspects special focus on healthy life styles, encouraging care within families, healthy aging during health and village sanitation day/camps.

Community Health Center
- **Geriatric clinic: Twice a week**
- **Rehabilitation services:** Physiotherapy and medical rehabilitation will be provided at CHC and for bed-ridden elderly patients, it will be given at home by rehabilitation worker.
- Data received from all the PHCs in jurisdiction of CHCs on elderly will be compiled and forwarded to the District Program Officer (NCD).
- Referral is done to District Hospitals/Medical Colleges as per need.

District Hospital
There will be special **Geriatric Unit** in District Hospitals with following services:
- OPD services to the Elderly for examination and management of their illnesses.
- Indoor services in **Geriatric Ward** (10-bedded); out of the 10 beds, 2 beds will be reserved for the bed-ridden.
- Facilities for laboratory investigations and provision of medicines
- It will give training to the Medical officers and paramedical staff of CHCs and PHCs.
- Provide referral services to the elderly patients referred from the lower level
- Conducting camps in PHCs/CHCs and other sites
- Referral services for severe cases to the higher level.

Note: There are 19 **Regional Geriatric Center** in India and at every center there will be two seats of MD (Geriatric Medicine).

Tertiary component of NPHCE is renamed as **Rashtriya Varishth Jan Swasthya Yojana (RVJSY)**.

BIBLIOGRAPHY

1. Govt. of India (2011), Operational guidelines for national programme for health care of the elderly, DGHS, Ministry of Health and Family Welfare, New Delhi. Available at: http://www.mohfw.nic.in/showfile.php?lid=2171

6.3 SCHEMES FOR WELFARE OF OLDER ADULTS

List of Schemes:

Department	Scheme
Department of Social Justice and Empowerment	Atal Vayo Abhyudaya Yojana (AVYAY)
Ministry of Rural Development	• National Social Assistance Programme (NSAP): IGNOAPS • Annapurna Scheme
Ministry of Health and Family Welfare	National Programme for the Health Care of Elderly (NPHCE)
Ministry of Finance	• Pradhan Mantri Vaya Vandana Yojana • Atal Pension Yojana (APY)
Ministry of Housing and Urban Affairs	Model Building Bye Laws, 2016 (MBBL)

ATAL VAYO ABHYUDAYA YOJANA

- **Vision:** A society in which senior citizens live a healthy, happy, empowered, dignified and self-reliant life along with strong social and inter-generational bonding.
- **Scope of the scheme** states that the State Government may establish and maintain such number of old age homes at accessible places, as it may deem necessary, in a phased manner, beginning with at least one in each district to accommodate in such homes a minimum of one hundred fifty senior citizens who are indigent.
- **Programme coverage:**
  - Shelter and health for senior citizens
  - Integrated Programme for Senior Citizens (IPSrC)
  - State Action Plan for Senior Citizens support (SAPSrC)
  - Health and nutrition support for indigent elders
  - Rashtriya Vayoshri Yojana (RVY)
  - Livelihood and Skilling for Senior Citizens (SHGs)
  - National Helpline, awareness, training and capacity building
  - Promoting silver economy
  - Channelization of CSR funds for elderly care.

Vayoshreshtha Sammans: A Scheme of National Award for Senior Citizens
- It was launched in 2005 and is dedicated to senior citizens.
- The scheme is funded by the central government.
- This scheme is applicable for eminent senior citizens and institutes involved in rendering distinguished services for the cause of elderly persons.

An Integrated Program for Older Persons
- **The main objective** of the scheme is to improve the quality of life of the older persons by providing basic amenities like shelter, food, medical care and entertainment opportunities and by encouraging productive and active aging through providing support for capacity building of Government/Non-Governmental Organizations/Panchayati Raj Institutions/local bodies and the community at large.
- **Approach:** Assistance under the scheme will be given the following purposes
  - Programmes catering to the basic needs of older persons particularly food, shelter and health care to the destitute elderly;
  - Programmes to build and strengthen intergenerational relationships particularly between children/youth and older persons;
  - Programmes for encouraging active and productive aging;
  - Programmes for proving institutional as well as non-institutional care/services to older persons;
  - Research, advocacy and awareness building programs in the field of aging; and
  - Any other programmes in the best interests of older persons.

Indira Gandhi National Old Age Pension Scheme
- Indira Gandhi National Old Age Pension Scheme (IGNOAPS), earlier called as "National Old Age Pension Scheme (NOAPS)" is a social sector scheme and forms part of the National Social Assistance Programme (NSAP) which came into effect from 15th August, 1995. This scheme provides social assistance for the old age persons.
- **Eligibility criteria:**
  - The age of the applicant (male or female) shall be 60 years or higher
  - The applicant must belong to a household below poverty line according to the criteria prescribed by the Government of India.
- **Pattern of assistance:**
  - The central assistance provided as pension is ₹ 200 per month for persons between 60 years and 79 years.
  - For persons who are 80 years and above the pension is ₹ 500 per month.
  - States are strongly urged to provide an additional amount at least an equivalent amount to the assistance provided by the Central Government so that the beneficiaries can get a decent level of assistance.

Annapurna Scheme
- It is scheme of Ministry of Rural Development.
- Beneficiary of the scheme are indigent Senior Citizens who are not getting pension under IGNOAPS.
- They are entitled to get 10 kg of food grains per person per month free of cost.

Pradhan Mantri Vaya Vandana Yojana

- Designed for senior citizens above 60 years of age.
- The policy term of this scheme extends to ten years.
- The pensioner can choose the frequency of the payment—monthly/quarterly/half-yearly/annually.
- They may earn interest of 8% per annum over this scheme.
- The minimum and maximum capping of pension are ₹3,000 per month and 10,000 per month, respectively.

Atal Pension Yojana

- The Atal Pension Yojana (APY) is a Government of India scheme which was launched on 9th May, 2015, with the objective of creating a universal social security system for all Indians, especially the poor, the under-privileged and the workers in the unorganized sector.
- It is for all citizens of India between 18–40 years of age having bank account in a bank or post-office.
- There are five pension plan slabs available under the scheme namely, ₹ 1000, ₹ 2000, ₹ 3000, ₹ 4000, and ₹ 5000 guaranteed by Government of India to the subscriber at the age of 60 years.
- On death of subscriber, same pension to spouse is guaranteed by Government of India.

NPHCE (Explained in Detail in the Chapter 6.2)

- The National Programme for Palliative Care (NPPC), National Programme for Control of Blindness and Visual Impairment (NPCBVI), National Mental Health Programme (NMHP), National Oral Health Programme (NOHP), National Programme for Prevention and Control of Deafness (NPPCD) and National Programme for Prevention and Control of Cancer, Diabetes, Cardiovascular Diseases and Stroke (NPCDCS) are the other programmes which also cater to health needs of elderly.
- Income tax Act, 1961 give some benefits in tax to a senior citizen.
- National policy on older person and health insurance is also formed.
- *Note:* Indian Railways concessions used to range from 25% to 100%, but with effect from March 20, 2020, the Railways indefinitely discontinued concessions for senior citizens and now available with to only four categories of Divyangjan, 11 categories of patients and students.

BIBLIOGRAPHY

1. https://pib.gov.in/PressReleasePage.aspx?PRID=1806506
2. https://www.seniority.in/blog/10-government-schemes-launched-for-the-benefit-of-senior-citizens/

6.4 ROLE OF FRONTLINE HEALTHCARE WORKERS IN GERIATRIC HEALTH

Role of ASHA

- Undertake household visits for community mobilization, risk assessment, counselling improved care seeking and increasing supportive environment in families and community.
- Generate awareness in the community about healthy lifestyle in the elderly to promote active and healthy aging.
- Identify elderly individuals in need of care in the community including mapping of elderly population.
- Provide support in family counselling and redressal of medical issues.
- Identify caregivers within or outside the family and link them to the nearest health care facility.
- Facilitate environmental modification, nutritional intervention and physical activities including yoga, lifestyle and behavioral changes at the family and individual level.
- Would work with Gram Sabha, ULB, SHG, VHSNC/MAS, JAS, RWA and local NGO to enable creation of facilitatory environment for elderly.
- Support caregivers in learning a range of practical skills like transferring a bed-bound elderly within house, support in daily routine activities like eating, bathing, etc.
- Facilitate services available for elderly at HWCs and referral centers.
- Home-based follow-up care for elderly discharged from higher facilities.

Role of ASHA Facilitator

- All elements of ASHA (as above)
- Deliver passive physiotherapy services to bed-bound elderly acting as a lay.
- Rehabilitation worker under the guidance of CHO and MPW from CHC.
- Supportive supervision to ASHA.

Role of ANM (FHW)/MPW-M

- Undertake initial screening using preliminary comprehensive geriatric assessment for all elderly twice in a year.
- Facilitate formation of elderly support groups named "Sanjeevini" and elderly caregiver support groups
- Reinforce healthy aging via adequate nutrition, physical activity, regular check ups and rehabilitative care.
- Undertake weekly visits to home-bound/bed-bound elderly.

Role of Community Health Officer

- Undertake comprehensive geriatric assessment twice a year
- Providing immediate/primary management of common ailments of elderly and referring to MO at PHC or conducting teleconsultation services and manage as per MO-PHC instructions.
- Develop and administer a personalized care plan for each elderly identified in the community in consultation with MO-PHC.

- Facilitate identification and provide guidance to caregivers regarding care given to bed bound elderly
- Develop elderly support groups named "Sanjeevini"
- Conduct periodic home visit to bedbound elderly, sick elderly and restricted mobile elderly
- Undertake preliminary assessment for the need of assistive devices.
- Support rehabilitative services for the elderly.

BIBLIOGRAPHY

1. https://nhsrcindia.org/sites/default/files/202106/Operational%20Guidelines%20for%20Elderly%20Care%20at%20HWC.pdf

CHAPTER 7

Mental Health

CHAPTER OUTLINE

7.1 Anxiety disorders
7.2 Depression
7.3 Psychosis including schizophrenia
7.4 Dementia
7.5 Suicide
7.6 Alcohol and other common substance abuse
7.7 Drug Deaddiction Programs
7.8 National Mental Health Policy
7.9 National Mental Health Program
7.10 The Mental Healthcare Act, 2017
7.11 Role of a community health nurse in mental health

7.1 ANXIETY DISORDERS

- Anxiety disorders are one of the most common psychiatric disorders.
- They have a very high prevalence in the society.
- They cause significant distress and dysfunction to the patient and affect healthy, productive community living.
- They are commonly comorbid with alcoholism and depression.
- **Cause:** Changes in serotonin and norepinephrine (neurotransmitters) transmission in the brain are currently understood to cause anxiety disorders. These changes may be triggered by life events in some cases.
- This is a group of disorders namely: All these disorders have distinct clinical features but pathological anxiety is common in all.
  - Phobias
  - Panic disorder

- Obsessive compulsive disorder (OCD)
- Generalized anxiety disorder
- Post-traumatic stress disorder (PTSD), etc.

❏ **Clinical features:**
- **Phobias** are characterized by excessive fear and avoidance of any particular object or situation, e.g.
  - **Claustrophobia:** Fear of closed spaces
  - **Agoraphobia:** Fear of going out of home alone, being in enclosed spaces (e.g., malls, cinemas, etc.), open spaces (e.g., bridges, vast playgrounds, etc.), using public transportation (e.g., trains, buses, planes, etc.)
  - **Social phobia:** Fear of social situations and excessive scrutiny by others. Marked fear and avoidance of social situations (e.g., interaction with strangers, meeting unfamiliar people, performing in front of others)
- **Panic disorder** are characterized by recurrent acute attacks of disabling anxiety coupled with autonomic symptoms like breathlessness, palpitations, sweating and an impending sense of doom. These attacks are not situation specific.
- In **generalized anxiety disorder** the patient has free floating anxiety triggered by everyday benign life situations and experiences constant muscular tension and worry. Chronic feeling of tension, apprehension, anxiety or worrying about a number of events or activities that involve every day routine life circumstances (e.g., work, school, health, finance, household chores, etc.)
- **OCD** includes obsessions which are recurrent, intrusive thoughts or images that are found inappropriate and difficult to resist by the patient and are often accompanied by Compulsions which are behaviors that the patient feels he must do to decrease his anxiety. Symptoms should last for at least 2 weeks to make diagnosis of OCD. **Example of recurrent and persistent unwanted thoughts:** unwanted sexual and blasphemous thoughts, fear of harming self or others, fear of contamination, doubts about daily activities, etc. and repetitive behaviors (e.g., excessive washing/cleaning, checking, ordering, etc.)
- **PTSD** occurs after a severely traumatic life event in which there has usually been a threat to life like a natural disaster, rape or war. Symptoms may occur anywhere between a few weeks to years after the event and include recurrent flashbacks and nightmares of the event with avoidance of talking about the event, emotional numbing, autonomic symptoms and depressive features.

Assessment

❏ Duration of anxiety
❏ Degree of distress, and impairment of day-to-day functioning
❏ Symptoms of depression
❏ Substance and alcohol misuse
❏ **Physical disorders:** Thyrotoxicosis, pheochromocytoma and hypoglycemia
❏ **Psychosocial factors:** Ongoing stress and other issues pertaining to work, family

Management

- **Psychoeducation:**
  - Reassurance
  - Explain symptoms are of anxiety/fear and mimic symptoms of physical illnesses, (e.g., heart attack)
  - Do not investigate excessively. Few investigations like ECG, ECHO maybe necessary in some patients
  - Discourage doctor shopping
  - Do not avoid triggers of panic attacks, (e.g., physical exertion, agoraphobic situations) and fear, (e.g., travelling by public transport).
  - Emphasize avoidance maintains fears and phobias.
  - **OCD:** Educate that the unwanted thoughts are a part of illness, and not a reflection of character or hidden intentions.
- **Psychotherapy:**
  - Cognitive behavior therapy
  - Relaxation therapy
  - Yoga and meditation.
- **Pharmacotherapy:** SSRIs are first line treatment in most anxiety disorders, e.g. paroxetine, sertraline, etc. SNRIs like venlafaxine are also effective. Benzodiazepines like diazepam, clonazepam and alprazolam are effective short-term treatment. In OCD a combination of psychotherapy and pharmacotherapy is beneficial.

BIBLIOGRAPHY

1. https://nhm.gov.in/images/pdf/programmes/NMHP/Training_Manuals/Hand_BookAssessment_and_Management_of_Mental_Health_Problems_in_General_Practice.pdf
2. https://stw.icmr.org.in/images/pdf/Psychiatry/Psychiatry_Anxiety_Disorder.pdf

7.2 DEPRESSION

- Depression is a mood disorder characterized by persistent sadness. It may be recurrent or chronic in few cases. It causes significant impairment in overall functioning and disability.
- Depressive disorders have a very high prevalence in the community (20–25%). They are considered to have the highest rank in global burden of diseases (higher than cardiovascular disease or infections). There is a significant loss of productive life years in patients suffering from depression along with a risk of suicide and self-harm. Around 15% of depressed patients attempt suicide. All these reasons make its treatment important and necessary.
- **Causes:** It is a biopsychosocial illness, currently understood as a neurochemical disturbance in the brain neurotransmitters (serotonin, norepinephrine and dopamine). Life stressors or drug abuse may precipitate or worsen the illness. Those with positive family history for depression have higher chances of getting the disorder.

Mental Health

- **Clinical features:**
  - Core symptoms:
    - Persistent low/depressed mood
    - Loss of interest and enjoyment
    - Easy fatigability/diminished activity
  - Additional symptoms:
    - Reduced concentration and attention
    - Reduced self-esteem and self-confidence
    - Ideas of guilt and unworthiness
    - Bleak and pessimistic views of the future
    - Ideas or acts of self-harm or suicide
    - Disturbed sleep
    - Diminished appetite
  - Symptoms must be present for at least 2 weeks to warrant diagnosis.
  - Illness may be of mild to severe grade. Following table would be helpful to decide the severity of the disease:

Severity of depression	Core symptoms	Additional symptoms
Mild depression	2	2 or more
Moderate depression	2	3 or more
Severe depression	3	4 or more

  - The overall socio-occupational functioning is affected in depression.
  - In some cases depression may be recurrent and in others may be followed by episodes of mania/hypomania, the latter case is then diagnosed as bipolar illness.

Investigations

- 'PHQ-2' (Patient Health Questionnaire) is part of CBAC form which is usually filled by ASHA.
- The purpose of 'PHQ-2' is to screen for symptoms related to depression.

PHQ–2					
Over the last 2 weeks, how often have you been bothered by the following problems?		Not at all	Several day	More than half the days	Nearly every day
1.	Little interest or pleasure in doing things?	0	+1	+2	+3
2.	Feeling down, depressed or hopeless?	0	+1	+2	+3
	Total Score				

Anyone with total score greater than 3 should be referred to CHO/MO (PHC/UPHC)

- After administering the PHQ-2, ASHAs will refer the individuals who have scored more than 3 to SHC-HWC. Community Health Officer (CHO) at SHC-HWC will ask the individuals more detailed questions to understand about the symptoms. CHO will ask questions from a detailed tool called 'PHQ-9' to these individuals and provide appropriate advice. The individual will be provided help at SHC-HWC or can be referred to PHC-MO by CHO.
- **Some basics investigations like:** • Hemogram • Thyroid function tests • Electrocardiogram • Electrolytes (Sodium) and some underlying causes of depression like hypothyroidism or use of anti-cancer drugs to be checked.

Management

- **Psychotherapy:** Trying to address the patients depressive cognitions and restructure them by CBT (cognitive behavior therapy) or addressing interpersonal stresses in IPT (interpersonal therapy), or supportive psychotherapy. In mild cases many times it is treatment of choice.
- **Antidepressant medication:** These correct the neurochemical disturbance said to be causative of depression. They may be given in all grades of depression and improve features of depression in 4-6 weeks. Many classes of antidepressants are available but SSRIs (Specific serotonin reuptake inhibitors) are most commonly prescribed as first line treatment. Drugs like Fluoxetine and Escitalopram are included in this group. Other drugs include SNRIs, Bupropion and Mirtazapine. TCAs (Tricyclic antidepressants) are used less frequently now due to the availability of other drugs with less side effects. Antidepressants are given for a period of at least 6 months to 1 year to prevent relapse and for longer periods in recurrent or more severe cases.
- **Electroconvulsive therapy (ECT)** may be required in very severe, treatment resistant or high risk suicidal cases

BIBLIOGRAPHY

1. https://nhm.gov.in/images/pdf/programmes/NMHP/Training_Manuals/Hand_BookAssessment_and_Management_of_Mental_Health_Problems_in_General_Practice.pdf
2. https://stw.icmr.org.in/images/pdf/Psychiatry/Psychiatry_Depression.pdf
3. https://nhsrcindia.org/sites/default/files/202111/MNS%20Training%20Manual%20for%20MPW.pdf

7.3 PSYCHOSIS INCLUDING SCHIZOPHRENIA

Broadly, psychiatric illnesses can be classified into two groups:
- 'Common mental disorders'(CMDs), e.g. depression, anxiety disorders
- 'Severe mental illnesses'(SMIs) which refers to a group of mental illnesses causing marked disruption in socio-occupational life, i.e. schizophrenia and bipolar disorder.

Basics of Psychosis

- Psychosis (Greek word, 'psyche" refers to mind/soul; and '-osis' refers to abnormal condition or derangement) means 'an abnormal condition of the mind'.
- Psychosis refers to a state characterized by an individual's loss of contact with reality. It may involve abnormality in thinking and perceptions, as well as disturbances in emotions. It is categorized as a severe mental disorder causing dysfunction in the life of the patient and family.
- It is common myth in general public to consider it due to religious and supernatural causes than illness, which often leads to delay in treatment seeking. Moreover, due to stigma attached to mental health services, there is often a delay in reaching to the psychiatrists.
- Psychosis is a major psychiatric illness. Psychosis is a disorder of thought and perception. Psychosis occurs in a number of psychiatric disorders, e.g. depression, bipolar disorder (manic-depressive illness), puerperal psychosis and sometimes with drug and alcohol abuse.

It can also occur in a number of medical and neurological conditions and caused due to medications.
- **It includes two categories:**
  1. Organic psychosis, which occurs due to brain disease or is a result of abuse of substances like alcohol or cannabis.
  2. Functional psychosis, which is a primary psychiatric disorder and includes schizophrenia, affective psychosis (bipolar disorder) and acute psychosis.
- **Clinical features:**
  - Abnormal/disorganized behavior/unusual appearance
  - Un-understandable talk/nonsensible speech
  - False beliefs (e.g., "people are planning to kill me")
  - False perception (e.g., hearing voices of people not around)
  - Social withdrawal
  - Neglect of usual responsibilities related to work/school/domestic chores
  - Talking to self
  - Violent/aggressive behavior
  - Restless and running here and there.
- **Clinical symptoms and signs can be divided into following two groups:**
  1. **Positive symptoms:** Hallucinations, delusion and formal thought disorder
  2. **Negative symptoms:** They include: Little/no drive to do things—lack of energy and interest—little display of feelings—speaking very less.

SCHIZOPHRENIA

- More than two symptoms of the following if present for more than one month duration causing disturbance in functioning:
  - Delusions
  - Hallucinations
  - Disorganized speech
  - Grossly disorganized or catatonic behavior
  - Negative symptoms
- Subtypes of schizophrenia:
  - **Paranoid schizophrenia:** Delusions; hallucinations (e.g. belief people are making plans to kill me or hearing of voices); most common subtype; better prognosis
  - **Catatonic schizophrenia:** Stupor; rigidity; mutism; maintaining odd postures for long time; good prognosis
  - **Hebephrenic schizophrenia:** Disorganized speech; self-care and behavior, e.g. vagabonds on street; poor prognosis
  - **Simple schizophrenia:** Negative symptoms; gradual onset; long lasting; poor prognosis
  - **Residual schizophrenia:** Earlier fulfill criteria for schizophrenia; partially attenuated form mainly as negative symptoms.

OTHER TYPES OF PSYCHOSIS

- **Acute psychosis:** It is characterized by appearance of psychotic symptoms within 2 weeks. It usually has rapidly changing clinical picture and complete improvement within 1 to 3 months, spontaneously or with effective treatment.

Mental Health

- **Persistent delusional disorder:** It is characterized by the presence of delusion, usually centered on one theme with absence of hallucinations. Person's social and occupational functioning in all areas other than the theme of delusion is unaffected. Delusion can be persecutory (e.g. suspicious or fearful of being harmed), grandiose (e.g. believes self to be in possession of extra power, worth knowledge, ability or identity) or somatic (e.g. false belief of having an abnormal somatic sensation or illness).

Treatment

- Antipsychotic medication, which forms the cornerstone of treatment of psychosis
- Education of the individual about his/her illness and treatment
- Family education and support
- Support groups and social skills training
- Rehabilitation to improve the activities of daily living
- Vocational and recreational support.

Nonpharmacological management of psychosis: Discuss with the patient and family regarding:
- The person's ability to recover
- The importance of continuing regular social, educational and occupational activities, as far as possible
- The suffering and problems can be reduced with treatment
- The importance of taking medication regularly
- The right of the person to be involved in every decision that concerns his or her treatment
- Importance of staying healthy (e.g. following healthy diet, staying physically active, maintaining personal hygiene).
- **Follow-up frequency:** Acute phase: Follow-up once or twice weekly. Maintenance phase: Follow-up every one to three month.

Referral: In following situations, consider need for referral to specialized mental health services:
- Nature of illness:
  - Severe level of symptoms and distress
  - Suicide or risk of harm to others
  - Marked violent aggressive behavior
  - Catatonic symptoms
  - Poor general medical status
  - Refusal to accept orally (meals/medications).
- Nature of treatment:
  - Partial or no response to treatment
  - Need to start modified electroconvulsive therapy
  - Need to start clozapine
  - Need of specific psychological therapies or vocational rehabilitation.
- Support system:
  - Poor social support system, (e.g. homelessness)
  - Family needs psychoeducation about nature of illness and need of treatment.

BIBLIOGRAPHY

1. http://clinicalestablishments.gov.in/WriteReadData/606.pdf
2. https://stw.icmr.org.in/images/pdf/Psychiatry/Psychiatry_Psychosis.pdf

7.4 DEMENTIA

- Forgetfulness related to ageing up to some extent happens almost with everyone.
- But dementia is different and is beyond the usual forgetfulness associated with aging.
- Dementia often starts with memory problems, but goes on to affect many other parts of the brain and leads to:
  - Difficulty in coping with day to day tasks
  - Difficulty in communicating
  - Changes in mood, judgment or personality.
- It is much more common in older people, but can start as early as 40.
- About 1 in every 20 person over-65s has dementia and by the age of 80 about 1 in 5 will have some degree of dementia.
- With increase in life expectancy, the elderly population in our country is growing.
- Dementia is one of the most debilitating illnesses in the elderly.

Clinical Features

- Progressive deterioration of intellectual functions like memory, intelligence and judgment, changes in the personality (behavior pattern), quick fluctuations in the emotional responses and stereotyped repetition of words or actions.
- As the illness progresses, patient is unable to take care of his personal needs and hygiene.
- Symptoms like restlessness, sleeplessness, wandering and suspiciousness may also develop.
- Learning new information becomes harder—patient cannot remember recent events, appointments or phone messages.
- Patient may forget the names of people or places and may struggle to understand or communicate with others.
- This can make patient frustrated and depressed.
- Patient may also have paranoid symptoms like ideas of being followed or criticized.
- Patients may also develop neurological symptoms like fits, difficulty in speech and motor movement coordination.

Causes

- Central nervous system (CNS) degenerative disorders like Alzheimer's disease **(commonest cause)**, vascular dementia, Parkinson's disease, Huntington's disease, etc. Damaged tissue builds up in the brain to form deposits called 'plaques' and 'tangles'. These cause the brain cells around them to die.
- CNS infections like tuberculosis, AIDS and cryptococcal meningitis.
  - Repeated trauma to the brain (e.g. in boxers)
  - Alcoholic dementia.

Mental Health

- Endocrine and metabolic causes (e.g. hypothyroidism, vitamin B_{12} deficiency)
- CNS space occupying lesions like tumors.
◻ About 10% of all dementia are treatable and reversible. Examples include dementia due to syphilis, tuberculosis of the brain, hypothyroidism, vitamin deficiency, normal pressure hydrocephalus and brain tumors.

Management

◻ These patients often need investigations and should be referred to a hospital.
◻ Treatable conditions (like—thyroid disorders, B_{12} deficiency, subdural hemorrhage) after full investigations should be managed on a priority.
◻ Counseling of the family members regarding the nature and course of the condition is very important.
◻ **Drugs for cognitive improvement:**
  - **Donepezil:** 5 mg once after breakfast × 1 month, then 10 mg after breakfast to continue. If any side effect/not tolerating then **Rivastigmine** to be used start dose 1.5 mg BD/1 month then 3 mg BD × 1 month, then 4.5 mg BD × 1 month, then 6 mg twice after meals only × 1 month.
  - **Memantine:** to be used in moderate to severe dementia 5 mg BD × 1 month, then 10 mg BD to continue.
  - **Sometimes patient may need anti-depressant drugs also.**
◻ Dementia patients require support from the family as well as the society.

BIBLIOGRAPHY

1. https://nhm.gov.in/images/pdf/programmes/NMHP/Training_Manuals/Hand_BookAssessment_and_Management_of_Mental_Health_Problems_in_General_Practice.pdf
2. https://stw.icmr.org.in/images/pdf/Neurology/Neurology_Dementia%20.pdf

7.5 SUICIDE

◻ Suicide is the termination of one's life intentionally.
◻ Suicide is the fourth leading cause of death among 15–29 year olds.
◻ Globally, more than 700,000 people die due to suicide every year.
◻ Every 3 second, one person attempts suicide and every 40 seconds one person die due to suicide.
◻ A suicidal patient needs emergent intervention as this can prevent a completed suicide.
◻ The prevalence of suicide is 10–15% in patients of depression, 10% in schizophrenia and this number rises when alcoholism complicates the picture.
◻ Ingestion of pesticide, hanging and firearms are among the most common methods of suicide globally. Other methods include slitting of wrist and overdose of sleeping pills.

Flowchart 7.1: Risk factors for suicide.

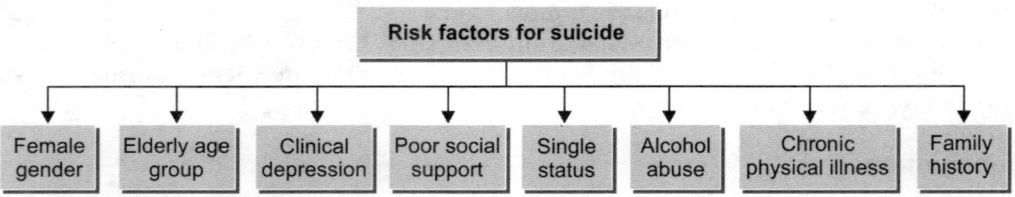

- **An individual can attempt suicide for many reasons like:**
  - An immediate negative event (such as failure in examination, intense shame or guilt for any happening)
  - Due to hopelessness caused by prolonged stressors (such as a chronic disease).
  - Having mental disorders like depression and substance dependence.
- **Warning signs of suicide:**
  - A person talks about death, threatens of committing or discusses suicide
  - Discusses different methods of suicide
  - A person mentions suicidal ideation
  - A person attempts any act of deliberate self harm
  - A person is seen making goodbye gestures or communications, writing of will or other acts suggestive of a suicidal plan
  - A person has suffered recent major loss of life or property
  - Hopelessness
  - Severe agitation/anxiety.

Note: A prior suicide attempt is the single most important risk factor for suicide in the general population.

Management
- A suicidal patient either thinks attempting suicide or has already attempted suicide.
- The goal of intervention is to prevent completed suicide.
- Suicide is preventable if intervention is done timely.
- Assessment of suicidal risk is important.

Flowchart 7.2: Steps in management of suicide.

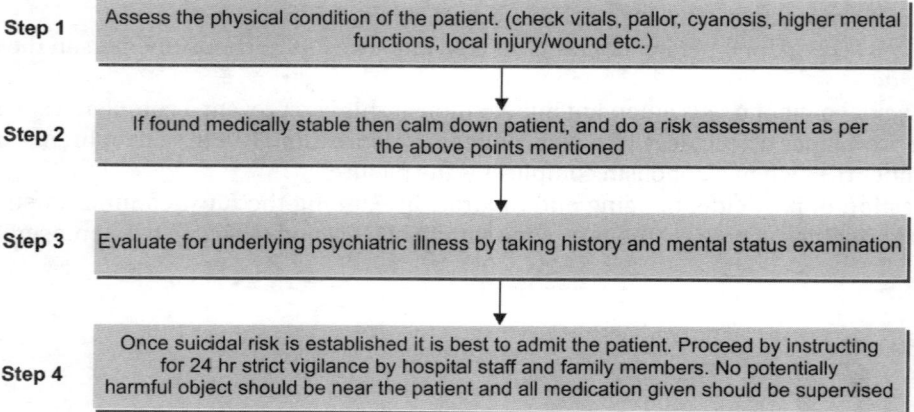

Mental Health

- **Protective factors for suicide:**
  - Children
  - Deterrent religious beliefs
  - Life satisfaction
  - Reality testing ability
  - Positive coping skills
  - Positive social support
  - Positive therapeutic relationship.

BIBLIOGRAPHY

1. https://nhm.gov.in/images/pdf/programmes/NMHP/Training_Manuals/Manual_for_Medical_OfficersAsswssment%20_and_Management_of_Mental_Health_Problems_in_General_Practice.pdf
2. https://www.who.int/news-room/fact-sheets/detail/suicide

7.6 ALCOHOL AND OTHER COMMON SUBSTANCE ABUSE

- Why do some people become addicted while others do not? No single factor can predict whether a person will become addicted to drugs.
- Risk for addiction is influenced by a combination of factors that include individual biology, social environment, and age or stage of development.
- The more risk factors an individual has, the greater the chance that the person will become dependent.
- Risk factors include:
  - The genes that people are born with—in combination with environmental influences—account for about half of their addiction vulnerability.
  - Additionally, gender, ethnicity, and the presence of other mental disorders may influence risk for drug abuse and addiction.
  - A person's environment includes many different influences, from family and friends to socioeconomic status and quality of life in general.
  - Factors such as peer pressure, physical and sexual abuse, stress, and quality of parenting can greatly influence the occurrence of drug abuse and the escalation to addiction in a person's life.
- Substance abuse largely affects the adolescent and young adult population which is the most productive group in society, hence its prevention and treatment is of utmost importance.
- Substance uses leads to health problems like acid/peptic disease, liver diseases, peripheral neuropathy, accidents and injuries, intoxicated behavior, memory deficits and drug abuse-related abnormal behavior.
- Tobacco intake in adolescents is the gateway to future drug abuse.
- Alcohol is the most common psychoactive substance used by Indians followed by Cannabis and Opioids.

COMMON SUBSTANCES OF ABUSE IN INDIA

- Cannabis (*Bhang, charas, hashish, ganja*)
- Alcohol
- Opioids like heroin/smack, spasmoproxyvon capsules, morphine, codeine containing cough syrups
- IV drugs like Avil injections, Buprenorphine injections
- Stimulants (Amphetamines)
- Hallucinogens (LSD, ecstasy, ketamine)
- Cocaine
- Tobacco (smoke and smokeless forms).

FEATURES OF ABUSE OR DEPENDENCE

- **Craving:** Irresistible desire to take the substance.
- Loss of control.
- **Tolerance:** A specified amount of alcohol/drug intake fails to give the required effect and the person increases the amount or switches to stronger drugs.
- Progressive neglect of family, work and social responsibilities.
- Deterioration of his moral and ethical standards.
- Neglect of alternative methods of recreation.
- Physical and mental health problems.
- **Withdrawal symptoms:** On stopping use or delay in intake symptoms like craving, tremors of hands, sleeplessness, aches and pains, restlessness, sweating, are reported.

Alcohol Dependence (Three of the Following Six Criteria to be Present for at Least One Month)

1. A strong desire or sense of compulsion to take alcohol
2. Difficulty in controlling alcohol use
3. Withdrawal state when alcohol use has stopped or been reduced or use of the alcohol (or benzodiazepines) to relieve or avoid withdrawal symptoms
4. Evidence of tolerance
5. Preoccupation with alcohol use
6. Alcohol use persisting despite clear evidence of harmful consequences.

Management

- **Identification:** Thorough clinical history and mental state examination, family interview and screening methods like AUDIT (Alcohol used disorders identification test) is useful for alcohol dependence.
- Inquire using open ended questions in a non-judgmental manner. Help patient to evaluate the risks versus the perceived benefits and to arrive at a decision to reduce or stop alcohol use.

Brief Intervention for Alcohol Dependence (FRAMES)
- **Feedback** about alcohol-related problems
- **Responsibility**—acknowledging that the patient is responsible for making the decision about their alcohol use
- **Advice** regarding the harms associated with continued use
- **Menu** of alternative change options (includes identifying alternative activities such as hobbies, involving the family in treatment)
- **Empathetic** attitude
- **Self-efficacy**—to encourage patients' confidence that they can make changes in their alcohol use and lifestyle
- **Motivation:** Check for motivation of the person to give up drugs.
- For **detoxification** of alcohol dependence, 30 mL of alcohol used requires either 5 mg of diazepam or 10 mg of chlordiazepoxide during detoxification. Therefore, if a person is using, let us say 300 mL of alcohol per day, will require 50 mg of diazepam or 100 mg of chlordiazepoxide on the first day of detoxification which should be gradually reduced and stopped at the end of 10 days. Give diazepam (50 mg) or chlordiazepoxide 100 mg in divided doses. Reduce diazepam 5 mg or chlordiazepoxide 10 mg a day from day 2. In addition, the person should be given vitamins. The detoxification phase usually lasts for 2 weeks and is followed by long-term maintenance treatment.

Referral: • History of withdrawal seizures/hallucinations • Additional psychiatric disorder • Recurrent failed attempts at treatment requires referral to secondary care.

For prevention of relapse: In motivated and consented patient drug disulfiram 250 mg OD with proper counseling could be very helpful in the prevention of relapse of alcohol abuse.

BIBLIOGRAPHY
1. https://nhm.gov.in/images/pdf/programmes/NMHP/Training_Manuals/Hand_BookAssessment_and_Management_of_Mental_Health_Problems_in_General_Practice.pdf
2. https://stw.icmr.org.in/images/pdf/Psychiatry/Psychiatry_Alcohol_Use_Disorders.pdf

7.7 DRUG DEADDICTION PROGRAMS
- The Constitution of India, under Article 47, enjoins that the state shall endeavor to bring about prohibition of the consumption of intoxicating drinks and drugs, which are injurious to health.
- The activities to reduce the drug use-related problems could broadly be divided into two categories:
  1. Supply reduction
  2. Demand reduction.
- The supply reduction come under the purview of the NCB under the MHA and the Department of Revenue as the administrator of the Narcotic Drugs and Psychotropic Substances (NDPS) Act, 1985 and the Prevention of Illicit Traffic in Narcotic Drugs and Psychotropic Substances (NDPS) Act, 1988.
- The demand reduction activities are run by the Ministry of Social Justice and Empowerment as the nodal Ministry and to some extent by the Ministry of Health and Family Welfare.

- Since 1988, Ministry of Health and Family Welfare is running a National 'Drug De-addiction Programme (DDAP)' with the objectives to provide affordable, easily accessible and evidence-based treatment for all substance use disorders through the government health care facilities and to build the capacities of health care staff in recognition and management of substance use disorders.
- AIIMS, New Delhi (NDDTC) is functioning as the National/Nodal center.
- The Drug Treatment Clinics (DTC) scheme is another strategy for enhancing the provision of treatment services coordinated nationally by the NDDTC, AIIMS and as of now, 27 DTCs are functional in different states in the country.
- Further, the Drug De-addiction Programme (DDAP) and National Programme for Tobacco Control (NTCP) has been renamed as **"National Program for Tobacco Control and Drug Addiction Treatment (NPTCDAT)"**.
- Ministry of Social Justice and Empowerment (MoSJE) implements National Action Plan for Drug Demand Reduction (NAPDDR).
- **Under this programme financial assistance is provided to:**
  (i) 'State Governments/Union Territory (UT) administrations for preventive education and awareness generation, capacity building, skill development, vocational training and livelihood support of ex-drug addicts, programs for drug demand reduction by states/UT, etc. and
  (ii) 'Non-Government-Organizations/Voluntary Organizations for running and maintenance of integrated rehabilitation centers for addicts (IRCAs), Community based peer led intervention (CPLI) for early drug use prevention among adolescents and outreach and drop in centres (ODIC) and addiction treatment facilities (ATFs) in Government Hospitals'.
- The MoSJE provides financial support for setting up of District De-addiction center (DDAC) in various districts all across India. For setting up of DDACs, preference is given to those districts, which do not have any facility of IRCA, CPLI, or ODIC.

NASHA MUKT BHARAT ABHIYAAN

- The Ministry of Social Justice and Empowerment is the nodal ministry for Drug Demand Reduction in the country and under its interventions it coordinates, implements and monitors several interventions like prevention, assessment of extent of the problem, treatment and rehabilitation of users, after care and follow-up, dissemination of information among the public and generation of awareness in the community,
- The Ministry of Social Justice and Empowerment launched "Nasha Mukt Bharat Abhiyaan (NMBA)" on 15th August 2020, in 272 districts identified as most vulnerable in terms of usage of drugs in the country.
- **Aim:** To tackle the issue of substance abuse and a vision to make India drug free
- Nasha Mukt Bharat Campaign is a three-pronged attack:
  - Supply curb by Narcotics Control Bureau
  - Outreach and awareness and demand reduction effort by social justice and empowerment
  - Treatment through Health Department.

BIBLIOGRAPHY

1. https://main.mohfw.gov.in/sites/default/files/drugs%20deaddiction%20programme.pdf
2. https://dmeo.gov.in/sites/default/files/202106/Department%20of%20Health%20and%20Family%20Welfare%20%2821-22%29.pdf
3. https://nmba.dosje.gov.in/about.php

7.8 NATIONAL MENTAL HEALTH POLICY

- **Vision:** The vision of the National Mental Health Policy is to promote mental health, prevent mental illness, enable recovery from mental illness, promote destigmatization and desegregation, and ensure socioeconomic inclusion of persons affected by mental illness by providing accessible, affordable and quality health and social care to all persons through their life-span within a rights-based framework.
- **Goals:**
  - To reduce distress, disability, exclusion morbidity and premature mortality associated with mental health problems across life span of the person.
  - To enhance understanding of the mental health in the country.
  - To strengthen the leadership in the mental health sector at the national, state and district levels.
- **Objectives of the policy:**
  - To provide universal access to mental health care.
  - To increase access to and utilization of comprehensive mental health services by persons with mental health problems.
  - To increase access to mental health care especially to vulnerable groups including homeless persons, persons in remote areas, educationally, socially and deprived sections.
  - To reduce prevalence and impact of risk factors associated with mental health problems.
  - To reduce risk and incidence of suicide and attempted suicide.
  - To ensure respect for rights and protection from harm of persons with mental health problems.
  - To reduce stigma associated with mental health problems.
  - To enhance availability and equitable distribution of skilled human resources for mental health.
  - To progressively enhance financial allocation and improve utilization for mental health promotion and care.
  - To identify and address the social, biological and psychological determinants of mental health problems and to provide appropriate interventions.

Cross Cutting Issues

- Stigma
- Rights-based approach
- Vulnerable populations
- Adequate funding
- Support for families

- Intersectoral collaborations
- Institutional care
- Promotion of mental health
- Research.

Strategic Directions and Recommendations for Action
- Effective governance and accountability of mental health
- Promotion of mental health
- Prevention of mental issues and reduction of suicide and attempted suicide
- Universal access to mental health services
- Improve availability of adequately trained mental health human resources to address the mental health needs of the community
- Community participation for mental health and development
- Research.

BIBLIOGRAPHY
1. https://nhm.gov.in/images/pdf/National_Health_Mental_Policy.pdf.

7.9 NATIONAL MENTAL HEALTH PROGRAM

Current Problem Statement
As per the National Mental Health Survey conducted by the National Institute of Mental Health and Neurosciences (NIMHANS), Bangalore in 12 states of the country, the prevalence of mental disorders including common mental disorders, severe mental disorders, and alcohol and substance use disorders (excluding tobacco use disorder) in adults over the age of 18 years is about 10.6%.

Major Findings of the Survey
- The prevalence of mental morbidity is high in urban metropolitan areas.
- Mental disorders are closely linked to both causation and consequences of several non-communicable disorders (NCD).
- Nearly 1 in 40 and 1 in 20 persons suffer from past and current depression, respectively.
- Neurosis and stress-related disorders affect 3.5% of the population and was reported to be higher among females (nearly twice as much in males).
- Data indicate that 0.9% of the survey population were at high-risk of suicide.
- Nearly 50% of persons with major depressive disorders reported difficulties in carrying out their daily activities.

Mental Health

About the Program
- The Government of India launched the National Mental Health Program (NMHP) in 1982, keeping in view the heavy burden of mental illness in the community, and the absolute inadequacy of mental health care infrastructure in the country to deal with it.
- The District Mental Health Program was added to the Program in 1996.
- The Program was re-strategized in 2003 to include two schemes, viz. Modernization of State Mental Hospitals and Up gradation of Psychiatric Wings of Medical Colleges/General Hospitals.

Objectives
- To ensure the availability and accessibility of minimum mental healthcare for all in the foreseeable future, particularly to the most vulnerable and underprivileged sections of the population;
- To encourage the application of mental health knowledge in general healthcare and in social development; and
- To promote community participation in the mental health service development and to stimulate efforts towards self-help in the community.

Strategies
- Integration mental health with primary health care through the NMHP;
- Provision of tertiary care institutions for treatment of mental disorders;
- Eradicating stigmatization of mentally ill patients and protecting their rights through regulatory institutions like the Central Mental Health Authority, and State Mental Health Authority.

THE DISTRICT MENTAL HEALTH PROGRAM (DMHP)
- DMHP was launched under NMHP in the year 1996.
- DMHP has been sanctioned for implementation in 704 districts for which support is provided through the National Health Mission.
- Facilities made available under DMHP at the Community Health Center (CHC) and Primary Health Center (PHC) levels, include outpatient services, assessment, counselling/psycho-social interventions, continuing care and support to persons with severe mental disorders, drugs, outreach services, ambulance services, etc.
- In addition to above services there is a provision of 10 bedded in-patient facility at the district level.
- The DMHP was based on **'Bellary Model'** with the following components:
  - **Early detection and treatment**.
  - **Training:** Imparting short-term training to general physicians for diagnosis and treatment of common mental illnesses with limited number of drugs under guidance of specialist. The health workers are being trained in identifying mentally ill persons.
  - **IEC:** Public awareness generation and also reduction stigma
  - **Monitoring:** The purpose is for simple recordkeeping.

Note: Government of India has launched the **National Tele Mental Health Programme** (Tele MANAS) on 10th October 2022 to provide access to mental health care services to all through a centralized toll-free helpline (14416 or 1800-891-4416).

BIBLIOGRAPHY

1. https://nhm.gov.in/index1.php?lang=1ANDlevel=2ANDsublinkid=1043ANDlid=359
2. https://pib.gov.in/PressReleasePage.aspx?PRID=1808230.

7.10 THE MENTAL HEALTHCARE ACT, 2017

- It was passed on 7 April 2017 and came into force from 7 July 2018.
- It shall extend to the whole of India.
- This Act superseded the previously existing Mental Health Act, 1987 that was passed on 22 May 1987.
- An Act to provide for mental healthcare and services for persons with mental illness and to protect, promote and fulfill the rights of such persons during delivery of mental healthcare and services and for matters connected therewith or incidental thereto.
- It differs from Mental Health Act, 1987 in the following points:
  - Decriminalizing the attempt to commit suicide
  - Empower persons suffering from mental illness and ensures every person shall have a right to access mental health care and treatment from mental health services run or funded by the appropriate government. It also guarantees free treatment for such persons if they are homeless or poor, even if they do not possess a Below Poverty Line card.
  - Aims to safeguard the rights of the people with mental illness, along with access to healthcare and treatment without discrimination from the government. Additionally, insurers are now bound to make provisions for medical insurance for the treatment of mental illness on the same basis as is available for the treatment of physical ailments.
  - The Mental Health Care Act, 2017 includes provisions for the registration of mental health-related institutions and for the regulation of the sector. These measures include the necessity of setting up mental health establishments across the country to ensure that no person with mental illness will have to travel far for treatment, as well as the creation of a mental health review board which will act as a regulatory body.
  - The Act has restricted the usage of electroconvulsive therapy (ECT) to be used only in cases of emergency, and along with muscle relaxants and anesthesia. Further, ECT has additionally been prohibited to be used as viable therapy for minors.
  - The Mental Health Care Act, 2017 has strong provisions to tackle stigma of mental illness.
  - 1987 Mental Act was institutionalized, while this Act is focused on the community.
  - Introducing proxy decision-making options and including opportunities to make advance directives (AD).
- **Determination of mental illness:**
  - Mental illness shall be determined in accordance with such nationally or internationally accepted medical standards (including the latest edition of the International Classification of Disease of the World Health Organization) as may be notified by the Central Government.

- No person or authority shall classify a person as a person with mental illness, except for purposes directly relating to the treatment of the mental illness or in other matters as covered under this Act or any other law for the time being in force.
- Mental illness of a person shall not be determined on the basis of:
    - Political, economic or social status or membership of a cultural, racial or religious group, or for any other reason not directly relevant to mental health status of the person;
    - Non-conformity with moral, social, cultural, work or political values or religious beliefs prevailing in a person's community.
- Past treatment or hospitalization in a mental health establishment though relevant, shall not by itself justify any present or future determination of the person's mental illness.
- The determination of a person's mental illness shall alone not imply or be taken to mean that the person is of unsound mind unless he has been declared as such by a competent court.

Rights of Person with Mental Illness

- Right to access mental healthcare
- Right to community living
- Right to protection from cruel, inhuman and degrading treatment
- Right to equality and non-discrimination
- Right to information
- Right to confidentiality
- Restriction on release of information in respect of mental illness
- Right to access medical records
- Right to personal contacts and communication
- Right to legal aid
- Right to make complaints about deficiencies in provision of services.

Offences and Penalties

- **Penalties for establishing or maintaining mental health establishment in contravention of provisions of this Act:**
    - Whoever carries on a mental health establishment without registration shall be liable to a penalty
        - For first contravention not be less than **five thousand rupees** but which may extend to **fifty thousand rupees**
        - For second contravention, a penalty which shall **not be less than fifty thousand rupees** but which may extend **to two lakh rupees**
        - For every subsequent contravention onwards, a penalty which shall **not be less than two lakh rupees** but which may extend to **five lakh rupees**
    - Whoever knowingly serves in the capacity as a mental health professional in a mental health establishment which is not registered under this Act, shall be liable to a penalty which may extend to **twenty-five thousand rupees.**

- **Punishment for contravention of provisions of the Act or rules or regulations made there under:**
  - Any person who contravenes any of the provisions of this Act shall
    - For **first contravention:** Punishable with imprisonment for a term which may extend to **six month**s, or with a fine which may extend to **ten thousand rupees** or with both, and
    - For **any subsequent contravention:** Imprisonment for a term which may extend to **two years** or with fine which shall not be less than **fifty thousand rupees but which may extend to five lakh rupees or with both**
- **Offences by companies:**
  - An offence under this Act has been committed by a company and it is proved that the offence has been committed with the consent or connivance of, or is attributable to, any neglect on the part of any director, manager, secretary or other officer of the company shall be deemed to be guilty of the offence and shall be liable to be proceeded against and punished accordingly.

BIBLIOGRAPHY

1. https://upload.indiacode.nic.in/showfile?actid=AC_CEN_12_13_00024_201710_1517807327874ANDtype=notificationANDfilename=MHA%202017%20notification.pdf
2. https://www.prsindia.org/uploads/media/Mental%20Health/Mental%20Healthcare%20Act,%202017.pdf
3. Kumar MT. Mental healthcare Act 2017: Liberal in principles, let down in provisions. Indian J Psychol Med 2018;40:101-7

7.11 ROLE OF A COMMUNITY HEALTH NURSE IN MENTAL HEALTH

- Mental health, according to the World Health Organization (WHO), is the state of well-being in which every individual realizes his or her own potentials, can cope with normal stressors of life, can work productively and fruitfully, and is able to make a contribution to his or her community.
- Mental illnesses are emerging as a major cause of morbidity in the country.
- These illnesses include depression, bipolar mood disorders, anxiety disorders, personality disorders, delusional disorders, substance use disorders, psychosexual disorders and sleep disorders, among others.
- It is estimated that at any point in time, 6% to 7% population in India suffers from some form of mental illness. WHO estimates that one in four persons will be affected by a mental illness at least once in their life time.
- Addressing mental illnesses by way of prevention, treatment and rehabilitation is necessary for achieving our health objectives.
- **Assessment of psychiatric patients:**
  - History-taking:

Mental Health

Crucial to establish and maintain rapport and be systematic in obtaining information

Begin with: Patient's name, age, gender, educational and marital status, occupation, religion, and circumstances of referral/reasons for attending the clinic

History of the present illness:
- Patient's complaints: in the patient's own words
- Duration, nature and progression of symptoms
- Precipitating, predisposing and perpetuating factors
- Degree of functional impairment: Effect on interpersonal relationships, work, family and other spheres of life
- Biological functions: Sleep and appetite

Family history:
- Parent's/sibling's age, occupations, relationships with the patient
- Enquiry into family history of psychiatric illness, suicide, alcohol and drug abuse, and mental retardation

Personal history:
- Early life and development
- Details of present circumstances: Accommodation, occupation, financial status
- Occupational history: Jobs, reasons for change, work satisfaction, relationships with colleagues
- Sexual practices, relationships, marriage
- In case of women: Menstrual pattern, contraception, miscarriage/termination of pregnancy

- **Mental state examination:** Mental state examination in psychiatric assessment of a person is as important as physical examination in a general medical condition.

Appearance and behavior:
- Careful observation of the patient's manner, rapport, eye contact, facial expressions, cleanliness, clothing, self-care, movements

Mood:
- Changes in the mood states: Depression, elation, euphoria, anxiety and anger

Speech:
- Rate, quantity (increased/decreased)
- Pattern: Spontaneity, coherence
- Abnormal words (neologisms)

Thought:
- Content: Delusions, preoccupations, obsessions, phobias, suicidal intentions
- Flow
- Abnormal form of throught may be deduced, for example where connections between statements are difficult to follow

Perception:
- Hallucinations, illusions

Sensorium and cognition:
- Consciousness, orientation (time, place, person)
- Concentration and attention
- Memory
- General fund of knowledge and intelligence
- Educational background must be taken into account

Mental Health

Management of patients with psychiatric illnesses: Treatment plan for the individual will be developed by MO/specialist. The key components of treatment include psychosocial interventions and pharmacological interventions. It is necessary that the mental disorders are treated by experts and their intervention. However, certain psychosocial interventions can be performed by anyone who trained in basic knowledge and skills. As a health worker, you can always extend basic care to the person dealing with mental disorder.

Psychosocial interventions comprise of:
- Psychoeducation
- **Psychological first aid:** To preserve life when a person may be a danger to him/herself or others, to provide comfort to the person and relieve for some symptoms and ensure further professional treatment
- Reducing stress and strengthening social support
- Promoting functioning in daily activities.

Service Delivery Framework

Care at community level	Care at SHC-HWC
IEC and community mobilization (MPW, CHO and ASHAs) • Promotion of mental health–through family enrichment programs, school health programs • Positive parenting, and physical activities initiative including yoga, balanced diet, exercise, sleep hygiene, and stress management (CHO and MPWs) • Screening and early detection using community informant decision tool (CIDT) (CHO/MPW/AF) • Screening using Patient Health Questionnaires 2 (PHQ2) as part of CBAC form administered by ASHAs • Follow-up care at home: Ensuring treatment compliance providing treatment adherence support and checking for side effects by ASHAs, MPW • Improving psychosocial competencies at individual and family level–Basic psychoeducation, psychological first aid, basic suicide risk assessment/management by MPW, CHO	**Community health officer** • Conducting individual level awareness and stigma reduction activities • Delivering psychosocial interventions • Identification/screening of MNS conditions • Referral to PHC or higher facilities for diagnosis and treatment • Administering Patient Health Questionnaire (PHQ) 9 for screening of depression • Tracking for improvement in PHQ 9 score during follow-up care • Emergency care for seizure/status epilepticus • Developing and implementing comprehensive life plan for persons with dementia • Dispensation of medicines prescribed by PHC-MO and specialists • Follow-up care checking for side effects and toxicities, for prescribed medications, monitoring for relapses and recurrences, checking for red flag signs, signs of abuse and neglect in patients with dementia • Facilitating community-based rehabilitation, family-based interventions, organizing meetings of self-help groups • Establish linkages with other programs, departments and NGOs for referral services

BIBLIOGRAPHY

1. https://nhm.gov.in/images/pdf/programmes/NMHP/Training_Manuals/Hand_BookAssessment_and_Management_of_Mental_Health_Problems_in_General_Practice.pdf
2. https://nhsrcindia.org/sites/default/files/202111/MNS%20Training%20Manual%20for%20MPW.pdf

CHAPTER 8

E-Health Including HMIS

CHAPTER OUTLINE
8.1 Basics of E-Health and National Digital Health Mission
8.2 E-Health: Reproductive and Child Health (RCH)
8.3 E-Health: Communicable diseases
8.4 E-Health: Noncommunicable diseases
8.5 Drugs and logistics
8.6 Management including Health Management Information System (HMIS)

8.1 BASICS OF E-HEALTH AND NATIONAL DIGITAL HEALTH MISSION

- **E-Health** or digital health is the use of information and communications technology (ICT) to improve health.
- **E-Health** innovations are key enablers for achieving and measuring universal health coverage. They can reduce healthcare costs to families, improve equitable access to quality services, and efficiently link health systems with social protection programs, and increase accountability and sustainability of health service delivery (WHO).
- **mHealth** is a component of eHealth.
- Global Observatory for e-Health (GOe) defined mHealth or mobile health as medical and public health practice supported by mobile devices, such as mobile phones, patient monitoring devices, personal digital assistants (PDAs), and other wireless devices.
- mHealth involves the use and capitalization on a mobile phone's core utility of voice and short messaging service (SMS) as well as more complex functionalities and applications including General Packet Radio Service (GPRS), third and fourth generation mobile telecommunications (3G and 4G systems), Global Positioning System (GPS), and Bluetooth technology.
- The eHealth initiatives have a vision to delivery better health outcomes in terms of:
  - Access
  - Quality

- Affordability
- Lowering of disease burden
- Efficient monitoring of health entitlements to citizens.

NATIONAL DIGITAL HEALTH MISSION (AYUSHMAN BHARAT DIGITAL MISSION)

- The Ayushman Bharat Digital Mission (ABDM) aims to develop the backbone necessary to support the integrated digital health infrastructure of the country.
- Based on recommendation of committee of Shri J. Satyanarayana.
- **National Digital Health Mission (NDHM)** has been launched on 27th September 2021.
- **National Health Authority (NHA)** under the Ministry of Health and Family Welfare will be the core implementing agency for the **National Digital Health Mission (NDHM)**.

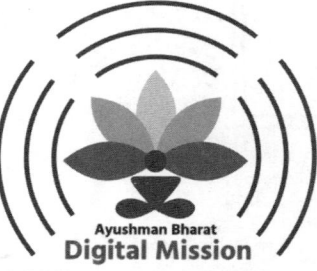

- Jan Dhan, Aadhaar and Mobile (JAM) trinity and other digital initiatives of the government, Ayushman Bharat Digital Mission will create a seamless online platform through the provision of a wide-range of data, information and infrastructure services, duly leveraging open, interoperable, standards-based digital systems while ensuring the security, confidentiality and privacy of health-related personal information.
- The mission will enable access and exchange of longitudinal health records of citizens with their consent.
- This mission will create interoperability within the digital health ecosystem, citizens will only be a click-away from accessing healthcare facilities.
- The NDHM is a complete **digital health ecosystem** comprising of five key features or components;
   1. Health ID/Ayushman Bharat Health Account (ABHA) number
   2. Personal health records
   3. Digi doctor
   4. Health facility registry
   5. Electronic medical record (EMR) web app
- It is also going to include **e-pharmacy and telemedicine** services in near future.
- The platform is based on both **app** and **website**.

1. Health ID/ABHA Number

- It is important to standardize the process of identification of an individual across healthcare providers.
- The national health ID will be **a repository of all health-related information** of every Indian.
- The health ID will be used for the purposes of uniquely identifying persons, authenticating them, and threading their health records (only with the informed consent of the patient) across multiple systems and stakeholders.
- **Various healthcare providers**—such as hospitals, laboratories, insurance companies, online pharmacies, telemedicine firms—will be expected to participate in the health ID system.

- Every patient who wishes to have their health records available digitally must create a **unique health ID,** using their basic details including demographic and location, family/relationship, and contact details and mobile or **Aadhaar** number.
- A digital health ID was proposed to "greatly reduce the risk of preventable medical errors and significantly increase quality of care".

2. Personal Health Records (PHR)

- The most salient feature of the PHR, and the one that distinguishes it from the EMR and EHR, is that the information it contains is under the control of the individual.
- Each health ID will be linked to a **health data consent manager,** which will be used to seek the patient's consent and allow for seamless **flow of health information from the Personal Health Records module.**
- The health ID will be **voluntary** and **applicable across states,** hospitals, diagnostic laboratories and pharmacies.

3. Digi Doctor (Doctors Directory)/Healthcare Professionals Registry (HPR)

- A single, updated repository of all doctors enrolled in nation with all the relevant details of the doctors such as name, qualifications, name of the institutions of qualifications, specializations, registration number with State medical councils, years of experience, etc. would be an essential building block of the digital health infrastructure of the country.
- The directory must be designed to be kept up-to-date as doctors gain skills via fellowships and map them to the facilities they are associated with.
- The **Digi Doctor** option will allow doctors from all over the country to enroll and enter their details like their contact numbers, etc.
- These enrolled doctors will also be **assigned digital signatures for free** which can be used for **writing prescriptions.**
  It will be **voluntary for the hospitals and doctors** to provide details for the app.

4. Health Facility Registry

- The Health Facility Registry is a single repository of all the health facilities in the country.
- he registry should be centrally maintained, store and facilitate the exchange of standardized data of both public and private health facilities in the country.
- The registry must allow health facilities to access their profile and update it periodically with specialties and services they offer, as well as provide a secure common platform to the facilities to maintain all essential information.
- Facilities should be able to e-sign documents such as patient records, apply for empanelment, have easier claims processing, as well as improve access to all healthcare ecosystem elements.

5. Electronic Medical Record (EMR) Web App

- An EMR is a digital version of a patient's chart.
- It contains the patient's medical and treatment history from a SINGLE health facility.
- EMRs helps service providers to identify which patients are due for screening, monitoring of certain indicators like blood pressure or due for vaccinations, etc.
- The EMR envisages to be the comprehensive view of the patients health information at a given facility.

Expected Outcomes of NDHM

- It will improve the efficiency, effectiveness, and transparency of health service delivery.
- Patients will be able to securely store and access their medical records (such as prescriptions, diagnostic reports and discharge summaries), and share them with healthcare providers to ensure appropriate treatment and follow-up.
- They will also have access to more accurate information on health facilities and service providers. NDHM will empower individuals with accurate information to enable informed decision making and increase accountability of healthcare providers.
- Patients will have the option to access health services remotely through tele-consultation and e-pharmacy.
- NDHM will provide choice to individuals to access both public and private health services, facilitate compliance with laid down guidelines and protocols, and ensure transparency in pricing of services and accountability for the health services being rendered.

BIBLIOGRAPHY

1. https://www.who.int/goe/publications/goe_mhealth_web.pdf
2. https://www.mygov.in/task/name-logo-and-tagline-contest-national-digital-health-mission-0/
3. https://www.drishtiias.com/daily-updates/daily-news-analysis/national-digital-health-mission
4. https://pib.gov.in/PressReleseDetail.aspx?PRID=1758248
5. https://ndhm.gov.in/abdm

8.2 E-HEALTH: REPRODUCTIVE AND CHILD HEALTH (RCH)

ANM ONLINE APPLICATION

- Auxiliary nurse midwife online (ANMOL) is a tablet-based application that allows ANMs to enter and updated data for beneficiaries of their workplace.
- This will ensure more prompt entry and updation of data as well as improve the data quality since the data is entered "at source" by providers of health services themselves.
- MCTS application—upgraded as RCH application—early identification and tracking of beneficiary—throughout the reproductive lifecycle.
- Reproductive child health (RCH) application helps in tracking of beneficiary for proper health care and promote family planning methods being adopted by them.
- Facilitates—timely delivery of antenatal, postnatal and delivery services
- Tracks children for complete immunization services including AEFI.
- RCH portal—designed to meet the requirements of the RMNCH program—incorporating additional functionality and features of the MCTS.
- Advantages of this application are shown in the following table:

E-Health Including HMIS

Feature	Advantage
Aadhaar enabled	Scan the QR code of Aadhaar card to register the beneficiary
Offline	Works in online and offline mode. Data gets auto sync to server whenever internet connectivity is available.
Dashboard	Ready available—registration and service delivery status for family planning, ANC, deliveries, PNC, immunization, critical indicator and KPI fact sheet, etc.
RCH register	On the fly generates—RCH register, EC register, PW register, ANC, Delivery and PNC register, High risk register, severe anemic register, child immunization, LBW child register, etc.
VHND	On selection of date and place generates—VHND due list, logistic planning and logistic used
Counseling	Empowers ANM with video and audio counselling, E-Book, e Tutorials, user manual, case focused counselling.
Work-plan	Sub-center-wise, village-wise, service-wise, ANM-wise, ASHA-wise, beneficiary-wise, high risk PW-wise, LBW child-wise
Update	Two-way transaction details from TAB to server both successful and failed
Connect	Directly connects to beneficiary through voice, SMS and can share counselling audio/video

KILKARI

- Kilkari means 'a baby's gurgle'.
- Kilkari is an interactive voice response IVR-based mobile service that delivers time-sensitive audio messages (voice call) about pregnancy and child health directly to the mobile phones of pregnant women, mothers of young children and their families.
- The service covers the critical time period—where the most maternal/infant deaths occur from the 4th month of pregnancy until the child is one year old.
- Families which subscribe to the service receive one prerecorded system generated call per week.
- Each call will be 2 minutes in length and serve as reminders for what the family should be doing that week depending on woman's stage of pregnancy or the child's age.
- This tool delivers free, weekly, time-appropriate 72 audio messages about pregnancy, child birth and child care directly to families' mobile phones from the second trimester of pregnancy until the child is one-year-old.
- Kilkari services will be available to states in regional dialect too.

MOBILE ACADEMY

- Mobile academy is an anytime, anywhere audio training course on interpersonal communication skills that the accredited social health activists (ASHA) can access from her mobile phone.
- Mobile Academy offers a training opportunity via their mobile phones, which reduces the need to travel and provides the flexibility in learning at their own pace and at times they find convenient.

- Mobile academy is being launched in Jharkhand, Madhya Pradesh, Rajasthan and Uttarakhand.
- It gives ASHAs tips on how to convince families to adopt priority RMNCH behaviors, while refreshing her existing knowledge.
- The course is 240 minutes long and consists of 11 chapters with 4 lessons each.
- At the end of each chapter, there is a quiz for them the ANM/ASHAs who pass the course will be provided with a certificate.

ICDS-CAS

- The Ministry of Women and Child Development has launched the information and communication technology enabled real time monitoring system (ICT-RTM) for improving the service delivery and ensuring better supervision of schemes by deploying the common application software (CAS) solution across the country covering all Anganwadi Centers (AWCs).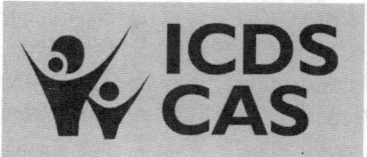
- ICDS-CAS replaces ~8.2 kg of paper registers with 173 gms of smartphone.
- ICDS-CAS is intended to use technology for furthering the objectives of the ICDS scheme.
- In the context of Anganwadi services, ICDS-CAS shall help in achieving the following objectives:
  - Improvement in efficiency and effectiveness of Anganwadi workers by embedding job aids and tools in their smart phones, e.g., pertaining to nutrition counseling of pregnant women, infant and young child feeding (IYCF) practices, etc.;
  - Individual child-based tracking for nutrition status;
  - Automated growth chart generation;
  - Automation of ICDS registers;
  - Monitor timeliness and quality of service delivered to the beneficiaries;
  - Provide reports and dashboards based on real time information and alerts to various stakeholders for prompt action and decision-making.
- **Household management:** Collect the information about children, women and other members of all the households in the feeder area of Anganwadi. Maintain this information and keep them updated.
- **Daily feeding:** Record daily attendance for children 3–6 years old. Do keep track of their activities and meals at the AWC.
- **Home visit scheduler:** Plan home visits to pregnant and lactating women, and children up to 2 years of age.
- **Growth monitoring:** Record the weight of children. The app shows underweight status automatically.
- **Take home ration:** Record the distribution of rations
- **Due list:** Creates a list of beneficiaries to be mobilized or notified for an upcoming VHSND to provide certain services. Record vaccination data during VHSND day.
- **AWC management**
  - Record infrastructure details, VHSND survey and visitor book details.
  - Watch video library
- **MPR List:** See monthly progress report (MPR).

BIBLIOGRAPHY

1. https://nhm.gov.in/images/pdf/in-focus/Kerala/Day-1/Session-2/ANMOL.pptx
2. https://main.mohfw.gov.in/sites/default/files/56987532145632566578.pdf
3. http://icds-wcd.nic.in/nnm/NNM-Web-Contents/LEFT-MENU/ICT-RTM/Training_Manual_MasterTrainers_English.pdf

8.3 E-HEALTH: COMMUNICABLE DISEASES

INDIA FIGHTS DENGUE

- It was launched in 2016.
- This App empowers the people to contribute towards prevention of dengue.
- **Features:**
  - User can check dengue symptoms.
  - User gets nearest Hospital/Blood bank information as per current geographical location.
  - User can share feedback via email.
  - Interactive and pictorial display for ensure dengue mosquito free area.
  - User can hear Shri Narendra Modi's Mann ki Baat audio.
  - User can check myths and facts for dengue application.
  - User can view Do's and Don'ts for prevention of dengue.
  - User can view dengue-related frequently asked Questions.
  - User can view Munnabhai video for fight against dengue.

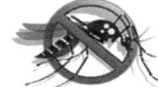

India Fights Dengue

NIKSHAY

- **NI-KSHAY**-(Ni = End, Kshay = TB) is the web enabled patient management system for TB control under the National Tuberculosis Elimination Programme (NTEP). It is developed and maintained by the Central TB Division (CTD), Ministry of Health and Family Welfare, Government of India, in collaboration with the National Informatics Centre (NIC), and the World Health Organization country office for India.
- Nikshay is used by health functionaries at various levels across the country both in the public and private sector, to register cases under their care, order various types of tests from labs across the country, record treatment details, monitor treatment adherence and to transfer cases between care providers. It also functions as the National TB Surveillance System and enables reporting of various surveillance data to the Government of India.

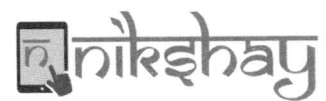

99 DOTS

- 99 DOTS is a low-cost approach for monitoring and improving TB medication adherence. It can be utilized either as a supplement to existing DOTS programs, or to enable remote observation of doses administered by patients or their family members.

- Using 99 DOTS, each anti-TB blister pack is wrapped in a custom envelope, which includes hidden phone numbers that are visible only when doses are dispensed.
- After taking daily medication, patients make a free call to the hidden phone number, yielding high confidence that the dose was "in-hand" and has been taken.

Other IT initiatives under NTEP:
- **Nikshay sampark: (1800-11-6666):** It is toll free, operational in 14 languages for information, for patient support, for service linkage and grievance redressal.
- **Nikshay patrika:** Quarterly publication of TB central division
- **Nutrition-TB App (N-TB App):** A mobile-based application to simplify nutritional assessment, counseling and care of patients with tuberculosis
- **TB Arogya Sathi:** Citizens using the TB Aarogya Sathi App will have access to common FAQs regarding TB, information on the symptoms of TB and side effects of anti TB drugs. Using the app, any user will be able to find the closest health facilities that can assist in diagnosis of TB. Patients registered with Ni-kshay will have access to update their treatment adherence and bank details using the app along with viewing the DBT details, adherence details and treatment progress.

BIBLIOGRAPHY

1. https://www.nhp.gov.in/mobile-app-dengue
2. https://nikshay.in/Home/AboutUs
3. https://www.99dots.org/About.html
4. https://tbcindia.gov.in/showfile.php?lid=3327

8.4 E-HEALTH: NONCOMMUNICABLE DISEASES

NHP SWASTH BHARAT MOBILE APPLICATION

- "Swasth Bharat Mobile Application" to empower the citizens to find reliable and relevant health information.
- The application provides detailed authentic health information regarding healthy lifestyle, disease conditions (A-Z), symptoms, treatment options, first aid and public health alerts.

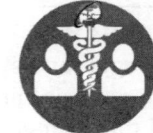

NHP Swasth Bharat

M-CESSATION

- It aims at reaching out to those who are willing to quit tobacco use.
- It supports them towards successful quitting through text messages sent via mobile phones.
- It uses two-way messaging between the individual seeking to quit tobacco use and program specialists providing them dynamic support.
- When offered along with traditional services, M-Cessation has been found to be cost-effective in comparison to traditional options for cessation support.
- The government has recently released version-2 of the "mTobaccoCessation" platform, which can deliver content through SMS or interactive voice response in 12 languages.

M-Diabetes Initiative

- The Ministry of Health and Family Welfare (MoHFW), Government of India in collaboration with the WHO country office for India and other partners, has launched a mobile health initiative for the prevention and care of diabetes—**mDiabetes**.
- This Initiative has been launched to provide information on diabetes and how to prevent and manage it.
- This information can be received with a missed call to 011-22901701.

CPHC-NCD

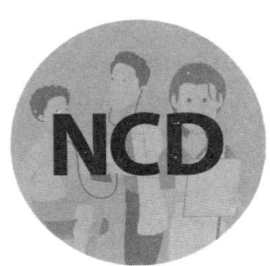

- The NCD-GoI ANM application allows the health-workers to do population enumeration of the community level, perform risk assessments for the enrolled population and screen the individuals for the five noncommunicable diseases—(1) hypertension, (2) diabetes, (3) oral, (4) breast and (5) cervical cancers.
- Based on the screening results, the individuals will be referred to higher facilities for further treatment and disease management.
- The application also allows the health-workers to follow-up with the individuals for treatment adherence and review self and sub-center's performance against targets.

BIBLIOGRAPHY

1. https://www.nhp.gov.in/mobile-app-swasth
2. https://www.drishtiias.com/daily-updates/daily-news-analysis/mobile-scheme-to-quit-tobacco
3. http://mdiabetes.nhp.gov.in/
4. https://play.google.com/store/apps/details?id=org.cphc.ncd.anmandhl=en_INandgl=USandpli=1

8.5 DRUGS AND LOGISTICS

E-RAKTKOSH INITIATIVE (CENTRALIZED BLOOD BANK MANAGEMENT SYSTEM)

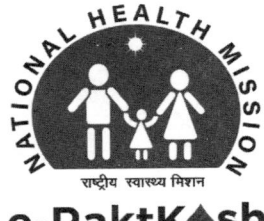
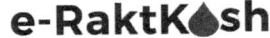

- It is an integrated Blood Bank management information system that is web-based mechanism interconnects all the Blood Banks of the State into a single network.
- An initiative by DoHFW to monitor:
  - Safe and adequate blood supplies
  - Reduced turnaround time
  - Networking of blood banks
  - Adherence to drug and cosmetic Act
  - Real time blood stock availability
  - State-wise/District-wise donor database
  - Reports to blood bank officials and administrators.

ELECTRONIC VACCINE INTELLIGENCE NETWORK (EVIN)

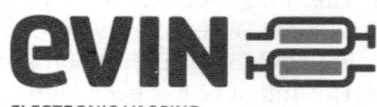

- eVIN is an integrated package of people, process and product.
- eVIN technology uses the smartphone, web-based application, temperature loggers and cloud-based server to digitize vaccine stock inventory and storage temperature from every vaccine store and cold chain points located at peripheral government health facilities.
- The technological innovation is implemented by the United Nations Development Programme (UNDP).
- eVIN is functional in 32 States and Union Territories (UTs) and in the remaining States and UTs of Andaman and Nicobar Islands, Chandigarh, Ladakh and Sikkim will also be rolled out.

COWIN (COVID VACCINE INTELLIGENCE NETWORK)

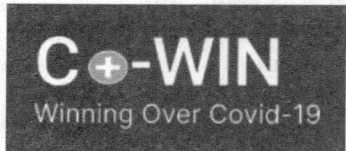

- A tech-based platform facilitating the planning, implementation, monitoring, and evaluation of COVID-19 vaccination in India **(Fig. 8.1)**.
- It was tech backbone of India to fight against the COVID-19.
- COWIN platform is based on principles like equitable and inclusive, single source of truth, evolvability and scalability, feedback and analysis.

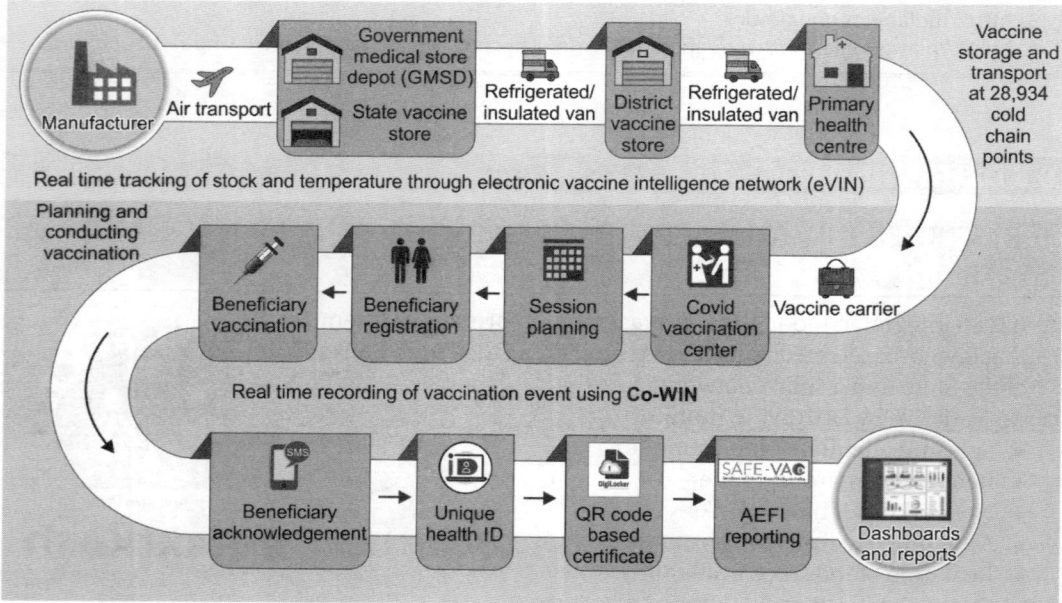

Fig. 8.1: COVID-19 vaccine delivery management system.

U-WIN

- After the success of the Co-WIN platform, U-WIN, the program to digitize India's Universal Immunization Programme (UIP) has been launched in a pilot mode in two districts of each State and Union Territory.
- It was launched on January 11 in 65 districts.
- Carrying vaccination cards of children and pregnant women, struggling to keep a tab on the next jab and other such hassles may soon become a thing of the past.
- The platform will be used to register and vaccinate every pregnant woman, record her delivery outcome, register every newborn delivery, administer birth doses and all vaccination events thereafter.
- The U-WIN is going to be the single source of information for immunization services, updating vaccination status, delivery outcome, planning of RI sessions and reports like antigen-wise coverage, etc.
- There will be digital registrations of all pregnant women and newborns for individualized tracking for vaccination, reminders for upcoming doses and follow-up of dropouts.
- "Healthcare workers and program managers will be able to generate real-time data of routine immunization sessions and vaccination coverage for better planning and vaccine distribution".
- This data will be linked to ABHA ID (Ayushman Bharat Heath Account).
- One of the best features of this platform is that people can check nearby ongoing routine immunization sessions and book appointments.
- "Once the whole immunization program is digitized, beneficiaries will get certificates on the spot, and they can also download them if they want to. These certificates will be stored in digilockers."

DRUG LOGISTICS INFORMATION AND MANAGEMENT SYSTEM (DLIMS)

- The basic aim of DLIMS is to maintain database of drugs stocks and medical equipment.
- It also handles procurement, storage and distribution of medicines and medical equipment.
- It enhances the operational efficiency of the healthcare services provided at PHC and sub-center level.

E-AUSHADHI

- This is supply chain management application that deals with purchase; inventory management and distribution of various drugs.
- The main aim of 'e-Aushadhi' is to ascertain the needs of various district drug warehouses such that all the required materials/drugs are constantly available to be supplied to the user district drug warehouses without delay.
- This includes classification/categorization of items, codification of items, quality check of these items, etc., and finally issuing drugs to the patients, who is the final consumer in the chain.
- It will help to implement a transparent system for procurement, storage and distribution of quality drugs, supplies, equipment, etc., required for the hospitals at reasonable competitive price.
- It is to ensure adequate savings in the drug budget by scientific forecasting system based on the preparation of essential drug list and its actual consumption.

FAMILY PLANNING-LOGISTICS MANAGEMENT INFORMATION SYSTEM (FP-LMIS)

- Supply chain involves many different personnel, departments, suppliers, agencies and procedures, hence managing family planning logistics becomes a complex task. At present, the top-down push system still prevails in the FP supply chain across the country. Moreover, the personnel at various levels lack skills in demand forecasting, inventory management and distribution processes, leading to either overstocking or stock outs across many public health facilities.
- An efficient supply chain and logistic system improves contraceptive availability, aids couples to avoid unplanned pregnancies and makes the Family Planning program more responsive to the clients' need. Government of India's Family Planning Logistic Management Information System (FP-LMIS) is a step towards ensuring effective, efficient and uniform management of family planning commodities across India.
- FP-LMIS is a web-based, mobile app-based, SMS-based application designed to assist in collection, processing, indenting and reporting of logistics to streamline the supply of FP commodities from national level to ASHA level. It will also enable real-time tracking and monitoring of the FP supplies, to assist program managers for appropriate and timely decision making.

BIBLIOGRAPHY

1. https://www.eraktkosh.in/
2. http://nhp.gov.in/electronic-vaccine-intelligence-network(evin)_pg
3. https://prod-cdn.preprod.co-vin.in/assets/pdf/CoWIN_Overview.pdf
4. https://www.business-standard.com/article/economy-policy/govt-launches-u-win-to-digitise-india-s-universal-immunisation-programme-123012300963_1.html
5. https://fplmismohfw.in/IMCS/hissso/Login.fp#

8.6 MANAGEMENT INCLUDING HEALTH MANAGEMENT INFORMATION SYSTEM (HMIS)

HEALTH MANAGEMENT INFORMATION SYSTEM

- Health management information system is an important building block for health system strengthening. A strong monitoring and evaluation system is a key to the success of any project, scheme or program. A good management information system (MIS) has many roles to perform like the decision support role, the performance monitoring role, and the functional support role, which in turn helps to improve performance and achieve results.

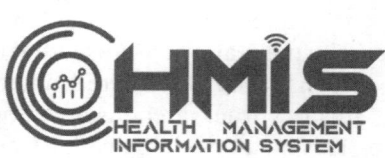

- Ministry of Health and Family Welfare, Government of India has put in place a web-based monitoring information system, health management information system (HMIS) in 2008 to monitor all its health program.

E-Health Including HMIS

- The new HMIS was launched on 28th December 2020 with data entry started since April 2020 onwards.
- The new portal has many new features which were earlier not available in HMIS (1.0). This includes person specific user credentials, real time data entry and real time monitoring, National Identification Number (NIN) and Local Government Directory (LGD) compliance, API (Application Program Interface), etc.
- This portal will be a gateway to wealth of information regarding the health indicators of India. The information available on this portal is derived data from data uploaded by the States/UTs.
- HMIS data specifically designed to support planning, management, and decision making based on grading of facilities, various indicators at Block, District at State as well as National level.
- Five types of health facilities viz. Sub-Centers (SCs), Primary Health Centers (PHCs), Community Health Centers (CHCs), Sub-District Hospitals (SDHs) and District Hospitals (DHs) report on HMIS. Medical colleges are mapped at SDH and DH level in respective States/UTs.
- Around 2.20 lakh health facilities, across all districts (735 districts), across all sub-districts (6858 sub-districts) of India are uploading data every month. HMIS generates huge amount of data (more than 3 Tb database size (Approx.) and captures more than 300 data items under service delivery and over 400 data items under infrastructure and HR.
- There are three types of data entry in HMIS portal:
  1. Daily
  2. Monthly service delivery
  3. Infrastructure and HR
- Data for the service delivery for a specific month are entered in the subsequent month. Facilities are supposed to enter the data by 5th of the subsequent month.
- Infrastructure data is entered on annual basis, facility is supposed to enter this data at the beginning of the financial year (by 30 April of that financial year) and update the information as and when required throughout the year.
- Daily data entry is to be done from PHC level to District Hospital level. Up to 2 days backlog can be entered in this module. Even nil reporting is mandatory in daily data entry.
- Monthly service delivery data entry has three parts:
  - Part A: For RCH related data (Antenatal care, intranatal care, postnatal care, child immunization, family planning) to be entered in M1 to M13 tab
  - Part B: Health facility services (M14 to M15)
  - Part C: Stock (M16 to M17)
- Monthly service delivery data to be done right from SC/HWC to DH.
- **Infrastructure and HR data:** There are different tabs like services, HR, investigations facilities, physical infrastructure, equipment and furniture and quality control.
- If there is no update in infrastructure and HR data, then just need to carry forward the previous month filled data.

STRATEGIC INFORMATION MANAGEMENT SYSTEM (SIMS)

- It is an integrated web-based reporting, data management and decision support system, with monthly reporting from almost all the program components of NACP comprising ICTC, TI, Blood banks, STI/RTI, IEC, laboratories.

- It is Web-based application for data entry at various levels including Reporting Unit (RU), District and State.
- It provides differential data management rights to various users
- Workflow similar to physical reporting system, but automatic aggregation to reduce manual error
- Both online and offline modes of data entry
- Once data is entered at the RU level, all higher levels can view the data in real time
- Ensures data quality checks across various reporting level
- Generates basic to advance reports using analytic tools (SAS, GIS).

INTEGRATED HEALTH INFORMATION PLATFORM (IHIP)

- The integrated health information platform is a web-enabled near-real-time electronic information system that is embedded with all applicable Government of India's e-Governance standards, information technology (IT), data and meta data standards to provide state-of-the-art single operating picture with geospatial information for managing disease outbreaks and related resources.
- **Key features of IHIP:**
  - Real time data reporting (along through mobile application); accessible at all levels (from villages, states and central level)
  - Advanced data modelling and analytical tools
  - GIS enabled graphical representation of data into integrated dashboard
  - Role and hierarchy-based feedback and alert mechanisms
  - Geo-tagging of reporting health facilities
  - Scope for data integration with other health programs.

MERA ASPATAAL (MA)

- Quality healthcare is an articulated commitment of MoHFW. The level of patient satisfaction is the litmus test for assessing quality of services provided by a healthcare facility.
- Mera Aspataal (My Hospital) is an ICT-based application for public and empanelled private hospitals to provide patient-centric care.
- A multichannel approach is used to collect information on patients' level of satisfaction, i.e., web portal, mobile application, short message service (SMS), and outbound dialing (OBD).
- The application allows feedback to be consolidated, analyzed and disseminated on a frequently updated dashboard which will improve quality of services in healthcare facilities.

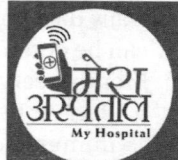

BIBLIOGRAPHY

1. https://hmis.nhp.gov.in/downloadfile?filepath=publications/Other/EBOOK_QTR1_2021-22.pdf
2. http://naco.gov.in/strategic-information-management
3. https://ihip.nhp.gov.in/idsp/#!/login
4. https://www.nhp.gov.in/mobile-mera-aspataal

CHAPTER 9

Delivery Mechanism of Community Health Services

CHAPTER OUTLINE

- 9.1 Rural healthcare delivery system
- 9.2 Urban healthcare delivery system
- 9.3 IPHS for SC/HWC, PHC, CHC
- 9.4 Financial and inventory management at public health facilities
- 9.5 Summary of different Indian systems of medicine (AYUSH)

9.1 RURAL HEALTHCARE DELIVERY SYSTEM

- Overall, there are three levels of the healthcare system: primary, secondary and tertiary level.
- **Primary level:** Subcenters/HWC and Primary health centers (PHCs).
- **Secondary level:** Community health centers (CHCs), FRUs, Subdistrict hospitals and district hospitals
- **Tertiary level:** Medical colleges and State level Institutions like center of excellence

HEALTHCARE DELIVERY SYSTEM IN RURAL AREA

Population norms	Plain area	Hilly/Tribal/Difficult area
Subcenter/HWC	5000	3000
Primary health center	30000	20000
Community health center	120000	80000

SUBCENTER/AB-HWCS

- **A subcenter** (SC) is the most peripheral and first contact point between the primary healthcare system and the community.

Delivery Mechanism of Community Health Services

- SCs provide services in relation to maternal and child health, family welfare, nutrition, immunization, diarrhea control and control of communicable diseases programs.
- **Type A** subcenter provides recommended services except that the facilities for conducting delivery. IPHS recommends two ANM (one essential and one desirable) and one Health Worker Male (essential).
- **Type B** subcenter provides all recommended services including facilities for conducting deliveries at the subcenter itself.
- For Type B subenters, IPHS recommends to provide two ANMs (essential) and one Health Worker Male (essential). One Staff Nurse or ANM (if staff nurse not available) is to be provided, if number of deliveries at the subcenter is 20 or more in a month.
- Sanitation services should be provided through outsourcing on part time basis at Type A and full-time basis at Type B.
- Ayushman Bharat - Health and wellness centers (AB-HWCs) are being set up as an upgraded version of existing health subcenters (HSC); primary health centers and urban primary health centers (UPHCs).

PRIMARY HEALTH CENTER (PHC)

- PHC is the first contact point between the village community and the medical officer.
- PHCs to provide integrated curative and preventive Healthcare to the rural population with emphasis on the preventive and promotive aspects of Healthcare.
- PHCs may be of two types depending upon the delivery case load—**Type A** and **Type B**. The PHCs with delivery case load of less than 20 deliveries in a month will be of Type A and those with delivery case load of 20 or more in a month will be of Type B.

COMMUNITY HEALTH CENTERS (CHCs)

- CHCs are established and maintained by the State Government under the MNP/BMS program in an area with a population of 120 000 people and in hilly/difficult to reach/tribal areas with a population of 80000. It serves as a referral center for PHCs within the block and also provides facilities for obstetric care and specialist consultations.
- An existing facility (**district hospital, sub-divisional hospital, CHC**) can be declared a fully operational **first referral unit (FRU)** only if it is equipped to provide round-the-clock services for emergency obstetric and newborn care, in addition to all emergencies that any hospital is required to provide.

Details of Services and Human Resources at AB-HWC

The Twelve Packages Envisaged under Comprehensive Primary Healthcare (CPHC)

1. Care in pregnancy and childbirth.
2. Neonatal and infant Healthcare services
3. Childhood and adolescent Healthcare services.
4. Family planning, contraceptive services and other reproductive Healthcare services
5. Management of communicable diseases: National health program
6. Management of common communicable diseases and outpatient care for acute simple illness and minor ailments
7. Screening, prevention, control and management of noncommunicable diseases
8. Care for common ophthalmic and ENT problems

9. Basic oral healthcare
10. Elderly and palliative healthcare services
11. Emergency medical services including burns and trauma
12. Screening and basic management of mental health ailments.

In addition to providing clinical services, HWCs are also to be utilized as a platform for teleconsultation and expanding the range of diagnostics.

ROLE OF COMMUNITY HEALTH OFFICER (CHO)

- Ensure that all households in the service area are listed, empaneled and a database is maintained—in digital format/paper format as required by the state.
- Provide clinical care as specified in the care pathways and standard treatment guidelines for the range of services expected of the Subcenter/sub health center (SHC).
- Clinical care provision would include coordinating for case management for chronic illnesses based on the diagnosis and treatment plan made by the Medical Officer/Specialists who will initiate treatment for chronic diseases, dispense drugs as per standing orders by the medical officer. Such coordination could be facilitated through telehealth.
- Focus attention in screening for chronic conditions, enabling suspected cases confirmed and initiating treatment according to guideline.
- Coordinate and lead local response to diseases outbreaks, emergencies and disaster situations and support the medical team or joint investigation teams for disease outbreaks.
- Support the team of MPWs and ASHAs in their tasks, including on the job mentoring, support and supervision and administrative functions of the HWC such as inventory management and management of untied funds.
- Support and supervise the collection of population-based data by frontline workers, collate and analyze data for planning and reporting of data to the next level in an accurate and timely fashion.
- Coordinate work with community platforms such as the VHSNC/MAS/SHGs
- Address issues of social and environmental determinants of health like safe potable water, sanitation, safe collection of refuse, etc.

ROLE OF MULTIPURPOSE WORKER-MALE (MPW-M) OF HWC-SHC

1. Clinical Work

- General OPD services and managing cases at HWC-SHC that are referred by ASHAs/or visit the health center with any illness or problem.
- **Identification, referral and follow-up:** Mobilize community members including children and guide them to nearest screening camps, health facilities/referral center, for registration, early identification of gestational diabetes and syphilis during pregnancy, STI/RTI, eye, ENT, TB, leprosy, noncommunicable diseases, vector-borne diseases, common mental conditions, substance use and epilepsy cases, delays in development and disability and other congenital anomalies.
- Referring of adolescents with anemia, underweight, issues related to nutrition, etc. to AB-HWCs.
- Follow-up of sick and malnourished children regarding their nutrition intake, especially those discharged from NRCs.

2. Public Health Work

Counseling and health education to the community on:
- Importance of institutional delivery, early and exclusive breastfeeding, seeking postnatal care, weaning and complementary feeding, consuming nutritious diet and where to go for delivery.
- Childhood and adolescent healthcare services including nutrition, personal hygiene, sanitation, vaccination and motivate to attend VHSND sessions related to adolescent health.
- Activities for prevention and early detection of hearing impairment/deafness, visual impairments at the level of health facility, community and schools.
- Sensitization of community regarding national health programs.
- Visit the family and perform activities like identify fever cases, collect the blood smear, mosquito control measure activities under National vector-borne disease control programme.
- Identify cases of TB, leprosy, diarrhea, AFP, measles, diphtheria, etc. and notify immediately to MO, CHO and health supervisor.
- Environmental sanitation activities like chlorination of water, distribution of chlorine tablet, educate community for sanitation and proper method of liquid and solid waste.
- Information and prevention of RTIs, STIs, HIV/AIDS through health education in the community.
- **Awareness generation:** Utilize meetings of the Village Health Nutrition and Sanitation Committee/Mahila Arogya Samiti (VHSNC/MAS) to raise awareness about the needs of palliative care patients, and mobilize individual and support.

3. Administrative Work

- Facilitate opening of Bank Account, Aadhar card registration of patients and ensure entry in portals such as Nikshay/TB notification register at health facility for DBT transfer.
- Maintain a record of cases in his area, who are under treatment for tuberculosis and leprosy and record of vital events.
- Coordinate and participate in the outreach activities of PHC/CHC/District Mobile clinic.
- Attending monthly meetings at PHC and supportive and supervisory function to ASHA.
- Support ASHA in active case detection of cases in the community and referral of suspected cases with skin patches to MO and also motivate the TB patients in taking regular treatment.

ROLE OF MULTIPURPOSE WORKER-FEMALE (MPW-F)/AUXILIARY NURSE MIDWIFE (ANM) OF HWC-SHC

1. Clinical Work

- General OPD services and managing cases at HWC-SHC.
- **Early registration of pregnancy:** Issuing of ID number and mother and child protection card and antenatal check-up and identifying high-risk pregnancies, child births and postpartum cases.
- Screening, referral of suspected cases and follow-up care in case of gestational diabetes and syphilis during pregnancy, STI/RTI, eye, ENT, TB, leprosy, communicable and non-communicable diseases, etc.
- Identification and support in management of anemia, nutritional deficiencies, and vaccine preventable diseases in children.

- Undertake diagnostic services: pregnancy test, hemoglobin, urine test, blood sugar, etc.
- Provide first aid treatment for obstetric emergencies, e.g., eclampsia, PPH, sepsis and prompt referral.
- Midwifery services in subcenters only where institutional deliveries have been allowed by the state governments and provide appropriate treatment or refer to higher centers in cases where ASHA is not able to manage with home-based care.
- Reviewing completed CBAC for cancer symptoms/epilepsy/COPD.

2. Public Health Work

- Undertake household survey with ASHAs for detailed mapping, enumeration and enrolment of population being covered in HWC
- Counseling and health education to the community on:
    - Danger signs during pregnancy, and teaching them importance of institutional delivery, early and exclusive breastfeeding, seeking postnatal care, weaning and complementary feeding, consuming nutritious diet and where to go for delivery.
    - Importance of complementary feeding, supplementary nutrition at AWCs and consuming iron-rich diet in children to avoid anemia.
    - Childhood and adolescent healthcare services including nutrition, personal hygiene, sanitation, menstrual hygiene management, healthy living, etc. in the community through home visits and through VHSNDs.
    - Family planning/education of children/dangers of sex selection/age at marriage
    - Information on/disease outbreak/disaster management/adolescent health.
    - Care during communicable and vector-borne disease infections.
    - Lifestyle modifications needed for noncommunicable diseases
    - Oral health education referral of cases with oral problems.
    - Motivation for quitting and referrals to Tobacco Cassation Center at District Hospital/Medical College.
    - Activities for prevention and early detection of hearing impairment/deafness, visual
    - Sensitization of community regarding government national health programs.

3. Field/Home Visits

- Prioritize visit to pregnant women who did not attend their regular ANCs in the monthly ANC clinics/VHSND
- Visits to postpartum mothers for home-based services and providing care-either as indicated by ASHA after a home visit, or if ASHA is not there, or if they failed to attend VHSND.
- Identify children who missed their immunization sessions
- Visit sick newborn/low birth weight babies and children who need referral but are unable to go
- Motivate families with whom ASHA is having difficulty in motivating for changing health-seeking behavior, adopting family planning methods and who did not come to VHSND.
- Patients having chronic illnesses, who have not reported for follow-up at the subcenter or VHSND and encourage them to attend special-day clinics
- Prioritized visits in areas where fever treatment depots/ASHAs have not been deployed—collecting blood smears or performs RDTs from suspected malaria cases during visits and providing treatment to positive cases.

- Distribution and utilization of LLIN bed nets; facilitate and ensure quality spray in households and insecticide treatment of community-owned bed nets.
- Verbal autopsy and/or at least preliminary inquiry into any maternal or child death.
- Surveillance for unusually high incidence of cases of any communicable disease and notify CHO and PHC-MO.
- Ensuring regular testing of salt at household level for presence of iodine through Salt Testing Kits by ASHAs.

4. Administrative Work

- In ensuring that the untied funds are utilized as per the rules and guidelines.
- Supportive and supervisory function to ASHA and replenishment of drugs in her kit.
- Survey in the community for nutritional deficiency among those who had experienced trauma/disaster/disease outbreak and spreading awareness on nutrition, lifestyle modification diet post trauma/disaster/disease outbreak.
- In coordinating for building convergence with women's group, self-help groups for generating awareness, counseling to promote behavior change at community level
- In coordinating for building convergence with ICDS (AWW) and conduct growth monitoring at AWC, counseling on nutrition, referral of cases (low weight babies, pregnant women with nutritional deficiency)
- Attending VHSND during disaster—in relief camps for awareness generation on nutrition, growth monitoring along with other service delivery.
- In community level care for emergency and coordination for first aid stabilization and follow up visit to patient.
- In organizing special "Day Clinics" to enhance attendance for ambulatory outpatient services.
- Support ASHA to ensure home-based care for newborn and young children.
- **Assisting ASHA:** Assist the ASHA/similar village health volunteer to motivate the TB patients in taking regular treatment.
- Functions of reporting and record maintenance.
- Register entries and housekeeping work, data entry; report preparation and review meetings.
- Support CHO in enabling every HWC to have a folder for every family.
- Attending monthly meetings at PHC
- Ensure timely documentation and registration of all births and deaths under the jurisdiction of subcenter.
- Attend VHSNC meetings maintain record
- Making and timely submission of reports for various programs i.e. RCH portal, NCD, HMIS, IDSP, NIKSHAY, etc.

Role of Accredited Social Health Activist (ASHA)

- One ASHA per 1000 population
- ASHA must primarily be a woman resident of the village married/widowed/divorced, preferably in the age group of 25–45 years.
- She should be a literate woman with due preference in selection to those who are qualified up to 10 standards wherever they are interested and available in good numbers. This may be relaxed only if no suitable person with this qualification is available.

- The ASHAs will receive performance-based incentives for promoting universal immunization, referral and escort services for reproductive and child health (RCH) and other healthcare programs, and construction of household toilets.
- ASHA will be the first port of call for any health-related demands of deprived sections of the population, especially women and children
- ASHA will be a health activist in the community who will create awareness on health and its social determinants and mobilize the community towards existing health services.
- ASHA will provide information to the community on determinants of health such as nutrition, basic sanitation and hygienic practices, healthy living and working conditions
- She will counsel women on birth preparedness, importance of safe delivery, breastfeeding and complementary feeding, immunization, contraception and prevention of common infections including reproductive tract infection/sexually transmitted infections (RTIs/STIs) and care of the young child.
- ASHA will mobilize the community and facilitate them in accessing health and health-related services available at the Anganwadi/subcenter/primary health centers, such as immunization, antenatal check-up (ANC), postnatal check-up, etc.
- ASHA conduct home visits for care of pregnant women, newborn, postpartum mother and undernourished children.
- She will act as a depot older for essential provisions like oral rehydration therapy (ORS), iron folic acid tablet (IFA), chloroquine, disposable delivery kits (DDK), oral pills and condoms, etc.
- Women's committees (like self-help groups or women's health committees), village health and sanitation committee of the Gram Panchayat, peripheral health workers especially ANMs and Anganwadi workers, and the trainers of ASHA and in-service periodic training would be a major source of support to ASHA.

As per Rural Health Statistics 2021-2022 (As on 31st March, 2022)

- **Subcenters (SCs):** As on 31st March 2022, there are a total of 161829 subcenters functioning both in rural and urban areas of India. These consist of 157935 SCs in rural areas and 3894 SCs in urban areas.
- **Primary health centers (PHCs):** Similarly, there are 31053 PHCs functioning in both rural and urban areas in India. These consists of 24935 PHCs in rural areas and 6118 PHCs in urban areas.
- **Community health centers (CHCs):** There are 6064 CHCs functional in the country, consisting of 5480 rural and 584 urban CHCs.
- **Subdivisional/district hospitals (SDH):** There are 1275 SDH functioning in the country which are catering to both rural and urban areas.
- **District hospital (DH):** There are 767 DH functioning in the country which are catering to both rural and urban areas.

Coverage of Rural Health Infrastructure (As on 31st March, 2022)

❏ Average rural population covered by health facility (based on the mid-year population as on 1st July 2022):

Health facility	Norm	Average rural population covered
Subcenter	300–5000	5691
Primary health center (PHC)	20000–30000	36049
Community health center (CHC)	80000–120000	164027

❏ Average rural area (sq. km) covered by:

Subcenter	19.55
Primary health center (PHC)	123.85
Community health center (CHC)	563.52

❏ Average radial distance (km) covered) by:

Subcenter	2.49
Primary health center (PHC)	6.28
Community health center (CHC)	13.39

❏ Average number of villages covered by:

Subcenter	4
Primary health center (PHC)	27
Community health center (CHC)	121

BIBLIOGRAPHY

1. https://nhm.gov.in/images/pdf/guidelines/iphs/iphs-revised-guidlines-2022/04-SHC_HWC_UHWC_IPHS_Guidelines-2022.pdf
2. https://nhm.gov.in/index1.php?lang=1 & level=1 & sublinkid=150 & lid=226

9.2 URBAN HEALTHCARE DELIVERY SYSTEM

Definition of Urban Area (As Per Census 2011)
❏ All places with a municipality, corporation, cantonment board or notified town area committee, etc.
❏ All other places which satisfy the following criteria:
  - A minimum population of 5,000
  - At least 75% of the male main working population engaged in nonagricultural pursuits; and
  - A density of population of at least 400 persons per sq. km.

Factors Contributing to Urban Vulnerability
❏ The harsh urban environment
❏ Lack of social networks/supports

Delivery Mechanism of Community Health Services

- Monetization of basic needs
- Limited access to social security schemes.

Healthcare Delivery System in Urban Area (Fig. 9.1)

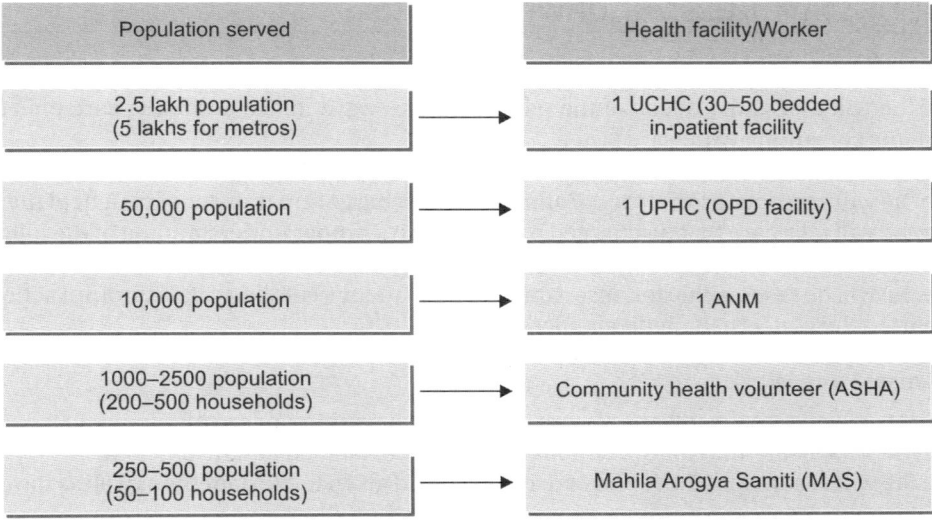

Fig. 9.1: Healthcare delivery system in urban area.

UPHC are being upgraded as UPHCs-HWCs. These centers would provide the same 12 packages of services which to be delivered by every Health and Wellness Centers. UPHCs with indoor beds already conducting deliveries can continue to function as 24 x 7 UPHCs-HWCs. Specialist UPHC/Polyclinic (Urban) are being built **(Fig. 9.2)**.

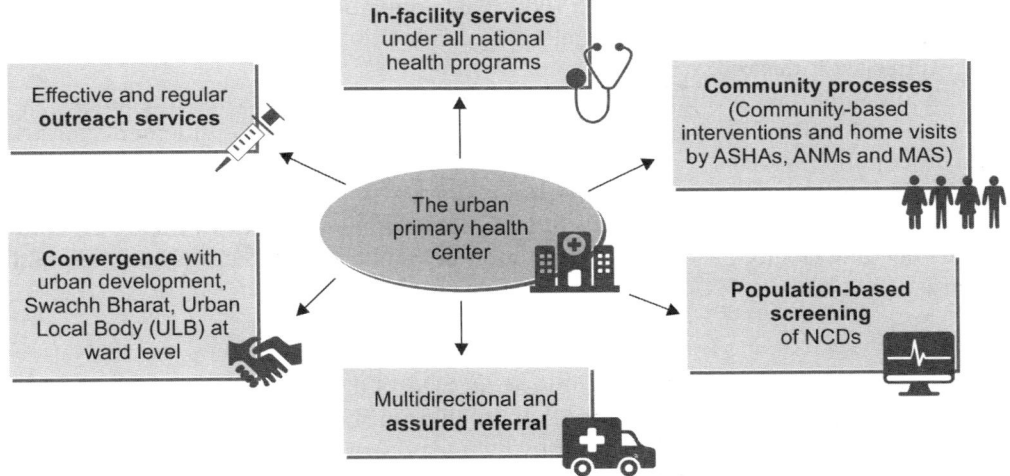

Fig. 9.2: Basic health services available at UPHC.

In addition to basic health services, the UPHC should also address social and environmental determinants in its catchment area through the ASHA and MAS, supported by the ANM and public health manager. The UPHC should also establish linkages with the ICDS system, homeless shelters, housing programs, and other relevant stakeholders so as to enable non-medical services, particularly for its vulnerable population.

ROLE OF STAFF NURSE OF UHWC

Clinical Work
- She/he will assess the needs of the patients in the ward, make a nursing care plan for all patients consulting with ward sister.
- She/he will give direct patient care and allotted responsibility to her/him by the ward sister.
- She/he will carry out procedures of admission, discharge and transfer of patient of the ward.
- She/he will take care that discharged patients have a proper understanding of the follow-up procedures and details of the diet, medication, exercise, etc.
- She/he will be responsible for observation of the patient's condition, take prompt action and report to the concerned medical officer.

Administrative Work
- She/he will ensure that all articles are sterilized, all equipment are maintained.
- She/he will ensure that the specimens are collected, labeled and dispatched.
- She/he will ensure that the reports are received and given to the patients as well as the doctor is informed.
- She/he will maintain all records and ensure the confidentiality of the patients.
- She/he will support and guide the ASHAs working in the HWC area.

URBAN ASHA
- Urban ASHA (USHA: Urban Social Health Activist)
- Each urban ASHA will cater area with 1000–2500 population. She preferably should be the resident of the "slum clusters" and belong to a vulnerable group. Formal education of at least 10th class is desired.
- She should undertake a vulnerability assessment of the households in her area.
- Her essential task to create awareness on social determinants and entitlements for health and other public services.
- She fulfills her role through **five activities**: Home visits, attending the Urban Health and Nutrition Day, visits to the health facility (to accompany pregnant women, sick child or others needing facility-based care), promotion of Mahila Arogya Samitis and maintaining records.

Role
- **Awareness generation:** Create awareness on factors that determine health status and entitlements related to health and other related public services, e.g. nutrition, basic sanitation and hygienic practices, healthy living and working conditions, information on existing health services and facilities and the need for timely access to health services.
- **Counseling:** Counsel women, families and adolescents on birth preparedness, the importance of safe delivery, breastfeeding and complementary feeding, immunization, contraception, substance misuse, prevention of domestic violence and sexual violence.

- **Curative care and supplies:** ASHA provides community level curative care for ailments such as diarrhea, fevers, childhood illnesses, nutrition, etc.
- **Community mobilization:** ASHAs mobilize the community and facilitate people's access to health services available at health centers for services including institutional delivery, immunizations, antenatal care (ANC), postnatal care (PNC) and related activities.
- **MAS coordination:** She will work with the Mahila Arogya Samiti to promote convergent action by the committee on the social determinants of health.
- **Information:** The ASHA will provide information on births and deaths in her area and any unusual health problems/disease outbreaks.

MAHILA AROGYA SAMITI (MAS)

- One MAS is group of 10–15 community women and it will be per 50–100 households. It is formed in slum and slum-like areas.
- MAS is coordinated by Urban ASHA.
- Addresses local issues related to health, nutrition, water, sanitation and social determinants of health at slum level.
- Groups will conduct monthly meetings to discuss issues faced by the community.
- To provide support and facilitate the work of community health workers like ASHA and other frontline Healthcare providers that form a crucial interface between the community and health institutions
- To organize or facilitate community level services and improve referral linkages to health services for maternal, newborn, child health and nutrition (MNCHN) issues and other related services for improved water, sanitation and hygiene (WASH), adolescent health, communicable and noncommunicable disease control.

BIBLIOGRAPHY

1. http://qi.nhsrcindia.org/cms-detail/nuhm-guidelines/MTA5
2. https://nhm.gov.in/index1.php?lang=1 & level=2 & sublinkid=1232 & lid=329
3. https://nhsrcindia.org/sites/default/files/202107/Guidelines%20for%20Organizing%20UPHC%20Services.pdf

9.3 IPHS FOR SC/HWC, PHC AND CHC

- To meet all these national and international commitments, it is essential for public health facilities to deliver quality services through defined standards known as the Indian Public Health Standards (IPHS).
- It provides guidance on the health system components such as infrastructure, human resource, drugs, diagnostics, equipment, quality and governance requirements for delivering health services at these facilities.
- IPHS implementation is the state's/UTs responsibility with technical support from MoHFW. IPHS does not define the implementation process.
- IPHS earlier launched in 2012 and now have been revised and launched in 2022.

Objectives of IPHS Standards

- To define uniform benchmark to ensure high quality services that are accountable, responsive, and sensitive to the needs of the community.
- To specify the minimum assured (essential) and achievable (desirable) services that are expected to be provided at different levels of public health facilities.
- To provide guidance on health systems strengthening components which includes architectural design of facilities, human resources for health, drugs, diagnostics, equipment, administrative and logistical support services to improve the overall health-related outcomes
- To achieve and maintain an acceptable standard of quality of care at public health facilities
- To facilitate monitoring and supervision of the facilities
- To provide guidance and tools for governance, leadership and evaluation.

The 2022 IPHS guidelines have been framed for:
- Sub-district Hospitals (SDH) and District Hospitals (DH)
- Community Health Centers (CHC)—rural and urban
- Health and wellness center—Primary health center (PHC)—rural and urban, including multispecialty UPHC (Polyclinics) in urban areas
- Health and wellness center—Sub-health center (SHC)—rural and urban.

Note: IPHS prescribes norms for allopathic services. However, AYUSH services have been retained in IPHS 2022 as desirable. The HRH, medicines, and other inputs required for AYUSH services shall be given by Ministry of AYUSH.

IPHS STANDARDS FOR HWC

Types/Categories of HWCs
- Health and wellness centers—primary health center:
  - HWC-PHC in rural areas
  - HWC- UPHC in urban areas
- Health and wellness centers—sub-health center:
  - Health and wellness center—sub-health center in rural areas
  - Urban health and wellness center in urban areas.

Population Norms for HWC-SHC and UHWC
- **HWC-SHC (rural):** In rural areas, one sub-health center is established for every 5000 populations in plain areas and 3000 populations in hilly/tribal/desert areas.
- **UHWC (urban):** In urban areas one Urban-HWC per 15,000-20,000 population caters predominantly to poor and vulnerable populations, residing in slums or other such pockets.
  - The healthcare services to be provided at these centers include health promotion, early identification, ensuring treatment adherence, follow-up care, ensuring continuity of care by appropriate referrals, optimal home and community follow-up, disease surveillance, and health promotion and prevention for the expanded range of CPHC services.
  - The twelve packages of CPHC are given in the Chapter 9.1.
  - In addition to providing clinical services, HWCs are also to be utilized as a platform for teleconsultation and expanding the range of diagnostics.

Infrastructure

- All the HWCs should be located in easily accessible area by the communities.
- Planning and provision of HWC-SHC and UHWCs takes into account factors affecting access such as geographical spread, access within the community, road connectivity and the 'time to care' approach (within 30 minutes of reach).
- The Urban HWCs should be located preferably within 1 kilometer radius from the periphery of under-served population in urban slums, vulnerable pockets, and temporary settlements in cities and peri-urban areas, which are the prime focus in the urban areas.

Waste Management

- Each healthcare facility should ensure that there is a designated central waste collection room situated within its premises for storage of biomedical waste till the waste is picked.
- Availability of dedicated biomedical waste disposal facility/deep burial pit along with septic tank and soaking pit should be ensured in the health and wellness centers. Panchayat/ULB should make arrangements for disposal of general/municipal waste. It should also be ensured that disposal of human anatomical waste, soiled waste and biotechnology waste is done within 48 hours.
- As per Biomedical Waste Management Rules and Guidelines 2016, deep burial pits need to be constructed only at such HWC-SHC/UHWCs where the common biomedical treatment plant is situated at a distance of more than 75 kms.

Oxygen Delivery Systems in HWC-SHC/UHWC

Sl. No.	Facility type	Bed capacity	B type (1500 L oxygen capacity) oxygen cylinder	Oxygen concentrator (10 LPM)
1	HWC-SHC/UHWC	2 (Day care)	3	1

HR at HWC-SHC

Sl. No.	Human resource required	Required numbers
1.	Community health officer (CHO)	1
2.	Multipurpose health worker	1 + Male + 1 Female

Sanitation and security services can be hired/outsourced.

There should be one ASHA per 1000 population or one ASHA per habitation in tribal, hilly and desert areas should be attached with the HWC as part of the entire team.

HR at UHWC

Sl. No.	Human resource	Required numbers
1.	Medical officer	1
2.	Staff nurse	1
3.	MPW (Male)	1
4.	Sanitary staff*	1
5.	Security staff**	1

*Sanitation and security services** can be hired/outsourced

One ASHA per 2000 population and one ANM per 10,000 population should be attached as part of the entire team in urban areas.

JAN AROGYA SAMITI

- The Jan Arogya Samiti (JAS) serves as an institutional platform of HWC in both rural and urban areas, for community participation in its management, governance and ensuring accountability, with respect to provision of healthcare services and amenities.
- They support AB-HWC team in working with VHSNCs/MAS, and serve as an umbrella, providing mentorship for Health Promotion and Action on Social and Environmental Determinants of Health, in community level activities of National Health Programs and other community interventions.
- JAS also act as Grievance Redressal Platform for families who access healthcare services at AB-HWCs, ensuring availability and accountability for quality services.
- JAS facilitate and support Gram Panchayats/Urban Local Bodies (ULBs) of the area in undertaking health planning.
- At the facility level, the JAS members will identify gaps related to physical infrastructure, services (essential and desirable), human resources for health, drugs, and diagnostics at HWC level based on the prescribed standards.
- Under the Ayushman Bharat, AB-HWC-SHCs are provided ₹ 50,000 as untied fund (increased amount from 20,000 to 50,000). This untied fund is to be managed by Jan Arogya Samiti.
- Rogi Kalyan Samiti at PHC level is also being reformed as JAS.

List of Diagnostic Tests and Equipment at HWC-SHC and UHWC

Essential

Hemoglobin, hCG, urine test, blood sugar, malaria test, HIV, dengue, cervical cancer, iodine, water testing for fecal contamination and chlorination, HbsAg test for Hep B, filariasis, syphilis, sputum for AFB, sickle cell rapid test, NESTROFT, solubility test.

Desirable

Screening test for G6PD enzyme deficiency, blood test for sickle cell anemia and thalassemia, clotting factor, lipid profile, test for diabetes like glucose tolerance test (GTT) and glycosylated hemoglobin (HbA1C), tests for TB, typhoid, cholera, diphtheria, kala-azar, tests for syphilis and other STIs, pap smear, troponin–I, kidney function test, liver function test, stool examination for ova/cyst and even occult blood.

IPHS STANDARDS FOR PHC/UPHC

Types/Categories of PHC/UPHC

- **HWC-PHCs:** Ideally, for rural areas, the states should aspire to make all PHCs functional as 24 × 7 facilities. However, there is a need to prioritize PHCs conducting deliveries to function as 24 × 7 HWC-PHCs. All other PHCs should continue to provide routine care along with health interventions services.
- **Urban HWC-PHCs:** In urban areas, assured round-the-clock emergency and secondary care services are readily available. Thus primary health centers are expected to provide routine OPD care along with preventive and promotive health interventions and function

Delivery Mechanism of Community Health Services

as UPHCs-HWCs. However, the UPHCs with indoor beds already conducting deliveries can continue to function as 24 × 7 UPHCs-HWCs.
- **Specialist UPHC/Polyclinic (Urban):** Multispecialty UPHC/Polyclinics in urban areas should be established with the aim to further reduce morbidity and mortality by providing specialist services on ambulatory/daycare basis. Such polyclinic services would be limited to outpatient care.

Population Norms for HWC-PHC

Sl. No.	Type of PHC facility	Plain (population)	Hilly and tribal areas (population)
1.	Rural PHC	30,000	20,000
2.	Urban PHC	50,000	–
3.	Polyclinic	2.5–3 lakh	–

Package of services and waste management-related norms similar to IPHS standards of HWC.

Bed Requirement at Primary Health Centers

	PHC		UPHC		24 × 7 PHC/UPHC	
No. of beds	Essential	Desirable	Essential	Desirable	Essential	Desirable
	2 beds	4 beds	2 daycare beds	4 daycare beds	6 beds	4 beds

Note: Desirable bed will be over and above the essential beds.

Oxygen Delivery Systems in Primary Health Facility-HWC

Sl. No.	Facility type	Bed capacity	B Type (1500 L oxygen capacity) cylinder	Oxygen concentrator (10 liters)
1.	Primary health center (Rural)	6	4	1
2.	Primary health center (Urban)	6 (Daycare)	4	1
3.	Primary health center/UPHC (24 × 7)	10	5	1

Human Resources

HR	PHC E	PHC D	UPHC E	UPHC D	Polyclinic E	Polyclinic D	24 x 7 PHC* E	24 x 7 PHC* D	24 x 7 UPHC* E	24 x 7 UPHC* D	Remarks
MO MBBS	1	1	2	–	2	–	2	1	2	1	*One doctor round the clock
MO Ayush	–	1	–	–	–	–	–	1	–	–	
MO Dental	–	1	–	1	1	–	–	1	–	1	
*Specialist for Medicine, Obstetrics and Gynecology, Pediatrics, Ophthalmology, Dermatology and Psychiatry	–	–	–	–	1*	#	–	–	–	–	* These specialists are on rotational basis # Option to add more specialties as per need and availability.

Delivery Mechanism of Community Health Services

HR	PHC E	PHC D	UPHC E	UPHC D	Polyclinic E	Polyclinic D	24x7 PHC* E	24x7 PHC* D	24x7 UPHC* E	24x7 UPHC* D	Remarks
Staff nurses	2	1	1	1	2	–	7*	–	7*	–	*1 in IPD in each shift including FP services +1 for labor deliver recovery in each shift +1 for OPD including NCD screening
Pharmacist	1	–	1	–	1	1*	1	1*	1	1*	1 Allopathy (Pharmacist) +1* Storekeeper
Medical laboratory technologist/lab technician	1	–	1	–	1	–	2	1	2	1	
Optometrist/ophthalmic assistant/vision technician	–	1	–	1	1	–	–	1	–	1	
Health worker (female)/ANM	1*	–	5**	–	5**	–	1*	–	5**	–	*For Subcenter of PHC ** 1 ANM for every 10,000 population
Health worker/health assistant (Male)	1	–	–	–	–	–	1	–	–	–	No male Health Assistant in urban areas
Health assistant (female)/lady health visitor	1	–	1	–	1	–	1	–	1	–	
Health educator/counsellor	–	1	–	1	1	–	–	1	–	1	
Dental assistant*	–	1	–	1	–	1	–	1	–	1	*Health assistant Male or any other staff can be trained to support dentists.
Cold chain/vaccine logistic assistant	–	1	–	1	–	1	1	–	1	–	If the PHC/UPHC is a cold chain point, there should be a cold chain/vaccine logistic assistant, or such work can also be handled by health worker or any other staff
Physiotherapist	–	–	–	–	1	–	–	1	–	1	
Public health manager	–	–	1	–	1	–	–	–	1	–	
Dresser	1	–	1	–	–	–	1	–	1	–	
LDC–1/Accountant	1	–	1	–	1	–	1	–	1	–	

Delivery Mechanism of Community Health Services

HR	PHC		UPHC		Polyclinic		24 x 7 PHC*		24 x 7 UPHC*		Remarks
	E	D	E	D	E	D	E	D	E	D	
Data entry operator	1	–	1	–	1	–	1	–	1	–	
Sanitation staff	1	–	1	–	2	–	4*	–	4*	–	*2 Morning+ 1 Evening + 1 Night–at least one female

Note:
- The number of HR indicated as desirable is over and above the HR indicated as essential.
- All the HR indicated under the support staff is to be only hired in-house, if the related services are not outsourced.

Compliance with Statutory Norms

The following needs to be adhered to:
- No objection certificate from the Fire Authority
- Compliance with state by-laws and the National Building Code (NBC) for all infrastructure
- Authorization under the revised Biomedical Waste (Management and Handling Rules), 2016 (amended in 2018).
- Seismic safety guidelines
- Registration of Births and Deaths Act
- Consumer Protection Act
- Drugs and Cosmetics Act
- Indian Medical Council Act and the Code of Medical Ethics
- Indian Nursing Council Act
- Pharmacy Act
- Medical Termination of Pregnancy Act
- Persons with disability Act
- PCPNDT Act
- Mental Health Act
- Narcotics and Psychotropic Substances Act
- Excise permit to store spirits
- Right to Information Act

List of Diagnostic Tests at Primary Health Center

Essential
- Hemoglobin, total leukocyte count, differential leukocyte count, platelet count, complete blood count, erythrocyte sedimentation rate, blood group and Rh typing, blood cross matching, peripheral blood film, reticulocyte count, absolute eosinophil count
- Bleeding time and clotting time
- Sickling test for screening of sickle cell anemia, sickle cell test rapid for screening of sickle cell anemia (strip test)
- NESTROFT Test for screening of thalassemia
- DCIP test for screening HbE hemoglobinopathy
- Screening test for G6PD enzyme deficiency

- MP slide method, Malaria rapid test
- Human chorionic gonadotropin (hCG) (urine test for pregnancy)
- Urine test for pH, specific gravity, leukocyte esterase, glucose, bilirubin, urobilinogen, ketone, protein, nitrite, urine microscopy, urine for microalbumin
- Stool for ova and cyst, stool for occult blood
- RPR/VDRL test for syphilis
- HIV test (antibodies 1/2 and HIV 1/2)
- Hepatitis B surface antigen test, HCV antibody test (anti HCV)
- Sputum, pus, etc. for AFB, typhoid test (IgM)
- Blood sugar, glucose tolerance test (GTT)
- S. bilirubin (T), S. bilirubin direct and indirect
- Serum creatinine, blood urea, SGPT, SGOT, S. alkaline phosphatase, S. total protein, S. albumin and AG ratio, S. globulin
- S. total cholesterol, S. triglycerides, S.VLDL, S.HDL, S. LDL, S. uric acid
- Glycosylated hemoglobin (HbA1C), serum calcium
- Wet mount and Gram stain for RTI/STD
- Throat swab (Albert stain) for diphtheria
- Stool for hanging drop for vibrio cholera
- Visual inspection acetic acid (VIA), Pap smear
- rK39 for Kala azar
- TB–Mantoux
- Troponin-I.

Desirable

D-Dimer, S. Sodium, S. Potassium, Magnesium, test for filariasis, S. TSH (including for newborn screening), CRP (including newborn).

IPHS STANDARDS FOR CHC

Types/Categories of CHC/UCHC

- **Non-FRU CHCs (rural):** Non-FRU CHCs are those that provide essential services including preventive, promotive, curative, palliative, and rehabilitative services, etc. Curative services include normal delivery, stabilization of common emergencies, etc. Non-FRU CHCs in rural areas will have 30 essential beds.
- **FRU CHCs (rural and urban):** FRU CHCs, in addition to the above services, provide specialized care which can be rendered through specialists (physicians, surgeons, obstetricians, pediatricians, and anesthesiologists) and the accompanying infrastructure (functional operation theatre and blood storage unit). Both elective and emergency surgical services of secondary level care shall be provided. FRU CHCs in rural areas will have 50 beds (30 essential and 20 desirable) while in FRU UCHCs in urban areas will have 50 beds for having 2.5 lakh population while 100 beds where having 5 lakh population.

Note:
- Thus, while CHCs in rural areas can be either non-FRU CHC or FRU CHC, the UCHC in urban areas will function only as FRU UCHCs.
- It is desirable to establish a 10 bedded NRC at FRU CHC and UCHC to manage the nutritional disorders in closer proximity of the community.

- A six bedded emergency area in 50 bedded FRU CHC/UCHC, 11 beds for 100 bedded FRU-UCHC and a four bedded emergency area in 30 bedded non-FRU CHC and FRU CHC should be established to manage the common emergencies.
- Blood storage units (BSUs) should be licensed and available in FRU-CHCs.

Population Norms for CHCs
- Community health center in rural areas (CHC) is to be established for a population norm of 80,000 (in hilly and tribal areas) and 1,20,000 (in plains) and/or time to care approach.
- The CHC in urban areas (UCHC) is set up as a secondary care referral center in metro cities with a population of 5 lakh and above and population of 2.5 lakh in non-metro cities.

BIBLIOGRAPHY
1. https://nhm.gov.in/images/pdf/guidelines/iphs/iphs-revised-guidlines-2022/04-SHC_HWC_UHWC_IPHS_Guidelines-2022.pdf
2. https://nhm.gov.in/images/pdf/guidelines/iphs/iphs-revised-guidlines-2022/03_PHC_IPHS_Guidelines-2022.pdf
3. https://nhm.gov.in/images/pdf/guidelines/iphs/iphs-revised-guidlines-2022/02-CHC_IPHS_Guidelines-2022.pdf

9.4 FINANCIAL AND INVENTORY MANAGEMENT AT PUBLIC HEALTH FACILITIES

FINANCIAL MANAGEMENT
- It is defined as a financial statement which is prepared and approved by the management in advance for a period of time, which determines all future actions of the organization.
- Budgets are broadly classified on the basis of time, function and flexibility.

Advantages of Budgeting
- Budgets are effective means of communication for all future organizational plans to all people, in monetary and financial terms.
- A pre-decided and approved budget serves as an effective tool for monitoring the ongoing operations.
- It reduces wastage and losses by identifying wasteful expenditures well in advance and rectifying them and help to control such activities.
- Budgets, when drawn up through participation, it encourage and develop team spirit which in turn results in collective responsibility towards excellence.
- It evaluates the performance of managers.

Cost
- It is the amount of expenditure (actual or notional) incurred on a thing.
- **Fixed costs:** The costs which remain constant and do not depend of the amount of output.
- **Variable costs:** Costs which are directly dependent on the quantity of output, such as cost of direct labor, direct material, etc.

- **Gross national income (GNI):** Also known as Gross National Product (GNP). It is gross income generated from within the country as also net income received from abroad.
- **Per capita income:** Average income earned per person in a given area in a specified year. It is calculated by dividing the area's total income by its total population.
- **Gross domestic product (GDP):** It is gross income generated within a country, i.e., it excludes net income received from abroad.
- **Purchasing power parity (PPP):** It is defined as the number of units of a country's currency required to buy the same amount of goods and services in the domestic market as one dollar would buy in the USA.
- **Pricing:** It is a process of fixing the value that a manufacturer will receive in the exchange of services and goods.
- **Types of pricing method:** The pricing method is divided into two parts
  1. **Cost-oriented pricing method:** It is the base for evaluating the price of the finished goods, and most of the company apply this method to calculate the cost of the product.
     - **Cost-plus pricing:** In this pricing, the manufacturer calculates the cost of production sustained and includes a fixed percentage (also known as mark-up) to obtain the selling price.
     - **Mark up pricing:** The fixed number or a percentage of the total cost of a product is added to the product's end price to get the selling price of a product.
     - **Target-returning pricing:** The company or a firm fix the cost of the product to achieve the rate of return on investment.
  2. **Market-oriented pricing method:** It is determined on the base of market research
     - **Value pricing:** The company produces a product that is high in quality but low in price.
     - **Perceived-value pricing:** In this method, the producer establishes the cost taking into consideration the customer's point of view.
     - **Going-rate pricing:** In this method, the company reviews the competitor's rate as a foundation in deciding the rate of their product.
     - **Differential pricing:** This method is applied when the pricing has to be differ according to the area, region, group, time, etc.
     - **Cost-benefit analysis:** In this method, the economic benefits of any program are compared with the cost of that program. The benefits are expressed in monetary terms to determine whether a given program is economically sound, and to select the best out of several alternate programs.
     - **Cost effective analysis:** This is a more important tool for application in the health field than cost-benefit analysis. It is similar to cost-benefit analysis except that benefit, instead of being expressed in monetary terms is expressed in terms of results achieved, e.g. number of lives saved or cases of disease detected.

Inflation

- It is a general rise in the price level of an economy over a period of time. When the general price level rises, each unit of currency buys fewer goods and services; consequently, inflation reflects a reduction in the purchasing power per unit of money.
- **Disinflation:** Reduction in the rate of inflation
- **Deflation:** Persistent decrease in the price level (negative inflation)
- **Reflation:** Price level increases when the economy recovers from recession based on value of inflation
- **Measurement** of inflation through different index.

- **Wholesale price index (WPI):** It is estimated by the Ministry of Commerce and Industry.
- **Consumer price index (CPI):** It is calculated by taking price changes for each item in the predetermined lot of goods and averaging them. (it is useful to calculate modified Prasad classification)
- **Producer price index:** It is based on the selling prices over time received by domestic producers for their output.

Steps in the Tendering System while Undertaking Purchases
- Specifications of the item to be purchased are established carefully.
- A vendor list is identified and competitive bids are invited from vendors through an open advertisement, which should also mention the technical specifications of the item, modalities of payment and any other terms and conditions.
- Comparative statement is drawn up of the quality, price and support services.
- Bids are evaluated and contract is awarded to lowest responsible bidder.
- Price negotiation with the selected vendor and issue of purchase order and supply of items.
- Inventory action (including inspection and issue to concerned department.

INVENTORY MANAGEMENT

Definition: It is method of maintenance of stock at a level at which purchasing and stocking costs are the lowest possible without interference with supply.
- Inventory control is a management tool which ensures that the optimal quantity of items is present at the facilities in accordance with the need and also at the most economical cost. It is also necessary to control that there are no stock outs or overstocking.
- In a Healthcare establishment some inventory of essential drugs, instruments and supplies has to be maintained to ensure that Healthcare to patients does not suffer.
- Techniques of inventory control are:
  - ABC analysis
  - VED analysis
  - SDE analysis
  - FSN analysis

ABC Analysis (Always Better Control)
- ABC analysis allows the management to decide which items require most efforts in controlling.
- Classification of items into A, B, and C is based on annual consumption unit.
- **"A" items:** 10% of items consuming 70% of budget
- **"B" items:** 20% of items consuming 20% of budget
- **"C" items:** 70% of items consuming 10% of budget

Class	Degree of control	Safety stock with more re-order
A	Tight	Low
B	Moderate	Moderate
C	Loose	Large stock with less frequent re-order

- Explanation: Class A items are the costliest item, so, it is required to monitor closely and kept under strict control.

- If such items are bought in large quantities then scarce finances will be used which ultimately leads to high operating cost of the hospital.
- It is very useful for allocation of funds and human resources and also maintenance of high inventory turnover rate.
- Here importance is only given to the money factor only and not to the other factors.

VED Analysis (V-Vital, E-Essential, D-Desirable)
- It is based on the criticality of the inventories.
- Sometimes item may be relatively inexpensive but may still be so important that the health service delivery may be critically impaired in its absence.
- **Vital (V):** The large stock of medicine in this group is maintained and must be available. These are critically needed for the survival of the patient.
- **Essential (E):** In this group drugs included which required during lower critically situations, so they may be available in the hospital.
- **Desirable (D):** These required only in minimum stock.
- **ABC-VED matrix analysis:** ABC-VED matrix is formulated by combining ABC and VED analysis which can be used for prioritization. It is better than individual analysis:

	V	E	D
A	AV	AE	AD
B	BV	BE	BD
C	CV	CE	CD

Intervention can be categorized into 3 groups.
- Category I: AV + AE + AD + BV + CV
- Category II: BE + CE + BD
- Category III: CD

- **Category I:**
  - It includes all the vital and costly items
  - Its shortage may affect the functioning of the hospital adversely, on the contrary over stocking may lead to financial loss.
  - It requires **strict management**.
  - It is high priority group, requires greatest attention.
- **Category II:**
  - It includes essential but less costly items
  - It is under **moderate management**.
- **Category III:**
  - This category is least costly so, under **simple management**.
  - Though medicines from this group are **desirable but would not affect** the functioning of the hospital (even medicines are not available for a long time).
  - **SDE analysis:** All inventories can be classified according to their availability into the three following groups and that will help us to manage the inventory accordingly.
    - S = Scare items
    - D = Different items
    - E = Easily available items

- Scare items require stringent control while easily available can be managed with simple management.
  - **FSN analysis:** It is based on quantity and rate of consumption. Fast moving items should be frequently reorder while slow or not moving items must be ordered cautiously to avoid overstocking and related other issues.
    - F = Fast moving items
    - S = Slow moving items
    - N = Not moving items

Reordering System

- **Fixed order size system** (Q-system): The size of order (Q) is fixed for but time between orders (interval) may vary.
- **Fixed order interval system** (T-system): The interval between orders is constant, while size of the order vary depending on the need.
  - Logistics management is defined as the systematic and scientific process of planning, implementing and controlling the efficient and effective flow and storage of resources (goods and services) from point of origin to the point of consumption in order to meet the customer's requirements.

Important Economic Terms in Inventory Control

- **Purchase cost:** It is the actual cost paid for the purchase of materials and stores, and the aim should be to reduce this as far as possible without compromising on the quality and quantity of items purchased
- **Ordering costs** are costs incurred by an organization in placing an order for material with a supplier
- **Inventory carrying cost** are the hidden costs and pertain to maintenance of a large inventory/stock.
  - For better understanding, one example for vaccine stock management is given in **Figure 9.3**.

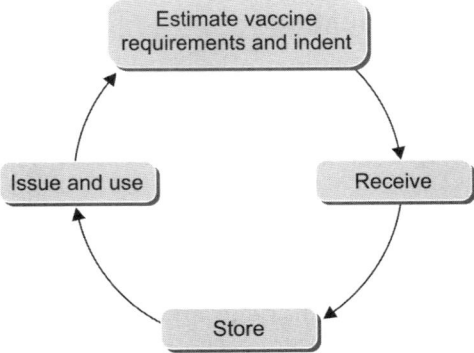

Fig. 9.3: Logistic management cycle.

Important Terminology

- **Stock out:** A condition when no stock of a vaccine or other supplies are available.
- **Inadequate stock:** Stock which is less than the buffer stock, i.e. less than 25% for vaccines and syringes.

- **Excess stock:** Stock which is more than the requirement for one month including the buffer stock, i.e. more than 125% for vaccines and syringes.
- **Lead time:** The time between ordering of new stock and its receipt. Lead time varies depending upon the speed of delivery, availability and reliability of transport and sometimes the weather.
- **Buffer stock:** It serves as a cushion or buffer against emergencies, major fluctuations in vaccine demands or unexpected transport delays. It is 25% extra for vaccines and syringes. Relationship between minimum, maximum and buffer stocks is shown in **Figure 9.4**.

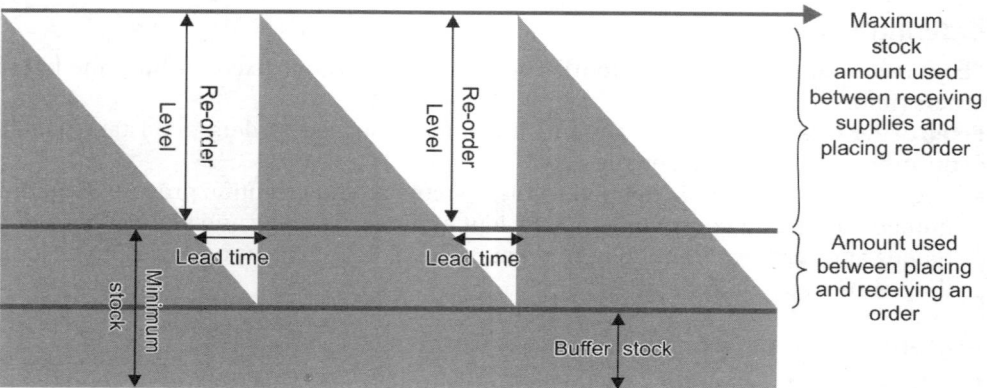

Fig. 9.4: Relationship between minimum, maximum and buffer stocks.

Example: If monthly requirement of pentavalent vaccine at a PHC is 380 doses and lead time is 1 week.
- Buffer stock = 95 doses (25% of requirement)
- Minimum stock (Re-order level) = lead time + buffer stock = 95 + 95 = 190 doses
- Maximum stock level = minimum stock + stock used between orders (3 weeks stock) = 190 + 285 = 475 doses.

Concept of Flow of Stores Accounting

- Issue of stock is of utmost importance in any Healthcare setup since the problems of obsolete items, expired medicines and old stocks are faced in a hospital.
- Different methods:
  - **First in, first out (FIFO):** Material from the oldest stock is issued first with the view to turn over the stock.
  - **Last in, first out (LIFO):** Materials which are received last are issued first in this case, but it is not recommended in Healthcare establishments.
  - **Specific cost method:** Provides the most realistic valuation of inventory stock and physical stock-taking of stores can be done any time of the year.
  - **Average cost method:** Average cost of each item issued from stores/received at stores is assessed and this value is taken for maintaining the cost of inventory held by the organization.

Role of Nurse in Inventory Control

- Keeping an adequate amount of equipment and supplies in the ward.
- Ensure timely supply and proper storage.

- Make sure that equipment and supplies are in good conditions and also put in a requisition for repair and maintenance when needed.
- To be observant of waste and misuse.
- Set a standard for the quantity of each item to be maintained in the ward all the time.
- Maintain stock register.

BIBLIOGRAPHY

1. Immunization Handbook for Medical Officers, 2017, Ministry of Health and Family Welfare, New Delhi, India.
2. Sikdar SK, Agarwal AK, Das JK. Inventory analysis by ABC and VED analysis in medical stores depot of CGHS, New Delhi. Health and Population. 1996;19(4):165-72.
3. Vaz FS, Ferreira AM, Kulkarni MS, Motghare DD, Pereira-Antao I. A study of drug expenditure at a tertiary care hospital: An ABC-VED analysis. J Health Manag. 2008;10:119–27.

9.5 SUMMARY OF DIFFERENT INDIAN SYSTEMS OF MEDICINE (AYUSH)

AYUSH

Ayurveda, Yoga and Naturopathy, Unani, Siddha, Homeopathy and Sowa Rigpa

Ayurveda

- Ayurveda means knowledge of life.
- It is derived from Atharveda.
- It is practiced throughout the India.
- Ayurveda conceives life as a perfect union of the body, mind, soul, and senses.
- The human body is seen as a complex matrix of interconnected systems in Ayurveda: a combination of the physiological entities, the humors, the structural components, the tissues, and the excretions, or waste materials.
- Thus, the living man is perceived as a conglomeration of the three humors (Vatta, Pitta and Kapha), seven basic tissues (Rasa or plasma/lymph fluid, Mansa or muscle, Meda or fat, Rakta or blood, Asthi or bone, Majja or marrow, and Shukra or semen) and the waste products of the body (Mala or stool, Mutra or urine, and Sweda or sweat).
- Panchamahabhutas are the five great elements that together make every element of this universe. These elements include Space, Wind, Fire, Water, and Earth.
- **Existence of these elements in the human body:**
    - **Air (Vayu):** It represents the gaseous form of matter present in the body. It also includes the energy formed by the several movements within the body like heartbeat, inspiration, and expiration. This element keeps the fire burning in the body.
    - **Space (Akasha):** It represents the hollowness of several parts like lungs, bones, mouth, etc. It helps in completing the process of transportation and communication.
    - **Fire (Tejas):** Fire helps in the transformation and conversion of various matters in the body. It is responsible to maintain the temperature of the body, metabolism, sight power, and mental power. It plays a major role in converting food to fats and muscle.

- **Water (Aap):** It represents various fluids or liquid elements in the body such as saliva, gastric juice, lymph, blood, and most importantly water. Water is one of the most basic and important elements that help in human survival.
- **Earth (Prithvi):** Everything solid in our body is represented by this element. Solid helps in stabilizing the water.
- A balance of several elements is required to avoid sickness and keep the human body healthy by restoring the balance of disturbed body-mind matrix with proper diet, right life-routine, administration of drugs, and resorting to preventive Rasayana and Panchakarma therapy.
- To bring back the balance of three doshas in the body, Ayurveda advises to follow various purification and medical processes called **"Panchakarmas"**.
- **Dhanvantri** is **God of Ayurveda**.
- **Atreya** is known as great Indian physician and teacher.
- **Charak** is **father of Indian Medicine**
- **Susruta** is **father of Indian Surgery**.

Yoga

- It aims to attain self-realization, by improving the inherent power of an individual in a balanced way.
- The very first mention of Yoga was in the Rig Veda, one of the oldest sacred texts. This spiritual discipline is based on a subtle science that aims to bring about harmony between the body and the mind.
- Yoga has been derived from the Sanskrit term 'Yuj' that means 'to yoke' or simply, 'to unite'. According to the Oxford Dictionary, the word Yoga means 'union'. Therefore, it is a union of the individual spirit with the universal spirit of God. Yoga is a combination of practices, which define the way we engage with the world to create harmony. Yoga, as a discipline means:
  - To engage
  - To participate
  - To get involved
  - To connect
- **The Father of Yoga, Maharishi Patanjali** combined multiple aspects of yoga and called them "Yoga Sutras" or aphorisms. He advocated "Ashtanga Yoga"; the eight-fold path of yoga that facilitates the all-round development of human beings.
- These components are Yama, Niyama, Pratyahara, Dharana, Asana, Pranayama, Dhyana and Samadhi.
- These components bring about physical discipline, help in the regulation of breath, restraining the sense organs, and promote contemplation and meditation.
- These techniques play an important role in the prevention of diseases such as psychosomatic disorders and promote overall health. It has benefited people at large and continues to blossom with each passing day.
- Yoga works on the mind, energy and emotional levels of an individual, thus promoting physical and mental well-being.
- **Types of Yoga:**
  - Japa Yoga
  - Karma Yoga
  - Gyana Yoga

- Bhakti Yoga
- Raja Yoga
- Swara Yoga
- Kundalini
- Nadi.

Naturopathy

- Relying on the healing power of nature, naturopathy stimulates the human body's ability to heal itself.
- It is the science of disease diagnosis, treatment, and cure using natural therapies including dietetics, botanical medicine, homeopathy, fasting, exercise, lifestyle counseling, detoxification, and chelation, clinical nutrition, hydrotherapy, naturopathic manipulation, spiritual healing, environmental assessment, health promotion, and disease prevention.
- The term Naturopathy was tossed by John Scheel in 1895 and was popularized by Benedict Lust. Known as the father of modern-day naturopathy.
- According to the manifesto of the British Naturopathic Association, "Naturopathy is a system of treatment which lays emphasis on the existence of the vital curative force within the body." Hence, it aids the human system to remove the cause of disease, i.e. toxins by eliminating unwanted and unused matters from the human body for curing diseases.
- **Some salient features of naturopathy:**
  - The basic cause of the disease is the accumulation of morbid matter in the body and the treatment of all the diseases is the elimination of morbid matter from the body.
  - It is to be believed under the naturopathy system of healing, acute diseases are self-healing efforts of the body. Chronic diseases are the result of incorrect treatment and the suppression of the acute disease.
  - Naturopathy relies on the fact that nature is the greatest healer. The human body possesses the power to protect itself from diseases and retrieve it.
  - In the process of cure, the entire human body is targeted to heal the disease.
  - Naturopathy successfully heals chronic ailments and is also effective in treating them in a comparatively lesser time.
  - In Naturopathy treatment, the suppressed diseases are brought to the surface and are eliminated permanently.
  - Naturopathy successfully treats all aspects of the human body like mental, physical, social, and spiritual.
  - In Naturopathy, it is to be believed that "food is the only medicine" and "no external medications are used."
  - Naturopathy believes that performing a prayer based on one's spiritual faith is an important part of treatment.
- **Techniques and benefits of different modalities of naturopathy**
  - Diet therapy
  - Fasting therapy
  - Mud therapy
  - Hydrotherapy
  - Masso therapy
  - Acupressure
  - Acupuncture

- Chromotherapy
- Air therapy
- Magnet therapy

Greek Medicine (Unani System of Medicine)

- The Unani system of medicine originated in Greece around 2500 years ago, and its foundation was laid by the Hippocrates.
- A tradition of Graeco-Arabic medicine, Unani medicine has a herbo-animo-mineral foundation.
- It was the Arabs who introduced the Unani system to India which acquired strong roots within no time.
- However, the system suffered a major setback during the British rule, with the introduction of the Allopathic system.
- At present, India is one of the leading nations that practice the Unani system of medicines and has the largest number of institutions that focus on Unani education, research, and healthcare.
- The Unani system of medicine provides treatment of diseases of the entire human body.
- Unani has proved to be highly effective for treating chronic ailments and diseases of the liver, skin, reproductive systems, musculoskeletal and immunological disorders.
- It focuses on promotive, curative, preventive, and rehabilitative healthcare.
- The four-humor theory of Hippocrates acts as the base for the Unani system of medicine.
- It presumes the presence of four humors in the human body that are: **phlegm, blood, black bile, and yellow bile.**
- The human body comprises seven core components which are as follows:
    1. *ARKAN (ELEMENTS):* There are four elements that make up the human body: Air, Earth, Fire, and Water.
    2. *MIJAZ (TEMPERAMENT):* In the diagnosis and treatment of the Unani system, temperament acts as the base. Mijaz in Unani helps characterize a person's physical, mental, and social state and also identifies the nature of a disease.
    3. *AKLAT (HUMORS):* Humors are the fluids in the human body that produce energy, and trigger growth, nutrition, and repair. The humors also perform the function of maintaining moisture in different organs of the human body.
    4. *AAZA (ORGANS):* Azaa are the various organs that account for the effective functioning of the human body. The health of each organ affects the overall health of the body, and any disease in the organs creates an imbalance in the health equilibrium.
    5. *ARWAH (SPIRIT):* Ruh or spirit is a gaseous matter that assists in all the metabolic activities of the human body. Obtained from the inspired air, it acts as the source of energy for the effective functioning of all the organs of the body. The Ruh burns the Akhlat Latifa and produces power (quwa).
    6. *QUWA (POWER):* There are three types of Quwa: Quwa Tabiyah (Natural Power), Quwa Nafsaniyah (Psychic power), Quwa Nafsaniyah and Quwa Haywaniyah (Vital power).
    7. *AFAAL (FUNCTIONS):* Afaal is the movement and proper functioning of all the organs of the human body. When the body is healthy, it means that all organs are in proper shape and are functioning efficiently.

- ***Diagnosis:*** The diagnosis in the Unani system of medicine depends on two factors: observation and physical examination.
- Unani emphasizes on the prevention of the ailment and promotes existing health by the way of six essential factors of life, which are also known as Asbab-e- Sittah Zarooriyah. The six factors are:
    1. Air (Al Hawa)
    2. Food and Drink (Al Maakool Wa Al Mashroob)
    3. Physical exercise and repose (Harkat Wa Sukoon-E-Badani)
    4. Mental exertion and repose (Harkat Wa Sukoon-E-Nafsaani)
    5. Sleep and wakefulness (Naum Wa Yaqza, Evacuation
    6. Retention (Istifraagh Wa Ehtebaas).

Homeopathic Medicine

- **Samuel Hahneman** was German physician and known as **Father of Homeopathy**.
- Homeopathy is a combination of two Greek words: Homois and Pathos.
- Homois means similar and pathos means suffering.
- Homoeopathic medicine is based on two alternative theories:
    1. **"Like cures like"**: It is the natural law of healing that says that a substance causing symptoms of a disease in a healthy individual would cure similar symptoms in a sick individual. This doctrine is also known as **similia similibus curentur**.
    2. **"Law of minimum dose"**: Homoeopathic products are mostly diluted to an extent that it eliminates the presence of the molecules of the original substance. It is believed that a lower dose of medication results in more effectiveness.
- Homeopathic products are made from plants such as mountain herbs, minerals like white arsenic, poison ivy, and animals like crushed bees.
- These homeopathic products take the form of sugar pellets, ointments, tablets, gels, creams, and drops.
- The treatments are tailored as per the needs of each individual. This means that people with different ailments who have the same conditions can receive different treatments.
- It is practiced almost everywhere across the globe and has gained a lot of popularity in India as well. The gentleness of its cure is what makes more than 100 million people of the Indian population depend on this treatment. And, India has around a quarter of a million registered homeopathic doctors who are more than other countries across the world.
- It follows a holistic approach towards achieving the inner balance of an individual on mental, physical, emotional, and spiritual levels. Homeopathy is a time-tested therapy and continues to spread its effectiveness around the world.
- **There are 4 principles of homeopathy**:
    1. **Similia similbus curentur:** A homeopathic drug produces same set of signs and symptoms that normally disease does.
    2. **Single remedy:** Only one homeopathic drug is given at one point of time.
    3. **The minimum dose:** Minimum possible dose of drug is used.
    4. **The potentized remedy:** Drug is diluted many times.

Siddha System of Medicine

- Siddha is one of the oldest medicinal systems originated in Tamil Nadu. The word 'Siddha' is derived from a Tamil word 'Siddhi' which means 'achievement' or 'perfection'.
- The Siddha medicinal system not just focuses on treating the disease but it also takes into account the patient behavior, environmental aspects, age, habits and physical condition.
- Siddha medicine focuses on making the human body perfect.
- Siddha system has close resemblance to Ayurveda.
- The Siddha system, has faith in the fact that all the substances in the universe along with the human body comprise the five basic elements which are known as **earth, water, fire, air, and sky**.
- The food and the drugs that the human body consumes everything is composed of these five elements.
- The Siddha system regards the human body as an assortment of three humors, seven basic tissues, and waste products of the body like sweat, urine, and feces.
- The food, which is regarded as the basic building material of the human body is what gets processed into body tissue, humors, and waste products. The equilibrium of humors is deemed as health and its imbalance or disturbance gives rise to illness or disorders.
- The Siddha system also copes with the theory of salvation in life. This system's advocates believe salvation can be attained by the means of meditation and medicines.
- This system is based on three physiological component as below:
  - Air (Vaadham)
  - Fire (Pitham)
  - Earth and water (Kabam)
- It is believed that success of the treatment is depends on environment, age sex and other factors.

Sowa-Rigpa

- "Sowa-Rigpa" is commonly known as the Amchi **system of medicine.**
- It is one of the oldest, Living and well documented medical traditions of the world.
- The term 'Sowa-Rigpa' is derived from the Bhoti language which means 'Knowledge of Healing'.
- Some scholars believe that it originated from India; some say China and others consider it to have originated from Tibet itself.
- Gyud-Zi (four tantra) is the fundamental textbook of this medicine.
- The four Tantras are as follows:
  1. Root tantra
  2. Exegetical tantra
  3. Instructional tantra
  4. Subsequent tantra.
- It has been popularly practised in Tibet, Magnolia, Bhutan, some parts of China, Nepal, a few regions of India, and a few parts of the former Soviet Union, etc.
- In India, this system has been practised in Sikkim, Arunachal Pradesh, Darjeeling (West Bengal), Lahoul and Spiti (Himachal Pradesh) and the Ladakh region of Jammu and Kashmir, etc.

- Traditionally the Amchis are trained under the traditional educational system either under private *guru-shishya* **tradition or under** *gyud-pa* (lineage) system in families in which the knowledge is passed down from father to son through generations.
- Although there is clear written instruction in the four Tantra, the oral transmission of medical knowledge still remains a strong element in Tibetan Medicine.
- Influence of Ayurveda:
    1. The majority of the theory and practice of Sowa-Rigpa is similar to "Ayurveda".
    2. The first Ayurvedic influence came to Tibet during the 3rd century AD but it became popular only after the 7th century with the approach of Buddhism to Tibet.

BIBLIOGRAPHY

1. https://main.ayush.gov.in/ayush-systems/

CHAPTER 10

Fundamentals of Leadership, Supervision, and Monitoring

CHAPTER OUTLINE
10.1 Leadership
10.2 Supervision
10.3 Monitoring

10.1 LEADERSHIP

Introduction
- Professor Warren G Bennis has said that 'Leaders are people who do the right thing; managers are people who do things right.' A leader is a person who creates an inspiring vision of the future, motivates and inspires people to engage with that vision, manages delivery of the vision and coaches and builds a team, so that it is more effective at achieving the vision. Leadership brings together the skills needed to do these things. Good leadership is important for the success of any organization.
- 'Leadership' is the quality of behavior of individuals whereby they guide people or activities for organized effort.

Qualities of a Good Leader
- High energy level and stress tolerance
- Self-confidence
- Internal locus of control
- Emotional maturity
- Personal integrity
- Honesty, passion, curiosity
- Achievement orientation
- Low needs for affiliation.

Difference Between Leader and Manager

Leader	Manager
Visionary	Planner
Strategist	Controller
Politician/advocate	Supervisor
Campaigner	Monitor
Team builder	Efficient use of resources
Change agent	Status quo: refers to current status

Leadership Style

- **Motivational style:** In this style leaders employ to motivate the group members to attain their objectives.
- **Orientation-based style:** Two types: Task-oriented and people-oriented.
- **Power-based style:** It is based on the way a leader express his power. There are three types:
  - Types of leaders:
    - Authoritarian/autocratic leader
    - Democratic leader
    - Laissez-faire leader
- **Situational style:** It depends upon the need of each situation/employee. Different situational approaches are: Directing, coaching, supporting and delegating.

Autocratic Leadership

- It is an appropriate type of leadership when decisions need to be taken quickly.
- Autocratic leaders generally take decisions without considering the views of their team members, even though their views would be useful, that is why this style can be demoralizing for other team members.
- No one challenges the decisions of autocratic leaders.
- Managers possess total authority and impose their will on employees.
- This leadership style benefits employees who require close supervision.
- This type of style gives quick decisions and might quick give results but may lead to more absenteeism and staff turnover also in some instances.

Democratic or Participative Type of Leadership

- Leaders of this style make the final decisions but at the same time they include team members and consider their inputs during the decision-making process.
- Due to participation of team members in the decision-making process this type of leadership is also known as participative type of leadership.
- They encourage creativity of the team members and get them involved in various projects.
- It causes team members to feel as if their opinions matter.
- Job satisfaction and high productivity is the best result of democratic leadership.
- Though this is one of the best leadership styles, but it is not a good choice to use when we need to make a quick decision.

Laissez-faire Leadership

- In this type of leadership, team members are free to decide the way of working and to set their deadlines.
- They give all the required resources and advices as needed but they do not get involved directly.
- This type of leadership can give high job satisfaction to the team members, but it can be damaging when team members start to misuse the autonomy like wasting of time or when team members do not have the knowledge, skills or when self-motivation is lacking.
- Laissez-faire leadership can occur spontaneously when leaders do not have control over their team members.
- A laissez-faire leader lacks direct supervision of employees and fails to provide regular feedback to those under his supervision.
- Laissez-faire leadership style is more feasible to use when team members are highly experienced and trained as they requiring little supervision.

Transactional Type of Leadership

- In this type of leadership, rewards or punishments to team members are given on the basis of the performance.
- Goals are set by leaders and team members together.
- Team members always follow the direction of the leader to achieve those goals.
- The leader reviews the results and guides employees accordingly.

Transformational Type of Leadership

- This type of leadership depends on high levels of communication between leaders and team members.
- Effective communication motivates employees and thus increases their enhance productivity and efficiency.
- It requires the involvement of management to achieve the goals.

Common Leadership Approach in Health Care Setting

- **Transformational leadership:** It requires leaders to communicate their vision in a manner that is meaningful, exciting, and creates unity and collective purpose.
- **Collaborative leadership:** Collaborative healthcare leadership requires a synergistic work environment; wherein multiple parties are encouraged to work together toward the implementation of effective practices and processes.
- **Shared leadership:** It results in individual staff members adopting leadership behaviors, greater autonomy, and improved client care outcomes.
- **Distributed leadership:** Here the work is distributed amongst staff members. The advantage is that individuals complement one another's strengths and offset one another's weaknesses.
- **Ethical leadership:** A good leader must have intentions, values, and behaviors that intend no harm and respect the rights of all stakeholders.

10.2 SUPERVISION

Introduction
Supervision is the process of guiding, helping and encouraging staff to improve their performance, so that they meet the defined standards of their organization. Supervision can be either traditional or modern/supportive.

Qualities of a Supervisor
- She/He should be very familiar with the health care system prevailing in his area.
- She/He should have the ability to address both administrative and programmatic issues of the health problems.
- She/He should be committed, responsible and have strong interpersonal skills.
- She/He should have the ability to train, motivate and support staff.
- She/He must be flexible, respectful and should have hard working attitude.
- She/He should have patience to listen carefully.
- She/He should probe into the problems, analyze the situations and formulate solutions to overcome it.
- She/He should have a good understanding about field situation and out of box thinking and innovative.
- She/He should have the ability to provide and receive feedbacks after each visit and write reports.

Importance of Supervision
- It provides an opportunity for learning to fill the gaps in the knowledge or skills of the service provider.
- It helps in understanding ground realities and challenges.
- It motivates the health worker.
- Supervision helps in team building.
- Identify mistakes and help works to correct.
- It helps to find the reason behind the poor performance and help to solve them.
- Supervision also helps in making the workers aware of new guidelines.
- Supervision helps the workers relate better to the community.

Differences Between Supervision and Monitoring

Supervision	Monitoring
• Supervision is overseeing or watching over an activity or task being done by someone and ensuring that it is performed correctly	• Monitoring is the continuous review of program implementation to identify and solve problems so that activities can be implemented correctly and effectively
• Supervision deals with the performance of the people working within the program including giving them support and assessing conditions in the health facility	• Monitoring involves regular collection and analysis of information/data on aspects of the program's activities
• Supervision usually having component of monitoring	• Monitoring does not often or automatically have a supervisory element

Types of Supervision

- **Traditional supervision:** The traditional supervision is effective to some extent only as it has several shortcomings. In the traditional way of supervising, there is no guidance given to the staff in problem-solving. Thus, performance improvement of the staff is not the objective of traditional supervision.
- **Supportive supervision:** Supportive supervision is a process that promotes quality at all levels of the health system by strengthening relationships within the system, focusing on the identification and resolution of problems, optimizing the allocation of resources, promoting high standards, teamwork and better two-way communication. Supportive supervision involves directing and supporting healthcare workers in order to enhance their skills, knowledge and abilities with the goal of improving health outcomes for the population they manage. It is an ongoing relationship between healthcare workers and their supervisors.
  - "Supportive supervision is a process of helping staff to improve their own work performance continuously. It is carried out in a respectful and non-authoritarian way with a focus on using supervisory visits as an opportunity to improve knowledge and skills of health staff."
  - Supportive supervision encourages open, two-way communication, and building team approaches that facilitate problem-solving.
  - It focuses on monitoring performance towards goals, and using data for decision-making, and depends upon regular follow-up with staff to ensure that new tasks are being implemented correctly.
  - Supportive supervision helps to make things work, rather than checking to see what is wrong.

Steps of Supportive Supervision

Setting up a supportive supervision system—3R
- **Right supervisor:** Training a core set of supervisors
- **Right tools:** Creating checklists and recording forms
- **Right resources:** Ensuring appropriate resources are available—vehicles, per diem, areas for collaboration with other programs

↓

Planning regular supervisory visits—3W
- **Where:** Using data to decide priority supervision sites
- **When:** Schedule supervision visits using a workplan
- **What subjects to train:** Identify training needs and skills that need updating

↓

Conducting supportive supervision visits
- Observation
- Use of data
- Problem-solving
- On-the-job training
- Recording observations and feedback

↓

Follow-up
- Follow-up on agreed actions by supervisors and supervised staff
- Regular data analysis
- Feedback to all stakeholders

Advantages of Supervision
- It helps healthcare workers to achieve work objectives by improving their performance.
- It ensures uniformity to set standards.
- It helps in identifying problems and solving them in a timely manner.
- It also identifies staff needs and provides opportunities for personal development.
- It reinforces administrative and technical links between high- and lower-level.

Supervisory methods: Field visits, review meeting, discussion with staff, review of records are different methods.

10.3 MONITORING
- Monitoring is the day-to-day follow-up of activities during their implementation to ensure that they are proceeding as planned and are on schedule.
- It is a continuous process of observing, recording, and reporting on the activities of the organization.
- It requires periodic collection and review of information on program implementation, coverage and identifying deviations and taking corrective action.

Monitoring Indicators (Fig. 10.1)
- There is a logical "flow" of indicators from inputs through impact.
- Plans should always include clear and measurable indicators that go beyond monitoring only the "process" to include also the "outcome", that is what the intervention should lead to as this is the main reason why certain activities have originally been planned.
- For example, a plan includes training courses for health providers on the management of a sick child.
- This is done—to improve health providers' case management skills of sick children—to improve how children are managed (outcome)—to improve child health, e.g., reducing child deaths (impact).

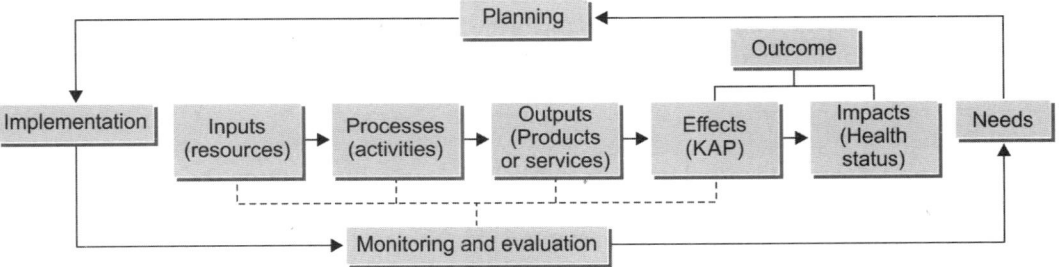

Fig. 10.1: Planning evaluation cycle.

Types

Input indicators
- These indicators refer to the resources needed for the implementation of an activity or intervention.
- Human resources, materials, financial resources, policies, legislation are example of input.

- **Example:** Inputs to conduct a training course may include facilitators, training materials, and funds.

Process Indicators
- Process indicators refer to indicators to measure whether planned activities took place. This indicator addresses the program issues.
- Examples include holding of meetings, conduct of training courses, distribution of medicines, development, and testing of health education materials.

Output Indicators
- Output indicators add more details in relation to the product ("output") of the activity.
- **Example:** The output of a training course on case management may be the number of medical assistants trained and, consequently, the number or proportion of them with improved knowledge and skills in case management.
- These indicators are useful management tools to monitor implementation and its quality. However, they do not provide information on the results and impact of the activity.

Outcome Indicators
- Outcome indicators refer more specifically to the objectives of an intervention that is its 'results', its outcome.
- These indicators refer to the reason why it was decided to conduct certain interventions in the first place. They are the result of both the "quantity" ("how many") and quality ("how well") of the activities implemented.
- **Example:** The outcome of a training of health providers in the integrated management of neonatal and childhood illness (IMNCI) should be improved management of sick children under 5 years old, e.g., the proportion of sick children correctly managed by the trained health providers.
- These indicators, therefore, allow us to know whether the desired outcome has been generated.
- It may take time before final outcomes can be measured. A number of intermediate outcome indicators should therefore be identified for all the intermediate changes that the intervention is expected to bring about and that will eventually lead to the final outcome. This helps us know whether we are progressing towards achieving the expected final outcome.

Impact Indicators
- Impact indicators refer to change in the health status of the target population due to the effects of interventions or activities—reduction in child mortality, reduction in child morbidity, improved child nutritional status.
- These indicators do not show progress over relatively short periods of time. It is then the logical flow of indicators described above which enables a more regular and frequent monitoring of changes.

BIBLIOGRAPHY

1. Different Types of Leadership Styles by Rose Johnson, available at: http://smallbusiness.chron.com/5-different-types-leadership-styles-17584.html, accessed on 25 September 2016.
2. http://www.emro.who.int/child-health/research-and-evaluation/indicators/Type-of-indicators.html
3. http://www.nihfw.org/doc/NCHRC-Publications/Module%20-%204.pdf
4. https://egyankosh.ac.in/bitstream/123456789/48005/1/Unit-3.pdf
5. Training for mid-level managers (MLM). Module 4: supportive supervision. Geneva: World Health Organization; 2008, republished 2020 under the license: CC BY-NC-SA 3.0 IGO.

CHAPTER 11

Disaster Management

CHAPTER OUTLINE
- 11.1 Introduction to disaster management
- 11.2 Disaster management cycle
- 11.3 Disaster impact and rescue
- 11.4 Epidemiologic surveillance and disease control

- **Disaster:** A catastrophe, mishap, calamity or grave occurrence in any area, arising from natural or man-made causes, or by accident or negligence which results in substantial loss of life or human suffering or damage to, and destruction of, property, or damage to, and degradation of, environment, and is of such a nature or magnitude as to be beyond the coping capacity of the community of the affected area.
- Thus, a disaster may have features like speed, unpredictability, unfamiliarity, urgency, uncertainty, and threat.
- Ingredients of any disaster includes:
  - A phenomenon or event which constitutes a trauma for a population/environment.
  - A vulnerable point/area that will bear the brunt of the traumatizing event.
  - The failure of local and surrounding resources to cope with the problems created by the phenomenon.
- **Vulnerability:** It is defined as "the extent to which a community, structure, service, and/or geographic area is likely to be damaged or disrupted by the impact of particular hazard, on account of their nature, construction and proximity to hazardous terrain or a disaster-prone area".
- **Hazard:** Hazards are defined as "Phenomena that pose a threat to people, structures, or economic assets and which may cause a disaster. They could be either man-made or naturally occurring in our environment."

- **Disaster risk** = Hazard + Vulnerability
- **Types of disaster:** According to the origin, disasters can be seen as different types:
  - **Climate-related:** Floods, droughts, cyclones, cloud bursts, hot and cold winds, forest wildfire, storms, and lightning fall.
  - **Geological:** Earthquake, landslide, rupture of the dam, fire in mine, volcano.
  - **Chemical, industrial and nuclear-related:** Chemical and industrial disaster and nuclear disaster.
  - **Accidental-related:** Fire, bomb, explosion, air, road and rail accidents, flooding in mines, collapse of main buildings.
  - **Biological disasters:** Epidemic (COVID-19), grasshopper invasion, animal pandemic, etc.
  - **Natural disasters:**
    - Earthquakes
    - Floods
    - Landslides
    - Cyclones
    - Tsunami
  - **Man-made disasters**
    - Nuclear and radiological disaster
    - Biological disaster
    - Chemical disaster
    - Terrorist attack
    - Bomb blast
    - Hijacking
    - Hostage situation
- India is vulnerable in varying degrees to a large number of natural as well as man-made disasters:
  - 58.6% of the landmass is prone to earthquakes of moderate to very high intensity. Out of these 12% is vulnerable.
  - Over 40 million hectares (12% of land) is prone to floods and river erosion.
  - Out of the 7,516 km long coastline, close to 5,700 km is prone to cyclones and tsunamis;
  - 68% of the cultivable area is vulnerable to drought and hilly areas are at risk from landslides and avalanches.
  - Further, the vulnerability to nuclear biological and chemical (NBC) disasters and terrorism has also increased manifold.
- Disaster risks in India are further compounded by increasing vulnerabilities. These include the ever-growing population, the vast disparities in income, rapid urbanization, increasing industrialization, development within high-risk zones, environmental degradation, climate change, etc.
- **General effects of disaster:**
  - Loss of life
  - Injury
  - Damage to and destruction of property.
  - Damage to and destruction of production.
  - Disruption of lifestyle
  - Loss of livelihood.
  - Disruption to essential services

- Damage to national infrastructure
- Disruption to governmental systems
- National economic loss
- Sociological and psychological after effect.

Morbidity Related to Disaster can be Classified into Four Group

1. Injuries
2. Emotional stress
3. Epidemic of disease; and
4. Increase in indigenous diseases
   - **Disaster-wise nodal ministry list:** Overall nodal ministry of disaster management is Ministry of Home Affairs **(Table 11.1)**.

Table 11.1: Nodal ministry/agency responsible for specific type of disasters.

Disaster	Nodal ministry/agency
Earthquake	Indian Meteorology Department (IMD)
Landslide	Geological Survey of India (GSI)
Flood	Central Water Commission
Aviation	Ministry of Civil Aviation
Epidemics/health	Ministry of Health and Family Welfare
Industrial and chemical accidents	Ministry of Environment and Forests
All other disasters	Ministry of Home Affairs

11.1 INTRODUCTION TO DISASTER MANAGEMENT

- Disaster management means a coordination and integrated process of planning, organizing, coordinating and implementing measures which are necessary or expedient for:
  - Prevention of danger or threat of any disaster
  - Mitigation or reduction of risk of any disaster or its severity or its consequences
  - Capacity building
  - Preparedness to deal with any disaster
  - Prompt response to any threatening disaster situation or disaster
  - Assessing the severity or magnitude of effects of any disaster
  - Evacuation, rescue, and relief
  - Rehabilitation and reconstruction
- Three fundamental aspects of disaster management:
  1. Disaster response
  2. Disaster preparedness
  3. Disaster mitigation

11.2 DISASTER MANAGEMENT CYCLE

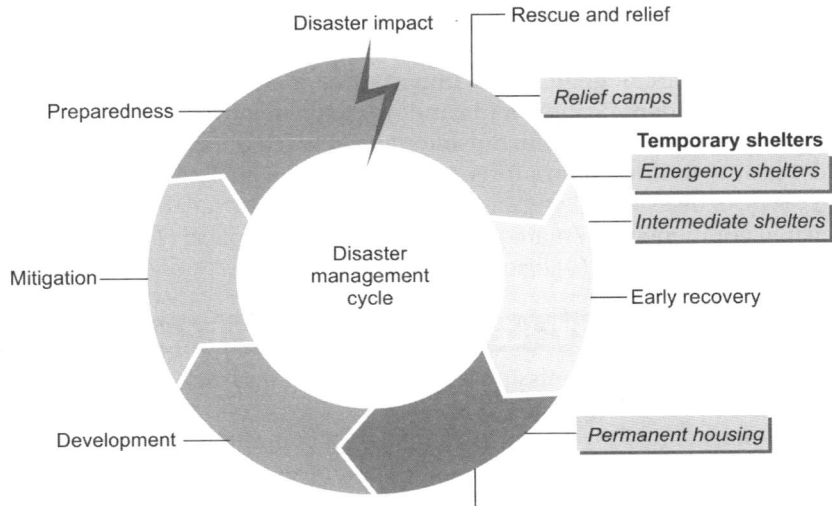

Fig. 11.1: Disaster management sequence.

- **Preparedness:** To combat the disaster, implement the training and disaster management plan to keep the people safe. Example: Plans, mock drill and warning systems.
- **Mitigation:** Mitigation refers to the structural and nonstructural measures which reduces the effect of disasters. Example: Building codes and zoning, vulnerability analysis, public education.
- **Response:** Conduct relief operations during the disaster. Example: Search and rescue, emergency operations, public warning systems.
- **Recovery:** Improve the state/condition of the affected life due to the disaster. Example: Temporary housing, counselling, long-term medical care **(Fig. 11.1)**.

11.3 DISASTER IMPACT AND RESCUE

- First few hours are very vital for emergency care.
- **Search, rescue, and first-aid:** Search and rescue to be done as we all know that immediate help comes from uninjured survivors.
- **Field care:** Stabilization of victims, providing proper care, increase availability of bed and surgical services, provision of food and shelter
- During emergency first come first treated principle is not followed instead we follow the triage system.
- **Triage:**
  - Triage consists of rapidly classifying the injured on the basis of the severity of their injuries and the likelihood of their survival with prompt medical intervention.
  - High-priority patients are those who can be saved with simple intervention while low-priority patients are who already moribund.
  - For doing triage the most common classification is four color code system.
    - Red—high priority treatment or transfer
    - Yellow—medium

- Green—ambulatory patients
- Black—dead/moribund patients
- **Tagging:** All patients should be identified with tags stating their name, age, place of origin, triage category, diagnosis and initial treatment.
- During disaster the care of **dead** is very important. It includes removal from disaster site, shifting to mortuary, identification, and handover to the relatives.
- **Relief:** Begins when assistance from outside starts to reach the disaster area.
- Type and quantity of humanitarian relief supplies are usually determined by two main factors: (1) Type of disaster (2) type and quantity of supplies available locally.
- Four principal components of managing humanitarian supplies: (1) acquisition of supply (2) transportation (3) storage (4) distribution.

11.4 EPIDEMIOLOGIC SURVEILLANCE AND DISEASE CONTROL

The communicable diseases transmission is increased after disasters through:
- Overcrowding and poor sanitation
- Population displacement may lead to introduction of communicable diseases
- Disruption of routine control programs
- Disruption and contamination of water
- Displacement of domestic and wild animals and zoonoses.
- Ecological changes favor breeding of vectors and increase in vector density population
- Provision of emergency food, water and shelter in disaster situation from different or new source may itself be a source of infectious diseases.

Principles of Preventing and Controlling Communicable Diseases After a Disaster

- Implement as soon as possible all public health measures
- Organize a reliable disease reporting system to identify outbreaks and to promptly initiate control measures
- Investigate all reports of disease outbreak rapidly.
- **Vaccination:** WHO does not recommend typhoid and cholera vaccines in routine in endemic areas. The best protection is maintenance of a high-level of immunity in the general population by routine vaccination. Polio and measles vaccination program should closely monitored after disaster.
- **Nutrition:** Affects the nutritional status by affecting one or more components of food chain depending on type, duration and extent of the disaster.
- **Important steps for effective food relief program:**
  - Assessing the food supplies after the disaster
  - Gauging the nutritional needs of the affected population
  - Calculating daily food rations and need for large population groups
  - Monitoring the nutritional status of affected population.
- **Rehabilitation**
  - Final phase in a disaster is a restoration of predisaster conditions.
  - First few weeks after disaster priorities shift from healthcare towards environment health measures.
- **Water supply:**
  - A survey of all public water supplies for distribution system and water source should be made.
  - During this situation microbial contamination of water may be happen. Chlorination is the best way to disinfect water.

- **Water sources require the protection like:**
  - Restrict access to people and animals
  - Ensure adequate excreta disposal at a safe distance from the water source
  - Prohibit bathing, washing, and animal husbandry
  - Upgrade wells
- **Food safety:** Kitchen cleanliness and personal hygiene of people involved in food preparation is important to prevent food-borne disease.
- **Sanitation and hygiene** are very important to prevent disease outbreaks. Proper bathing, washing and cleaning facilities and sanitary disposal of excreta should be provided. All preventive measure requires to control vector-borne disease like malaria, dengue, plague, typhus, leptospirosis, and rat bite fever.

Disaster Mitigation
Aim of mitigation is to reduce the vulnerability of the system.

Disaster Preparedness
- It includes long-term development activities whose goals are to strengthen the overall capacity and capability of a country to manage efficiently all types of emergency.
- It is a multisectoral activity. It includes: (a) evaluate the risk, (b) organize communication and warning system, (c) follow standard and regulation, (d) ensure coordination and response mechanism, (e) develop public education program, (f) financial resource, (g) coordinated information with media
- Reason for community preparedness are: Community is the first-level respond at the time of disaster, resources are easily pooled at community level and sustained development is achieved through community.

Role of Community Health Nurse in Disaster
- Occupational health nursing need to practice the principle of triage while managing the disaster. Postdisaster nursing intervention are also critical e.g., identifying the ongoing disaster-related health needs of the workers and community residents, collecting epidemiological data, and assessing the cause and the necessary steps to prevent a recurrence.
- During disasters, the role of nurse is to coordinate plan and implement, communication, working with people within the work setting and in the community to develop a workable plan and management.

Disaster Management Act
- On 23 December 2005, the Government of India (GoI) took a defining step towards holistic DM by enacting the DM ACT, 2005.
- However, it came into force in January 2006.

Aim
To manage disasters, including preparation of mitigation strategies, capacity-building and more.

Features

- **Nodal agency:** The Act designates the Ministry of Home Affairs as the nodal ministry for steering the overall national disaster management.
- **Institutional structure:** It puts into place a systematic structure of institutions at the national, state, and district levels.
- **National level important entities (Fig. 11.2):**
  - **The national disaster management authority (NDMA):** It is tasked with laying down disaster management policies and ensuring timely and effective response mechanisms. The National Disaster Management Authority (NDMA) under the DM Act is the nodal central body for coordinating disaster management, with the Prime Minister as its Chairperson.
  - **The national executive committee (NEC):** It is constituted to assist the NDMA. The NEC is responsible for the preparation of the National Disaster Management Plan for the whole country and to ensure that it is "reviewed and updated annually".
  - **The national institute of disaster management (NIDM):** It is an institute for training and capacity development programs for managing natural calamities.
  - **National disaster response force (NDRF):** It refers to trained professional units that are called upon for specialized response to disasters.
- **State and district level:** The Act also provides for state and district level authorities responsible for, among other things, drawing plans for implementation of national plans and preparing local plans.
  - State disaster management authority
  - District disaster management authority

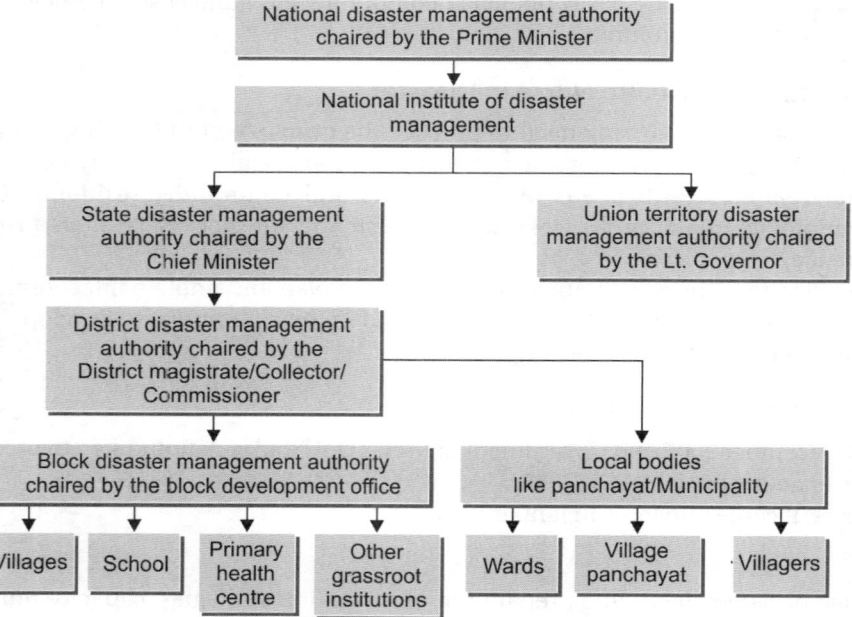

Fig. 11.2: Organogram for disaster management.

- **Finance:** It contains the provisions for financial mechanisms such as national disaster response fund and similar funds at the state and district levels.
- **Civil and criminal liabilities:** Under Section 51 of the Act, anyone refusing to comply with orders is liable for punishment with imprisonment up to one year, or fine, or both. In case this refusal leads to death of people, the person liable shall be punished with imprisonment up to two years.
- **Challenges:** One of the most glaring inadequacies in the Act is the absence of a provision for declaration of 'disaster-prone zones'. Almost all disaster-related legislations in the world have mapped out disaster-prone zones within their respective jurisdictions. The state cannot be expected to play a proactive role unless an area is declared 'disaster-prone'. Classification helps in determining the extent of damage as well.

Note: Lockdown imposed during COVID-19 pandemic was done under the ambit of the disaster management Act.

BIBLIOGRAPHY

1. https://puducherry-dt.gov.in/disaster-management/
2. https://www.witpress.com/Secure/elibrary/papers/DMAN11/DMAN11008FU1.pdf
3. https://www.researchgate.net/publication/291757440_A_Study_on_Flash_Floods_and_Landslides_Disaster_on_3rd_August_2012_along_Bhagirathi_Valley_in_Uttarkashi_District_Uttarakhand
4. https://sdma.cg.gov.in/raipur%20english.pdf
5. https://ndma.gov.in/sites/default/files/PDF/DM_act2005.pdf
6. http://www.mati.gov.in/docs/Academic%20Module%20-%202/PDF%20(3rd%20November%202021)/DDMA%20SWKH%20mawkyrwat.pdf

CHAPTER 12

Biomedical Waste Management

CHAPTER OUTLINE

12.1 Overview of biomedical waste
12.2 Biomedical Waste management at community level and health facility level
12.3 Biomedical Waste Management Act

12.1 OVERVIEW OF BIOMEDICAL WASTE

PROBLEM STATEMENT

- Health and environmental risks arise out of poor infection control practices and unsound environment management systems such as inappropriate disinfection and poor biomedical waste handling, treatment, and disposal. These hazards can never be underestimated and the outcome is often irreversible.
- In India the quantity of hospital waste is estimated to be 1–2 kg per bed per day in a hospital and 600 g per day per bed in a clinic.
- Around 85% of the hospital waste is non-hazardous, 15% is infectious/hazardous.
- Mixing of non-hazardous waste with hazardous waste results in contamination and makes the entire waste hazardous.
- Hence there is necessity to segregate, treat and proper disposal.
- Improper disposal increases risk of infection and also increase chances of the recycling of prohibited disposables and expired drugs.
- **Definition:** Biomedical waste means any waste, which is generated during the diagnosis, treatment or immunization of human beings or animals or research activities pertaining thereto or in the production or testing of biological or in health camps, including the categories mentioned in the BMW rules.

HAZARDS

- The hazardous nature of Biomedical wastes is due to the presence of the following:
  - Presence of infectious agents
  - Presence of used sharps
  - Presence of cytotoxic compounds
- Nurses are the most vulnerable to needle stick injuries among the health care staff:

Prone to needle stick injury	Relative of injuries
Staff nurses	34.6%
Interns	15.7%
Residents	11.7%
Trainee nurses	8.5%
Technical staff	6%
Workers responsible for waste management/cleaning	19%
Others	4.5%

- **Hazards due to infectious waste and sharps:** Hepatitis B, Hepatitis C and HIV infection. It can be entering through an abrasion or cut in the skin.
- Hazards due to **genotoxic waste**
- **Hazards due to chemical and pharmaceutical waste:** It is due to chemical nature of radioactive, explosive, corrosive and genotoxic nature.
- **Hazards due to radioactive waste:** It depends upon type and duration of exposure.

Overview of Hospital Waste (Fig. 12.1)

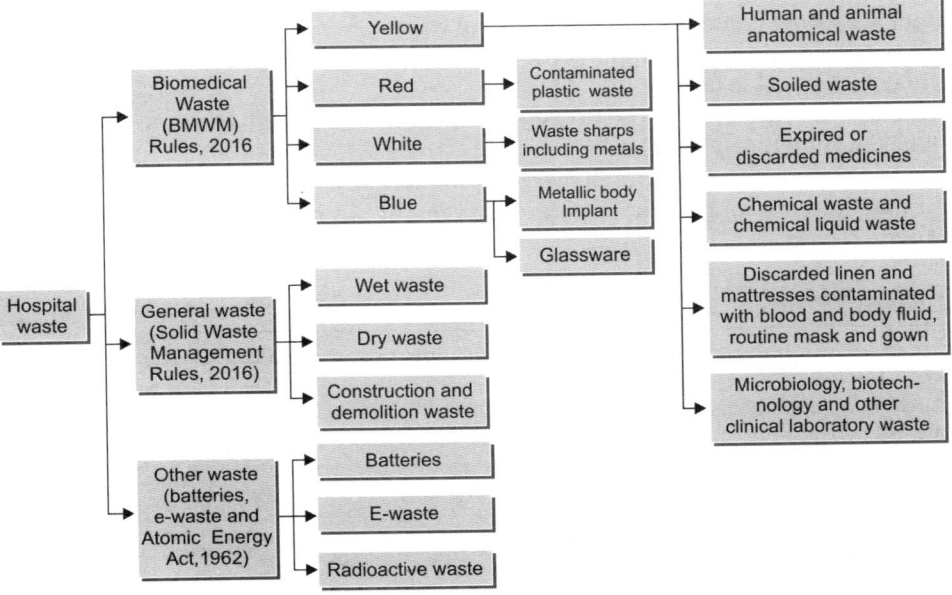

Fig. 12.1: Overview of hospital waste.

Segregation, Packing Storage and Transportation

- No untreated biomedical waste shall be mixed with other wastes.
- The biomedical waste shall be segregated into containers or bags at the point of generation prior to its storage, transportation, treatment and disposal.
- The containers or bags shall be labeled as specified in BMW Act.
- The vehicles used for transportation of biomedical waste shall comply with the conditions if any stipulated by the State Pollution Control Board or Pollution Control Committee in addition to the requirement contained in the Motor Vehicles Act, 1988 (59 of 1988), if any or the rules made there under for transportation of such infectious waste.
- Untreated human anatomical waste, animal anatomical waste, soiled waste and, biotechnology waste shall not be stored beyond a period of 48 hours.
- Microbiology waste and all other clinical laboratory waste shall be pre-treated by sterilization before packing and sending to the common biomedical waste treatment facility.
- If required to store beyond 48 hours, the occupier shall ensure that it does not affect human health and inform the SPCB with reason.
- During COVID-19 pandemic, the biomedical waste generated during COVID-19 testing, at isolation centers or during quarantine period, those all wastes to be labeled as COVID-19 waste and its separation, storage and handling should be done in separation from the routine biomedical waste management.
- The laboratory waste should be collected in double layered red bags and its carrying bin should be disinfected with 1% sodium hypochlorite before disposal while waste generated in quarantine wards will be collected in yellow color bags.

ROLE OF COMMUNITY HEALTH NURSE

- Proper follow the guideline for segregation of waste
- Disinfect all contaminated equipment
- Disinfect all reusable items
- Daily clean the surfaces in close proximity to patient and patient area
- Follow the guideline of standard precaution
- In case of risk, use personal protective equipment (PPE)
- Maintain different source wise and ward wise register
- Maintain record.

BIBLIOGRAPHY

1. https://www.mohfw.gov.in/pdf/National%20Guidelines%20for%20IPC%20in%20HCF%20-%20final%281%29.pdf
2. https://meghealth.gov.in/docs/MANUAL%20FOR%20BIOMEDICAL%20WASTE%20MANAGEMENT.pdf
3. https://cpcb.nic.in/uploads/Projects/Bio-Medical-Waste/Guidelines_healthcare_June_2018.pdf

12.2 BIOMEDICAL WASTE MANAGEMENT AT COMMUNITY LEVEL AND HEALTH FACILITY LEVEL

BIOMEDICAL WASTE MANAGEMENT AT COMMUNITY LEVEL (VHND/RI SESSIONS/HEALTH CAMPS)

Segregation

Category	Type of waste	Color of bag/container	Job responsibility	Standard precautions
Yellow	Placenta (home delivery by SBA)	Yellow	ANM/MLHP	3 ply mask, gloves, hand hygiene
Yellow	Soiled waste including cotton swabs	Yellow bag	ASHA, ANM, SW	3 ply mask and gloves, hand hygiene
Red	Syringes, gloves	Red bag	ANMs/MLHPs	3 ply mask and gloves, hand hygiene
Blue	Used/broken diluent ampoules	Card box	ANMs/MLHPs	3 ply mask and gloves, hand hygiene
White	Needles	Hub cutter	ANMs/MLHPs	3 ply masks and gloves, hand hygiene

Collection and Transportation

Yellow Category

- At the end of RI sessions at VHND platform, the yellow bag is secured with a tie and assigned health worker collects and carries the yellow bag back to the sub-center.
- Upon arrival at the sub-center the ANM/MLHP records the weight of the waste and dispose of the waste into the deep burial pit located in the sub-center compound.
- ANM/MLHP conducting delivery at home to take the yellow bag containing placenta and carry it back to sub-center, records the weight, and to dispose the waste into the deep burial pit of the sub-center
- The ANM/MLHP discards the empty yellow bags into a red bag for treatment and disposal by the PHC
- If deep burial pit is not available, assigned health worker carry the wastes to the PHC for disposal by deep burial
- ANM/MLHP to collect all disinfecting fluid/housekeeping liquid in a housekeeping bucket and record the quantity, treat the fluid with 1% chlorine solution and discharge into a soakage pit.

Deep Burial (Fig. 12.2)

It is allowed only in remote rural area where there is no access to common biomedical waste treatment facility (CBMWTF).

- A pit or trench should be dug about two meters deep.
- It should be half filled with waste, then covered with lime within 50 cm of the surface, before filling the rest of the pit with soil.
- Every time, when wastes are added to the pit, a layer of 10 cm of soil shall be added to cover the wastes.
- The deep burial site should be relatively impermeable and no shallow well should be close to the site.
- The pits should be distant from habitation, and located so as to ensure that no contamination occurs to surface water or ground water. The area should not be prone to flooding or erosion.

Burial must be performed under close and dedicated supervision. The institution shall maintain a record of all pits used for deep burial.
- Covers of galvanized iron or wire meshes may be used. So, we prevent the access of animal.

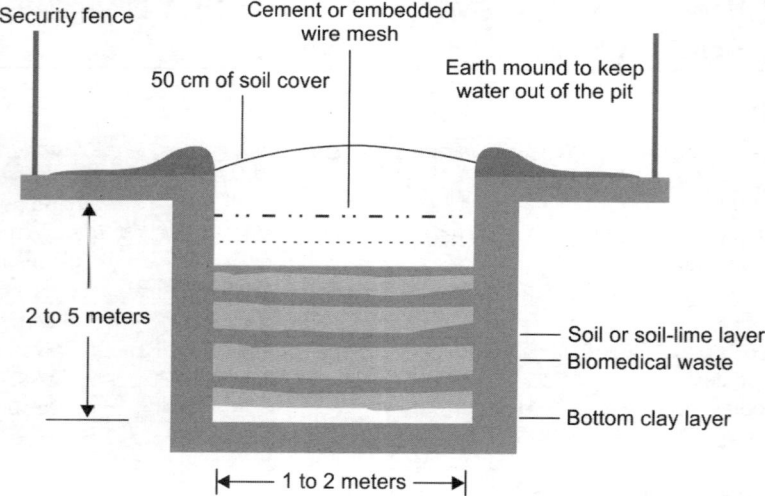

Fig. 12.2: Layout of deep burial pit.

Sharp Pit/Tank (Fig. 12.3)
- For disposal of treated needles and broken vials, pit is used.
- Rectangular or circular pit can be dug and lined with brick, masonry or concrete rings. It should be covered with a heavy concrete slab, which is penetrated by a galvanized steel pipe projecting about 1.5 meters above the slab, with an internal diameter of up to 50 millimeters or 1.5 times the length of vials, whichever is more.
- The top opening of the steel pipe shall have a provision of locking after the treated waste sharps has been disposed in. When it is full it can be sealed completely and another has been prepared.

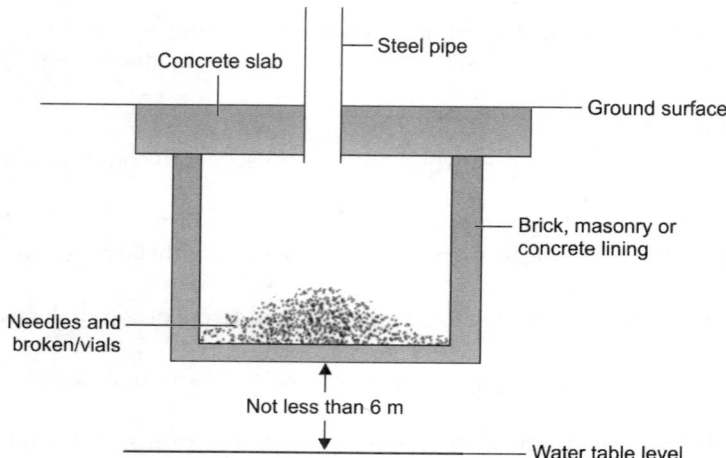

Fig. 12.3: Layout of sharp pit/tank.

Red Category and White Category

- At the end of RI sessions at a VHND platform, assigned health worker collects and carries the red bag secured with a tie and the hub cutter along with the vaccine carrier to the PHC.
- Upon arrival at the PHC waste storage room he/she informs the sister on duty and hands over the red bag.
- Sister on duty records the weight and makes entry in the PHC Waste Logbook.
- The needles in the hub cutter are emptied into a sharps bin in the PHC waste storage room and the hub cutter is disinfected with 1% chlorine solution for 30 minutes. The hub cutter is hand back to the assigned health worker.

Blue Category

At the close of the session the assigned health worker collects the broken diluent ampoules, in a blue container, and take back to the PHC waste storage room.

Biomedical Waste Management at Health Facility Level

- As mention above, for SC/PHC/CHC/District hospital we have to follow the guideline for segregation, collection, transportation and disposal of biomedical waste.
- More detail on this topic given in the Chapter 12.3.

BIBLIOGRAPHY

1. https://www.mohfw.gov.in/pdf/National%20Guidelines%20for%20IPC%20in%20HCF%20-%20final%281%29.pdf
2. https://meghealth.gov.in/docs/MANUAL%20FOR%20BIOMEDICAL%20WASTE%20MANAGEMENT.pdf

12.3 BIOMEDICAL WASTE MANAGEMENT ACT

BMW MANAGEMENT RULES, 2016

- **Nodal Ministry:** Ministry of Environment Forest and Climate Change
- **Scope of the rule:** These rules shall apply to all persons who generate, collect, receive, store, transport, treat, dispose, or handle biomedical waste in any form including hospitals, nursing homes, clinics, dispensaries, veterinary institutions, animal houses, pathological laboratories, blood banks, AYUSH hospitals, clinical establishments, research or educational institutions, health camps, medical or surgical camps, vaccination camps, blood donation camps, first aid rooms of schools, forensic laboratories and research laboratories.
- These rules shall not apply to:
  - Radioactive wastes
  - Hazardous chemicals covered under the Manufacture, Storage and Import of Hazardous Chemicals Rules, 1989
  - Solid wastes covered under the Municipal Solid Waste Rules, 2000
  - The lead acid batteries
  - Hazardous wastes covered under the Hazardous Wastes Rules, 2008

- E-waste
- Hazardous microorganisms, genetically engineered microorganisms and cells.

The major salient features of BMW Management Rules, 2016 include the following:
- The scope of the rules has been expanded to include vaccination camps, blood donation camps, surgical camps or any other healthcare activity.
- Pretreatment of the laboratory waste, microbiological waste, blood samples and blood bags through disinfection or sterilization on-site in the manner as prescribed by WHO or NACO.
- Provide training to all healthcare workers and others involved in handling of biomedical waste at the time of induction and thereafter at least once in a year and immunize all health workers regularly especially for hepatitis and tetanus.
- Report major accidents that happen at any stage of biomedical waste management; and forward a report within twenty-four hours in writing regarding the remedial steps taken in Form I.
- Existing incinerators to achieve the standards for retention time in secondary chamber (retention time was 1 sec in BMW Rules 2011 that is now 2 sec in BMW Rules 2016) and Dioxin and Furans standards added for the first time in BMW rules and all these standards to be achieved within two years.
- These new standards for incinerator are more stringent and thus it will help to reduce the emission of pollutants in environment.
- Biomedical waste has been classified into 4 categories instead 10 categories to improve the segregation of waste at place of origin.
- Procedure to get authorization for bedded healthcare facilities (HCFs) been simplified.
- One time Authorization for Non-bedded HCFs also been made compulsory. (Non-beded hospitals were not needed to be registered in the earlier version of the BMW rules).
- State Government to provide land for setting up common biomedical waste treatment and disposal facility.
- No occupier shall establish on-site treatment and disposal facility, if a service of common biomedical waste treatment facility is available within distance of 75 kilometer.
- Untreated human anatomical waste, animal anatomical waste, soiled waste and, biotechnology waste shall not be stored beyond a period of 48 hours.

The salient features of BMW Management Rules, 2018 and 2019 include the following:
- Biomedical waste generators will have to phase out chlorinated plastic bags (excluding blood bags) and gloves by March 27, 2019.
- Operators of common biomedical waste treatment and disposal facilities shall establish bar coding and global positioning system for handling of biomedical waste in accordance with guidelines issued by the Central Pollution Control Board by March 27, 2019.
- All bedded health facility should maintain detailed biomedical waste management register on daily basis and monthly summary to be uploaded on their website.
- All bedded health facility should upload annual report of biomedical waste management.

Biomedical Waste Management

There are 4 schedules and 5 forms in the BMW Act 1998, that are included with some changes in the BMW rules 2016 which are as follows:

Schedule I

Biomedical wastes categories and their segregation, collection, treatment, processing and disposal options:

Category	Type of waste	Type of bag or container to be used	Treatment and disposal options
Yellow	1. Human anatomical waste	Yellow colored non-chlorinated plastic bags	Incineration or plasma pyrolysis or deep burial
	2. Animal anatomical waste	Same as above	Same as above
	3. Soiled waste (e.g., blood or body fluids contaminated dressings, plaster cast or cotton swabs)	Same as above	If above facilities are not available then autoclaving or microwaving followed by shredding can be considered.
	4. Expired or discarded medicine	Same as above	Can be sent to pharmaceuticals companies for incineration or can be incinerated at common waste treatment plants.
	5. Chemical waste	Same as above	Disposed of by incineration or plasma pyrolysis or encapsulation
	6. Chemical liquid waste	Separate collection system leading to effluent treatment system	Chemical liquid must be pretreated before mixing with other waste water
	7. Discarded linen, mattresses, beddings contaminated with blood or body fluid	Yellow colored non-chlorinated plastic bags	Incineration or plasma pyrolysis or for energy recovery. In absence of above facilities, shredding or mutilation or combination of sterilization and shredding.
	8. Microbiology, biotechnology and other clinical lab waste	Autoclave safe plastic bags or containers	Pre-treat first as per guidelines of NACO or WHO.

Biomedical Waste Management

Category	Type of waste	Type of bag or container to be used	Treatment and disposal options
Red	Contaminated waste red colored (recyclable)	Red colored non chlorinated plastic bags or containers	Autoclaving or microwaving followed by shredding. Then this treated waste will be sent to authorized recyclers to make fuel or road.
White	Sharp wastes including metals	Puncture proof, leak proof, tamper proof containers	Autoclaving or dry heat sterilization followed by shredding then disposal to iron foundries.
Blue	Glassware (e.g., medicine ampoules or vials)	Cardboard boxes with blue colored markings	Disinfection or autoclaving or microwaving then sent for recycling
	Metallic body implants	Cardboard boxes with blue colored markings	–

Schedule II
Standards for treatment and disposal of biomedical wastes
In this schedule, standards have been given for incineration, microclaving, chemical disinfection, etc.

Schedule III
List of prescribed authorities and the corresponding duties
In this schedule, authorities and duties right from the national level up to the district level has been mentioned for timely and correctly management of the biomedical waste and for the monitoring of the whole process.

Schedule IV
Schedule IV has been divided into two parts:

Part A: Label for biomedical waste containers or bags.

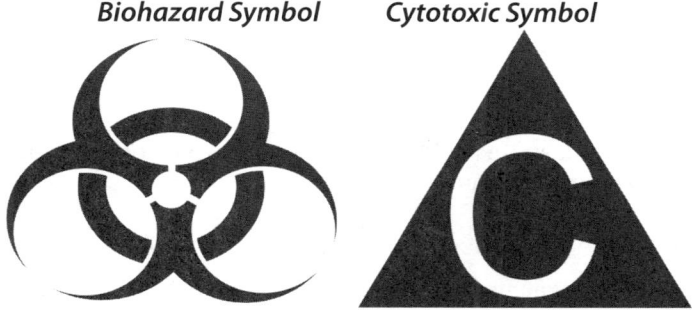

Biohazard Symbol   Cytotoxic Symbol

Part B: Label for transporting biomedical waste bags or containers
- Day ....Month ....
- Year ....
- Date of generation ....
- Waste category number ....
- Waste quantity.............
- Sender's Name and Address: Receiver's Name and Address:
- Phone Number ....   Phone Number ....
- Fax Number...............   Fax Number ....
- Contact Person ....   Contact Person ....
- In case of emergency please contact:
- Name and Address:
- Phone No.
- (Note: Label shall be non-washable and prominently visible.)

List of the forms that to be filled for particular purpose as follows:
- Form–I: Accident reporting
- Form–II : Application for authorization or renewal of authorization
- Form–III: Authorization
- Form–IV: Annual report
- Form–V: Application for filing appeal against order passed by the prescribed authority

STANDARDS FOR TREATMENT OF BIOMEDICAL WASTES

Part I: Standards for Autoclaving of BMW

Type of autoclave	Temperature	Pressure	Exposure/residence time
A-class (Gravity driven)	121°C	15 psi	60 minutes or more
	135°C	31 psi	45 minutes or more
	149°C	52 psi	30 minutes or more
B-class (Pre-vacuum)	121°C	15 psi	45 minutes or more
	135°C	31 psi	30 minutes or more

*Conduct a weekly spore test (biological indicator) and maintain records

Part II: Standards for Chemical Disinfection

Chemical disinfection methods shall demonstrate a 4 Log10 reduction or greater for Bacillus Subtilis (ATCC 19659) in chemical treatment systems.

Part III: Standards for Liquid Waste

The treated effluent liquid waste should have achieved the certain parameters to the following limits before discharge into the sewer:

Parameters	Permissible limit
pH	6.5–9
Suspended solids	100 mg/L
Oil and grease	10 mg/L
BOD	30 mg/L
COD	250 mg/L
Bio-essay test	90% survival after 96 hours in 100% effluent

Part IV: Standards for Deep Burial

Details given in Chapter 12.2

Part V: Standards for Incineration

- Combustion efficiency (CE) shall be at least 99%.
- (CE): $\% CO_2 / (\% CO_2 + \% CO) \times 100$
- The temperature of the primary chamber shall be a minimum of 800°C and the secondary chamber shall be minimum of 1050°C ± 50°C.
- The secondary chamber gas residence time shall be at least two seconds with minimum 3% oxygen in the stack gas.

BIBLIOGRAPHY

1. https://meghealth.gov.in/docs/MANUAL%20FOR%20BIOMEDICAL%20WASTE%20MANAGEMENT.pdf
2. The gazette of India. The Bio-Medical Waste Management Rules, 2016.

13 CHAPTER

National and International Agencies Related to Health

CHAPTER OUTLINE

- 13.1 World Health Organization (WHO)
- 13.2 United Nations Children's Fund (UNICEF)
- 13.3 Important UN Agencies (UNDP, UNFPA), World Bank, FAO and ILO
- 13.4 International Bilateral Agencies or NGOs (CARE, Ford Foundation, Rockefeller Foundation, SIDA, DANIDA, Colombo Plan)
- 13.5 National Health Agencies

13.1 WORLD HEALTH ORGANIZATION (WHO)

- WHO came into existence on 7th April 1948 and because of that 7th April is celebrated as a world health day.
- WHO is UN's specialized nonpolitical agencies which has own constitution.
- Main Headquarter: Geneva
- WHO has six regional organizations and details of them are as follows:

Sl. No.	Name of region	Headquarter
1.	Africa	Brazzaville, Republic of Congo
2.	Europe	Copenhagen, Denmark
3.	South-East Asia	New Delhi, India
4.	Eastern Mediterranean	Cairo, Egypt
5.	Western Pacific	Manila, Philippines
6.	The Americas	Washington DC, USA

- India is the member of South East Asia region organization.
- There are total 11 countries in SEARO. Those eleven countries are: Bhutan, Bangladesh, India, Indonesia, Maldives, Myanmar, Korea, Nepal, Sri Lanka, Thailand and Timor-Leste.

Objectives

- **Main objective:** "The attainment by all peoples of the highest level of health".
- To act as the directing and coordinating authority on international health work.
- To establish and maintain effective collaboration with the United Nations, specialized agencies, governmental health administrations, professional groups and such other organizations as may be deemed appropriate.
- To provide assistance to the Governments, upon request, in strengthening health services.
- To promote cooperation among scientific and professional groups which contribute to the advancement of health.

Administration of WHO

Three main Division: World health assembly, Executive board, Secretariat

- **World health assembly:** It determines overall the policy of organization and also supervise financial policies and activities. It is constituted by delegates representing member countries. Delegates are usually the most qualified and competent person in the field of health. They usually meet once a year.
- **Executive Board:** Three or more members from each WHO region are in the executive board. Currently there are 34 members in the executive boards. They usually meet at least twice a year. The main task of the Board is to execute and implement and the decisions and policies of the Assembly. The Board can take action on its own during time of emergency.
- **Secretariat:** It is headed by the Director General. Director General provides technical and managerial support to the member states. Director General is appointed by the World Health Assembly.

Activities

- **Prevention and control of specific diseases:** Epidemiological surveillance of communicable diseases is the important activity of WHO. They usually communicate about diseases important from IHR point of view through an Automatic Telex Reply Service (ATRS) and the "Weekly Epidemiological Record" (WER). 8th May, 1980 small pox eradication day is the one of the greatest achievement of WHO. WHO has been doing commendable job for polio and measles elimination. WHO also working for noncommunicable diseases like cancer, cardiovascular diseases, genetic disorders, diabetes, blindness, mental disorders, drug addiction, and dental diseases.
- **Family health:** It includes maternal and child health care, human reproduction, nutrition and health education. The core target is to improve the quality of life of the family.
- **Development of comprehensive health services:** WHO helps every member nation to develop their national health policy and various comprehensive national health program. Main focus has been strengthening primary care with help of appropriate technology.
- **Environmental health:** WHO has issued various standardized criteria for the protection of the quality of water, food, air, standard related to economics, radiation protection and early identification of new hazards originating from new technological developments. So far for the improvement of the environmental health WHO has introduced 'WHO Environmental Health Criteria Programme' and 'WHO Environmental Health Monitoring Programme'.

- **Health literature and information:** WHO serves as a main source of information for various health issues. So far, WHO has published hundreds of titles on a wide variety of health subjects. Public information service is available both at headquarters and regional offices.
- **Health statistics:** WHO publishes data related to morbidity and mortality through open access platform for wider dissemination. Details of publication as follows:
  - Epidemiological Record: Weekly
  - World Health Statistics: Quarterly and
  - World Health Statistics: Annually.
  - International Classification of Diseases (Current version is ICD 11): Every 10th year.
- **Biomedical research**: During COVID-19 pandemic WHO facilitated conduction of solidarity trial. Six tropical diseases (malaria, schistosomiasis, trypanosomiasis, filariasis, leishmaniasis and leprosy) are the target of the WHO special program for research and training in tropical diseases to develop new tools, strengthen research institutions and training workers in the countries affected.
- **Cooperation with other organizations**: WHO works in cooperation with UN allied and other international agencies with maintaining degrees of working relationships.

Three Billion Plan by WHO

- A billion more people have universal health coverage,
- To protect a billion more people from health emergencies, and
- Provide a further billion people with better health and well-being.

SEARO (including INDIA) has following eight key areas:
1. Measles and rubella elimination;
2. Preventing noncommunicable diseases; reducing maternal mortality;
3. Under-five and neonatal mortality;
4. Universal health coverage with a focus on human resources for health and essential medicines;
5. Combating antimicrobial resistance;
6. Scaling up capacities for emergency risk management;
7. Eliminating neglected tropical diseases
8. Accelerating efforts to end TB.

13.2 UNITED NATIONS CHILDREN'S FUND (UNICEF)

- UNICEF is the United Nations Children's Fund, formerly United Nations International Children's Emergency Fund.
- It was established on 11th December 1946 and in 1953 the emergency word removed from UNICEF.
- It is known to reach the most disadvantaged children and adolescents for protection of the rights of every child, everywhere.
- UNICEF supports child health and nutrition, safe water and sanitation, quality education and skill building, HIV prevention and treatment for mothers and babies, and the protection of children and adolescents from violence and exploitation. It is the world's largest providers of vaccines.

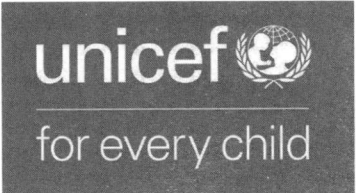

National and International Agencies Related to Health

- **UNICEF Regional Offices Details (overall Headquarter: New York)**

Sl. No.	Name of the UNICEF regional office	Headquarter
1.	The Americas and Caribbean	Panama City (Panama)
2.	Central and Eastern Europe, Commonwealth of Independent States	Geneva (Switzerland)
3.	East Asia and the Pacific	Bangkok (Thailand)
4.	Eastern and Southern Africa	Nairobi (Kenya)
5.	Middle East and North Africa	Amman (Jordan)
6.	South Asia	Kathmandu (Nepal)
7.	West and Central Africa	Dakar (Senegal)

- UNICEF collects data to monitor the situation of children and young people around the world.

ADMINISTRATION OF UNICEF

UNICEF Executive Board
- It is the governing body of UNICEF.
- It is a 36-member board which is made up of government representatives elected by the United Nations Economic and Social Council, usually for three-year terms.
- Executive board that establishes policies, approves programs, and oversees administrative and financial plans.
- It is providing intergovernmental support and oversight to the organization, in accordance with the overall policy guidance of the United Nations General Assembly and the Economic and Social Council.

Activities
- **Child health:** Production of vaccines and sera in many countries. UNICEF has supported India's BCG vaccination program. It has also assisted for penicillin plant, donated a DDT plant; two plants for the manufacture of triple vaccine and iodized salt. It has also assisted environmental sanitation programs emphasizing safe and sufficient water for drinking and household use in rural areas. Currently, providing primary health care to mothers and children. Main core area of work is immunization; infant and young child care; family planning aspects of family health; safe water and adequate sanitation.
- **Family and child welfare:** To improve the care of children, both within and outside their home's activities like parent education, day-care centers, child welfare and youth agencies and women's clubs is started.
- **Child nutrition:** In mid-1950, supplementing child feeding started through low-cost protein-rich food mixtures. "Applied nutrition" programs is started in collaboration with FAO which help through community development, agricultural extension, schools, and health services. To combat nutritional deficiency started intervention like provision of large doses of vitamin A in Xerophthalmia prevalent areas; enrichment of salt with iodine in areas of endemic goiter; provision of iron and folate supplements to combat anemias and enrichment of foods.

National and International Agencies Related to Health

- **Education—formal and nonformal:** UNICEF is assisting India for improvement of teaching science, science laboratories' equipment, workshop tools, library books, and audio-visual aids in collaboration with UNESCO.
  - UNICEF is promoting **GOBI FFF** campaign to encourage four strategies for a 'child health revolution":
    - G for growth charts to better monitor child development;
    - O for oral rehydration to treat all mild and moderate dehydration;
    - B for breastfeeding; and
    - I for immunization against measles, diphtheria, polio, pertussis, tetanus, and tuberculosis
    - F for female education
    - F for family spacing
    - F for food supplements
- **WASH:** Water, sanitation and hygiene strategy has been launched by UNICEF for ensuring clean water and reliable sanitation.

13.3 IMPORTANT UN AGENCIES (UNDP, UNFPA), WORLD BANK, FAO AND ILOS

United Nations agencies	Bilateral agencies
UNICEF	USAID
UNDP	The Colombo plan
UNFPA	SIDA
FAO	DANIDA
ILO	
World Bank	

UNITED NATIONS POPULATION FUND (UNFPA)

- Earlier it was known as the **United Nations Fund for Population Activities** but formally known as United Nation Population Fund. It came into existence in 1969.
- UNFPA is an UN agency for delivering a world where every pregnancy is wanted, every childbirth is safe and every young person's potential is fulfilled.

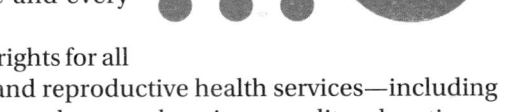

- UNFPA calls for the realization of reproductive rights for all and supports access to a wide range of sexual and reproductive health services—including voluntary family planning, maternal health care and comprehensive sexuality education.
- Headquarter: New York USA.

Functions

- To develop national capability for production of contraceptives.
- To develop population education programs.
- To undertake organized sector projects.
- To strengthen program management as well as to improve the productivity of grass-root level health workers.

- To introduce innovative approaches to family planning and MCH care.

In 2018 UNFPA has launched efforts for three core objectives like ending unmet need for family planning, ending preventable maternal death and ending gender-based violence and harmful practices.

UNITED NATIONS DEVELOPMENT PROGRAM (UNDP)

- Established in 1965 by merging United Nations expanded program of technical assistance and United Nation special fund.
- UNDP mandate is to end poverty, build democratic governance, rule of law, and inclusive institutions.
- It helps poorer nations to develop their human and natural resources through providing funds to technical assistance.
- It helps every economic and social sector—agriculture, industry, education and science, health, social welfare, etc.
- Its work is concentrated in three focus areas; sustainable development, democratic governance and peace building, and climate and disaster resilience.

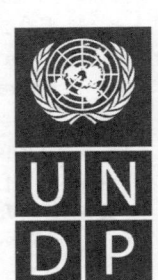

WORLD BANK

- Motto of world bank is world free from poverty
- Established in 1944.
- Headquarter: Washington D.C., USA
- It is a group of five institutions namely IBRD (187 member countries), IDA (173 member countries), IFC, MIGA, and ICSID. Out of which IBRD and IDA are forming the World Bank while the other three are private sectors.
- The World Bank commitment is for reducing poverty (reduction of extreme poverty to 3% by 2030), increasing shared prosperity (by increasing income of the poorest 40% of people in every country) and promoting sustainable development.
- It loans to poor countries for projects like electric power, roads, railways, agriculture, water supply, education, family planning, nutrition, etc.
- Currently Bank Group's work focuses nearly every sector that is important to fighting poverty, supporting economic growth, and ensuring sustainable gains in the quality of people's lives in developing countries.

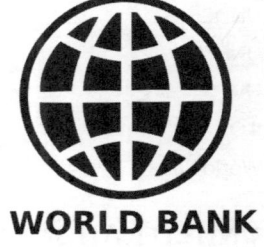

FOOD AND AGRICULTURAL ORGANIZATION OF THE UNITED NATIONS (FAO)

- Established in 1945
  - Goal: To achieve food security.
  - Headquarter: Rome, Italy.
  - Tag line of FAO "*FIAT PANIS*" means "let there be bread".
  - Codex alimentarius was created jointly by FAO and the World Health Organization in 1961.
  - At present FAO has 194 member states.

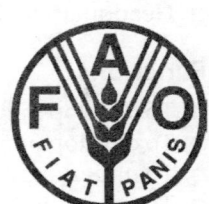

Objectives
- To help nations to raise living standards.
- To improve nutrition level of the people of all countries.
- To enhancing the efficiency of farming, forestry and fisheries.
- To enhance the production and distribution of food and agriculture products.
- To improve the condition of rural people.
- To improve knowledge and administration in nutrition, food, and agriculture.

INTERNATIONAL LABOR ORGANIZATION (ILO)

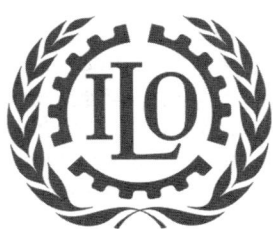

- It is the UN agency for the world of work.
- It is the first specialized UN agency working since 1919 and currently it has 187 member states.
- It set labor standards, develop policies and devise programs promoting decent work for all women and men.
- The main aims of ILO are:
  - To promote rights at works
  - To encourage decent employment opportunities
  - To enhance social protection
  - To strengthen dialogue on work-related issue
- **Aim:** To establish peace by promoting social justice, to improve economic stability, to improve labor conditions and standard of living.
- Headquarter: Geneva, Switzerland.

13.4 INTERNATIONAL BILATERAL AGENCIES OR NGOs (CARE, FORD FOUNDATION, ROCKEFELLER FOUNDATION, SIDA, DANIDA, COLOMBO PLAN)

COOPERATIVE FOR ASSISTANCE AND RELIEF EVERYWHERE (CARE)

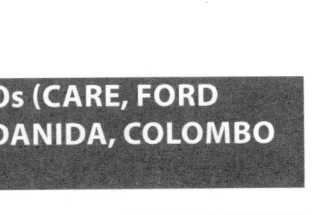

- CARE was founded in North America in the wake of the Second World War in the year 1945.
- Earlier CARE was "Cooperative for American relief everywhere" and since 1993 it is known as "Cooperative for Assistance and Relief Everywhere".
- It is one of the world's largest independent, nonprofit, nonsectarian international relief and development organizations.
- CARE provides emergency aid and long-term development assistance.
- CARE began its operation in India in 1950. Till the end of 1980s, the primary objective of CARE—India was to provide food for children in the age group of 6–11 years.
- From mid 1980s, CARE-India focused its food support in the ICDS program and in development of programs in the areas of health and income supplementation.

Functions
Emergency response, advocacy, climate change, maternal health education, HIV and AIDS, economic development, food security, water sanitation and hygiene, focus on women and girls and COVID-19 response also.

Key projects for maternal and child health are:
- Stop Stunting, Gift Every Child a Great Start in Life
- Khushaal Madhepura
- Elimination of Kala Azar-BTSP
- Ensuring Newborn Survival Through Intervention in The Community and Facilities
- Improving Treatment for Child Health
- Reproductive and Child Health Nutrition and Awareness (RACHNA)
- Briddhi
- Family Health Initiative in Bihar (FHI).

FORD FOUNDATION

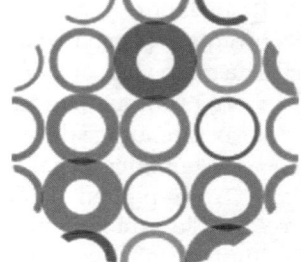

- Rural health services and family planning services are two main field area of this organization.
- It has been working in India since 1922.
- Following **projects in India:**
  - **Orientation training centers:** It is established at Singur, Poonamallee and Najafgarh. They provide training courses in public health for medical and paramedical personnel from all over India.
  - **Research cum-action projects:** Aim of this project to solve basic problems in environmental sanitation, e.g., designing and construction of hand-flushed acceptable sanitary latrines in rural areas.
  - Pilot project in rural health services, Gandhigram (Tamil Nadu): It is useful model for health administrators for coordinated type of health service in the country.
  - Establishment of NIHAE: National Institute of Health Administration and Education established at Delhi. The Institute provides senior staff college type training for health administrators.
  - Calcutta water supply and drainage scheme: Plan for water supply, sewerage and drainage for the city of Calcutta was prepared in collaboration with other international agencies.
  - **Family planning program:** The Foundation helps for research in reproductive biology and in family planning fellowship programs.

ROCKEFELLER FOUNDATION (RF)

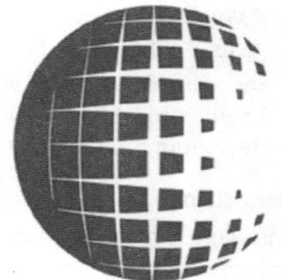

- It is established in 1913 by Mr John D Rockefeller.
- **Aim:** To promote the well-being of mankind throughout the world.
- Initially it helps work for public health and medical education and later on the advancement of life sciences, the social sciences, the humanities and the agricultural sciences.
- Their work in India began in 1920 with a scheme for the control of hookworm disease in the Madras Presidency.
- The establishment of the All India Institute of Hygiene and Public Health at Kolkata was in a large measure due to the cooperation of the Rockefeller Foundation.

- It helps in establishment of London School of Hygiene and Tropical Medicine (UK), Johns Hopkins School of Public Health (US), Harvard School of Public Health (US) and School of Hygiene (Canada).

The Foundation's **program** includes:
- Training of competent teachers and research workers;
- Training abroad of candidates from India through fellowships and travel grants;
- Providing grants-in-aid to selected institutions: Development of medical college libraries; population studies;
- Assistance for the development of the institutions like National Institute of Virology at Pune, field demonstration area (Ballabgarh) in connection with a department of preventive and social medicine and All India Institute of Medical Sciences (AIIMS).

SWEDISH INTERNATIONAL DEVELOPMENT AGENCY (SIDA)

- Since 1979, it is assisting the National Tuberculosis Control Programme.
- It assists mainly for procurement of supplies like X-ray units, microscopes and antituberculosis drugs.

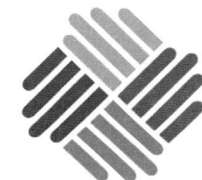

DANIDA

- Since 1978, The Government of Denmark is providing assistance for the development of services under National Blindness Control Programme.
- They also work for eradication of poverty and ensuring sustainable development.

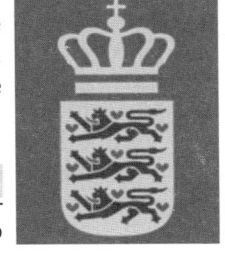

THE COLOMBO PLAN

- At a meeting of the commonwealth Foreign Ministers at Colombo in January 1950, a program was drawn up for cooperative economic development in South and South East Asia.
- The aim of Colombo plan is seeking to improve living standards of the people of the area by reviewing developmental plans and coordinating development assistance.
- Membership comprises 20 developing countries within the region and six nonregional members—Australia, Canada, Japan, New Zealand, UK and USA.
- It assists industrial and agricultural development, also provide support to health promotion, mostly through fellowships. The AIIMS at New Delhi was established with financial assistance from New Zealand.

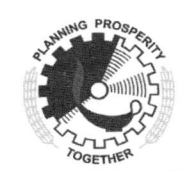

THE COLOMBO PLAN

13.5 NATIONAL HEALTH AGENCIES

INDIAN RED CROSS SOCIETY

- It is a voluntary humanitarian organization.
- There are more than 1,100 branches across the nation providing relief during disaster or any emergency. It also promotes health of vulnerable communities.
- It is part of the International Red Cross and Red Crescent Movement.

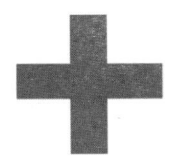

Indian Red Cross Society

- It was established in 1920 by under the Indian Red Cross Society Act. Honorable President of India is the President and Hon'ble Union Health Minister is the Chairman of the Society. Vice chairman is elected by members of the managing body.
- The three **objectives** of the improvement of health, prevention of disease, and mitigation of suffering.
- **Principles:** Humanity, impartiality, neutrality, independence, voluntary services, unity, and universality.
- In peacetime, the society provides military hospitals with such amenities as newspapers, periodicals, musical instruments and other comfort goods.

Activities

- Social emergency response volunteers (SERV)
- Blood Bank
- Livelihood program
- First aid
- Education and training program
- Tuberculosis (TB) program
- Family news service
- Youth program
- Partners for resilience
  - The **JUNIOR RED CROSS** is one of the most active sections of the society. It provides an opportunity to millions of boys and girls all over India to work for the village uplift, first aid, antiepidemic work and building up of an international fraternity of youth, thus promoting international friendliness, understanding, and cooperation.
  - **Nursing services:** MCW unite teach Home nursing skills to different cadre of nursing fraternity.

INDIAN COUNCIL FOR CHILD WELFARE (ICCW)

- Established in 1952.
- ICCW is affiliated to the International Union for Child Welfare.
- It is working for disadvantaged children for issue like child labor, child abuse, female infanticides, child education, and training.

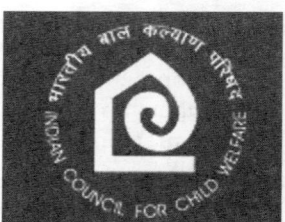

Activities:
- Sponsorship for school education of under-privileged children
- Honoring children for bravery
- Honoring child artists
- National integration camps/adventure camps
- Advocating children's rights
- Scrutiny of adoption cases
- Rehabilitation of abandoned children
- Creches for children
- Programs with special focus on the girl child
- Training programs for child care workers
- Projects for street and working children
- Institutional and daycare services for differently abled children

FAMILY PLANNING ASSOCIATION OF INDIA

- Established in 1949.
- Headquarter: Mumbai
- FPA India was key agency in advocating for family planning to be introduced in the country's first Five Year Plan (1952). And as a result of that, India became the first country in the world to have a family planning program.
- It generates awareness of small family norms, runs family planning clinics and trains the health staff and social workers.
- Currently, FPA India delivering essential health services focusing on sexual and reproductive health in 18 states and UTs.

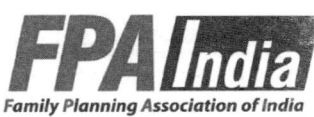

TUBERCULOSIS ASSOCIATION OF INDIA

- Established in 1939
- Headquarter at New Delhi

Objectives

- The prevention, control, treatment, and relief of tuberculosis.
- The encouragement of and assistance in the establishment throughout India of State Associations having objectives similar in whole or in part to those of the Association.
- The undertaking of the Research and Investigation on subjects concerning tuberculosis and allied chest diseases.

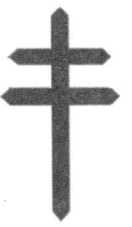

Activities: Every year organize TB seal campaign to raise funds, train staff and social worker in anti TB work, health promotion, and education.

HIND KUSHT NIVARAN SANGH (HKNS)

- Established in 1950.
- Headquarter in New Delhi.
- Its predecessor was the Indian Council of the British Empire Leprosy Relief Association, which was dissolved in 1950.
- The objectives of serving leprosy afflicted individuals, removing stigma of leprosy from the society and promoting social and research activities in the field of leprosy in India.

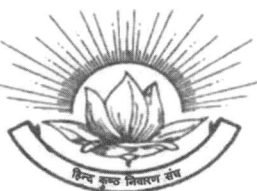

Activities of HKNS

- Help leprosy homes and clinics.
- Health education through publication and publicity.
- Training of health personnel.
- Field diagnosis and research.

- Arranging leprosy worker's conference and publication of quarterly "Leprosy India".
  - Celebrate Anti-Leprosy Day on the 30th of January every year to create mass awareness about leprosy.
  - Rehabilitation of leprosy patients.

CENTRAL SOCIAL WELFARE BOARD (CSWB)

- Established in 1953
- It is an independent organization under the general administrative control of the Ministry of Education.

Functions

- Identify needs and requirements of voluntary welfare organizations in the country.
- Promote and establish social welfare organizations on a voluntary basis.
- Ender representation of financial aid to deserving existing organizations and institutions.

Activities

- Social education, literacy classes, maternity help for women, distribution of milk, Balwadis and organization of play centers for children.
- Started industrial cooperative scheme for women in urban area belongs to lower-middle-class to supplement their income by doing paid work.

BLIND PEOPLE'S ASSOCIATION OF INDIA

- It is a professional organization which provides equal opportunities to all categories of people with disabilities.
- The blinds, deaf, mentally retarded, orthopedically impaired, mentally ill, multiple disability, aged peoples, etc., Are covered under mission of BPA.
- Employment plays an essential part in the life of a person because it gives him status and binds him to the society.
- It works for providing education, employment opportunities, equal rights, and quality life for them.

ALL INDIA WOMEN'S CONFERENCE

- Established in 1926
- It is the only voluntary women's welfare organization in the country.
- **Vision:** Emancipation, education, and empowerment of women.
- It gives special contribution in running of maternal, child health clinics, health centers, family planning clinics, and milk centers. It also makes arrangements for adult education.

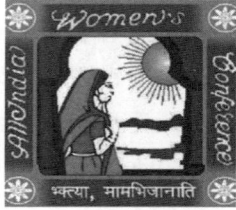

LIST OF IMPORTANT INDIAN PUBLIC HEALTH INSTITUTIONS WITH THEIR HEADQUARTERS

Sl. No.	Name of public health institution	City/Headquarter
1.	Central Research Institute	Kasauli
2.	All India Institute of Hygiene and Public Health	Kolkata
3.	National Centre for Diseases Control	Delhi
4.	Central Drugs Laboratory	Kolkata
5.	Central Institute of Psychiatry	Ranchi
6.	Medical Stores Organization (total 7)	Mumbai, Kolkata, Chennai, Hyderabad, Guwahati, Karnal, and New Delhi
7.	B.C.G. Vaccine Laboratory	Guindy, Chennai
8.	Central Food and Standardization Laboratory	Ghaziabad
9.	All India Institute of Physical Medicine and Rehabilitation	Mumbai
10.	National Tuberculosis Institute	Bengaluru (Bangalore)
11.	Central Leprosy Teaching and Research Institute	Chengalpattu
12.	All India Institute of Medical Sciences	Delhi
13.	All India Institute of Speech and Hearing	Mysuru (Mysore)
14.	National Institute of Mental Health and Neuroscience	Bengaluru (Bangalore)
15.	International Institute of Population Sciences	Mumbai
16.	Indian Council of Medical Research	Delhi
17.	National Institute of Nutrition	Hyderabad
18.	National Institute of Virology	Pune
19.	National Environmental Engineering Research Institute	Nagpur
20.	Central Japanese Leprosy Mission for Asia (JALMA)	Agra
21.	All India Institute of Medical Sciences	Delhi
22.	Central Drug Research Institute	Lucknow
23.	Haffkine Institute	Mumbai
24.	LRS institute of TB and allied diseases	Delhi
25.	Tuberculosis Research Center	Chennai
26.	National Institute of Occupational Health (NIOH)	Ahmedabad
27.	National Institute of Epidemiology (ICMR)	Chennai
28.	National Institute of Research in Reproductive Health	Mumbai
29.	Center for Research in Medical Entomology (VCRC)	Madurai

BIBLIOGRAPHY

1. http://www.who.int/en/
2. http://unicef.in/
3. https://www.undp.org/
4. https://www.unfpa.org/
5. https://www.worldbank.org/en/about
6. http://www.fao.org/home/en/
7. https://www.ilo.org/global/lang--en/index.htm
8. https://www.careindia.org/
9. https://www.fordfoundation.org/about/about-ford/mission/
10. https://www.rockefellerfoundation.org/
11. https://www.sida.se/en/about-sida
12. https://www.unicef.org/chad/danida
13. https://colombo-plan.org/history/
14. https://indianredcross.org/ircs/index.php/
15. https://www.iccw.co.in/aboutus.html
16. https://fpaindia.org/
17. http://www.tbassnindia.org/index.html
18. http://hkns.in/
19. https://www.cswb.gov.in/
20. https://bpaindia.org/
21. http://www.aiwc.org.in/about_us.html
22. K Park. Park's Textbook of Preventive and Social Medicine, 25th ed. Jabalpur: Bhanot Publishers; 2019.

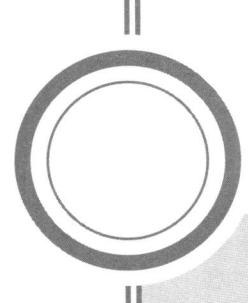

Annexures

CHAPTER OUTLINE

1. Knowing your population
2. Incentives of ASHA
3. APGAR score
4. Partograph
5. Objective structured clinical examination (OSCE)

1. KNOWING YOUR POPULATION

DEMOGRAPHIC STRUCTURE

As grass root healthcare worker, to understand, predict and cater to the health needs of your population, you need to first understand—what constitutes your population. So, following table would help to estimate the number of population from different age group.

Age groups	Percentage	Formula	Total population in a catchment area of 5000
0–1 year of age	3	3 × 5,000/100	150
0–4 year of age	9.7	9.7 × 5,000/100	485
1–5 year of age	11.2	11.2 × 5,000/100	560
5–9 year of age	9.2	9.2 × 5,000/100	460
10–14 year of age	10.5	10.5 × 5,000/100	525
0–14 year of age	29.5	29.5 × 5,000/100	1,475
10–19 year of age	18.4	18.4 × 5,000/100	920
15–49 year women of reproductive age group	24	24 × 5,000/100	1,200

Age groups	Percentage	Formula	Total population in a catchment area of 5000
15–59 years of age	62.5	62.5 × 5,000/100	3,125
30 years and above	37	37 × 5,000/100	1,850
60 years and above	8	8 × 5,000/100	400
65 years and above	5.3	5.3 × 5,000/100	265

(% of each age group based on census 2011)

CALCULATING THE BENEFICIARIES

Estimated Number of Pregnant Women in HWC Area
- For example, birth rate of your area is 20.2/1,000 population.
- Population under each SHC-HWC is 5,000
- Therefore, expected number of live-births = (20.2 × 5,000)/1,000 = 101 births
- Correction factor = 10% of live births [i.e. (10/100) × 101] = 10.1. As some of the pregnancies may not result in a live-birth (i.e., abortions and stillbirths may occur), the expected number of live births is an underestimation of the total number of pregnancies. Hence, a correction factor of 10% is required.
- Therefore, total number of expected pregnant women in a year under one HWC = 101 + 10.1 = 111.1 = 111 per year.

Number of Live Births/Estimated Newborns in HWC Area
- Expected number of live-births = (20.2 × 5,000)/1,000 = 101 births
- Hence number of newborns per month = 101/12 = 8–9/month in a population of 5,000.

Estimated Number of Pregnant Mothers with Complications
- Estimated maternal complications is 15% approx.
- Hence number of mothers with complications in pregnancy, delivery and postpartum are: Number of pregnant women × 15%.
- Number of pregnant women with under one HWC-SHC = 111
- Number of pregnant women with complications = 111 × 15% = 16 to 17 annually.

Eligible Couples: 17% of Total Population
Total number of eligible couples in HWC-SHC = (5,000 × 17/100) = 850 eligible couples/5,000 population.

Sick Newborns: 10–12% of Total Live Births
- Total number of live-births in SHC-HWC = 101 births
- Number of sick newborns in SHC-HWC = (101 × 12/100) = 12–13 sick newborns.

Estimation of Beneficiaries for Common Noncommunicable Diseases
- Population above 30 years is 37% of the total population, i.e., 1850
- No. of men above 30 years 51% of the total above 30 age group = 944
- No. of women above 30 years 49% of the total above 30 age group = 906

Annexures

- For hypertension and diabetes cases annually = 1,850
- For oral cancer –for men and women per year = 370
- Breast cancer and cervical cancer per year = 182

Number of Neonatal/Infant Deaths

- For example, IMR in your area: 33/1,000 live births
- NMR can be approximately calculated as 2/3rd of the IMR
- Hence NMR: 2/3 × 33 = 22 approx.
- Annual live births in a year at 5,000 population or under one HWC-SHC = 101
- Hence, the number of infant's deaths is equal to number of births annually × IMR divided by 1,000 = 101 × 33/1,000 = 3.33; thus 3–4 infant deaths annually at a HWC-SHC.
- Total number of births annually × NMR and divided by 1000 = 101 × 22/1,000 = 2.2
- Thus, 2–3 neonatal deaths annually at a HWC-SHC.

Antenatal Care Coverage

Percentage of pregnancies in the area that received ANC: = (No. of pregnancies received ANC/Total number of pregnancies) × 100.

BIBLIOGRAPHY

1. http://www.nrhmorissa.gov.in/writereaddata/Upload/Documents/Induction%20Training%20Module%20for%20CHOs.pdf

2. INCENTIVES OF ASHA

Sl. No.	Activities	Amount in ₹/case
I	**Maternal Health**	
1.	JSY financial package (₹600 for rural and ₹400 for urban area)	
a.	For ensuring antenatal care for the woman	₹300 for rural areas and ₹200 for urban areas
b.	For facilitating institutional delivery	₹300 for rural areas and ₹200 for urban areas
2.	Reporting death of women (15–49 years age group) by ASHA to PHC Medical Officer/THO	₹200 for reporting and ₹1,000 if within 24 hours of occurrence of death by phone
3.	e-PMSMA	₹300 (₹100 per visit for three visit) and ₹500 on 45th day after delivery
II	**Child Health**	
1.	Undertaking home visit for the care of the newborn and postpartum mother Six visits in case of institutional delivery (Days 3rd, 7th, 14th, 21st, 28th, and 42nd) Seven visits in case of home deliveries (Days 1st, 3rd, 7th, 14th, 21st, 28th, and 42nd)	₹250

Sl. No.	Activities	Amount in ₹/case
2.	Undertaking home visits of young child for strengthening of health and nutrition of young child through home visits—(recommended schedule- 3rd, 6th, 9th, 12th and 15th months)—(₹50 × 5 visits) follow-up of low-birth-weight babies and newborns discharged after treatment from specialized new-born care units are also included in it	₹50/visit with total ₹250/per child for making 05 visits. If ASHA does visit between 3–5 then eligible to get ₹125 and if less than 3 then nothing will be given.
3.	Child death review for reporting child death of children under 5 years of age	₹50
4.	For mobilizing and ensuring every eligible child (1–19 years out-of-school and nonenrolled) is administered Albendazole.	₹100/ASHA/Bi-annual
5.	ASHA incentive for prophylactic distribution of ORS to families with underfive children during IDCF	₹1 per ORS packet for 100 under five children
6.	Mother's absolute affection (MAA) program promotion of breastfeeding—quarterly mother meeting	₹100/ASHA/quarterly meeting
III	**Immunization**	
1.	Full immunization for a child under one year	₹100, some states giving ₹150
2.	Complete immunization per child up to two years age	₹75, some states giving ₹90
3.	Mobilizing children for OPV immunization under Pulse Polio Program	₹150/day (Break up: ASHA-25, AWW-50, AWH-50, Other-25)
4.	DPT booster at 5–6 years of age	₹50
IV	**Family Planning**	
1.	Ensuring spacing of 2 years after marriage	₹500
2.	Ensuring spacing of 3 years after birth of 1st child	₹500
3.	Ensuring a couple to opt for permanent limiting method after 2 children	₹1,000
4.	Counseling, motivating and follow-up of the cases for Tubectomy	₹200 in 11 states with high fertility rates (UP, Bihar, MP, Rajasthan, Chhattisgarh, Jharkhand, Odisha, Uttarakhand, Assam, Haryana, and Gujarat) ₹300 in 146 MPV districts ₹150 in remaining states
5.	Counseling, motivating and follow-up of the cases for Vasectomy/ NSV	₹300 in 11 states with high fertility rates (UP, Bihar, MP, Rajasthan, Chhattisgarh, Jharkhand, Odisha, Uttarakhand, Assam, Haryana and Gujarat) and 400 in 146 MPV districts and ₹200 in remaining states

Sl. No.	Activities	Amount in ₹/case
6.	Female postpartum sterilization	₹300 in 11 states with high fertility rates (UP, Bihar, MP, Rajasthan, Chhattisgarh, Jharkhand, Odisha, Uttarakhand, Assam, Haryana, and Gujarat) and 400 in 146 MPV districts
7.	Social marketing of contraceptives—as home delivery through ASHAs	₹1 for a pack of 03 condoms, ₹1 for a cycle of OCP, ₹2 for a pack of ECPs
8.	Escorting or facilitating beneficiary to the health facility for the PPIUCD insertion	₹150/per case
9.	Escorting or facilitating beneficiary to the health facility for the PAIUCD insertion	₹150/case
Mission Parivar Vikas—in selected 146 districts in six states-(57 in UP, 37 in Bihar, 14 in Rajasthan, 9 in Jharkhand, 2 in Chhattisgarh, and 2 in Assam)		
10.	Injectable contraceptive MPA (Antara program) and a nonhormonal weekly centchroman pill (Chhaya)—incentive to ASHA	₹100 per dose
11.	Mission Parivar Vikas campaigns block level activities—ASHA to be oriented on eligible couple survey for estimation of beneficiaries and will be expected to conducted eligible couple survey- maximum four rounds	₹150/ASHA/round
12.	Nayi Pahel—a FP kit would be given to the newly wed couple by ASHA (In initial phase ASHA may be given 2 kits/ASHA)	₹100/ASHA/Nayi Pahel kit distribution
13.	Saas Bahu Sammelan—mobilize Saas Bahu for the Sammelan—maximum four rounds	₹100/per meeting
14.	Updating of EC survey before each MPV campaign- Note: updating of EC survey register incentive is already part of routine and recurring incentive	₹150/ASHA/quarterly round
V	**Adolescent Health**	
1.	Distributing sanitary napkins to adolescent girls	₹1/pack of 6 sanitary napkins
2.	Organizing monthly meeting with adolescent girls pertaining to menstrual hygiene	₹50/meeting
3.	Incentive for support to peer educator (for facilitating selection process of peer educators)	₹100/per PE
4.	Incentive for mobilizing adolescents for adolescent health day	₹200/per AHD
VI	**Incentive for Routine Recurrent Activities**	
1.	Mobilizing and attending VHND or (outreach session/ urban health and nutrition days)	₹200 per session
2.	Convening and guiding monthly meeting of VHSNC/ MAS	₹150

Sl. No.	Activities	Amount in ₹/case
3.	Attending monthly meeting at Block PHC/SU-PHC	₹150
4.	• Line listing of households done at beginning of the year and updated every six months • Maintaining records as per the desired norms like– village health register • Preparation of due list of children to be immunized updated on monthly basis • Preparation of due list of ANC beneficiaries to be updated on monthly basis • Preparation of list of eligible couples updated on monthly basis	₹1,500
VII	**Participatory Learning and Action- (In selected 10 states that have low RMNCH+A indicators—Assam, Bihar, Chhattisgarh, Jharkhand, MP, Meghalaya, Odisha, Rajasthan, Uttarakh, and and UP)**	
1.	Conducting PLA meetings—2 meetings per month- Note: Incentive is also applicable for AFs @ ₹100/- per meeting for 10 meetings in a month	₹100/ASHA/per meeting for 02 meetings in a month
VIII	**Revised National Tuberculosis Control Programme/NTEP**	
	Honorarium and counselling charges for being a DOTS provider	
1.	For drug sensitive TB patients	₹1,000
2.	For drug resistant TB patients	₹5,000
3.	For notification if suspect referred is diagnosed to be TB patient by MO/Lab	₹100
IX	**National Leprosy Eradication Programme**	
1.	Referral and ensuring compliance for complete treatment in pauci-bacillary cases of Leprosy—for 33 states (except Goa, Chandigarh and Puducherry)	₹250 (for facilitating diagnosis of leprosy case) + ₹400 (for follow-up on completion of treatment)
2.	Referral and ensuring compliance for complete treatment in multi-bacillary cases of Leprosy—for 33 states (except Goa, Chandigarh, and Puducherry)	₹250 (for facilitating diagnosis of leprosy case) + ₹600 (for follow-up on completion of treatment)
X	**National Vector Borne Disease Control Programme**	
A.	**Malaria**	
1.	Preparing blood slides or testing through RDT	₹15/slide or test
2.	Providing complete treatment for RDT positive Pf cases	₹75/- per positive cases
3.	Providing complete radical treatment to positive Pf and Pv case detected by blood slide, as per drug regime	
4.	For referring a case and ensuring complete treatment	₹300
B.	**Lymphatic Filariasis**	
1.	For one time line listing of lymphoedema and hydrocele cases in all areas of nonendemic and endemic districts	₹200

Annexures

Sl. No.	Activities	Amount in ₹/case
2.	For annual mass drug administration for cases of lymphatic filariasis	₹200/day for maximum three days to cover 50 houses and 250 persons
C.	**Acute Encephalitis Syndrome/Japanese Encephalitis**	
1	Referral of AES/JE cases to the nearest CHC/DH/medical college	₹300 per case
D.	**Kala Azar elimination**	
1.	Involvement of ASHAs during the spray rounds (IRS) for sensitizing the community to accept indoor spraying	₹100/- per round during Indoor residual spray, i.e., ₹200 in total for two rounds
2.	ASHA incentive for referring a suspected case and ensuring complete treatment.	₹500/per notified case
E.	**Dengue and Chikungunya**	
1.	Incentive for source reduction and IEC activities for prevention and control of dengue and chikungunya in 12 high endemic states (Andhra Pradesh, Assam, Gujarat, Karnataka, Kerala, Maharashtra, Odisha, Punjab, Rajasthan, Tamil Nadu, Telangana and West Bengal)	₹200/- (1 Rupee/House for maximum 200 houses PM for 08 months–during peak transmission season). The incentive should not be exceed ₹1,600/ASHA/Year
XI	**National Iodine Deficiency Disorders Control Programme**	
1.	ASHA incentive for salt testing	₹25 a month for testing 50 salt samples
XII	**Incentives under Comprehensive Primary Health Care (CPHC) and Universal NCDs Screening**	
1.	Maintaining data validation and collection of additional information—per completed form/family for NHPM-Ayushman Bharat	₹5/form/family
2.	Filling-up of CBAC forms of every individual—one time activity for enumeration of all individuals, filling CBAC for all individuals 30 or >30 years of age	₹10/per form/per individual as one time incentive
3.	Follow up of patients diagnosed with hypertension/diabetes and three common cancer for initiation of treatment and ensuring compliance	₹50/per case/Bi-annual
4.	Delivery of new service packages under CPHC component	₹1,000/ASHA/PM (linked with new packages of activities)
XIII	**Drinking water and sanitation**	
1.	Motivating households to construct toilet and promote the use of toilets	₹75 per household
2.	Motivating households to take individual tap connections	₹75 per household

To improve the financial security of ASHAs, the Government of India has already taken several steps in addition to routine and recurring incentives, which inter-alia includes:

- Pradhan Mantri Jeevan Jyoti Bima Yojana (premium of ₹330 contributed by GOI).
- Pradhan Mantri Suraksha Bima Yojana (premium of ₹12 contributed by GOI).

- Pradhan Mantri Shram Yogi Maan Dhan (PM-SYM) (50% contribution of premium by GOI and 50% by beneficiaries).
- The government has also approved a cash award of ₹20,000/- and a citation to ASHAs who leave the program after working as ASHAs for minimum of 10 years, as acknowledgement of their contribution.

BIBLIOGRAPHY

1. https://pib.gov.in/Pressreleaseshare.aspx?PRID=1606212.

3. APGAR SCORE

- It was originally developed by Virginia Apgar (Anesthesiologist) in 1952.
- It was developed to address the need for a standardized way to evaluate infants shortly after birth.
- The Apgar score is a quick tool for healthcare providers to assess the health of all newborns at 1 and 5 minutes after birth and in response to resuscitation.
- APGAR is acronym for **A**: Activity, **P**: Pulse, **G**: Grimace, **A**: Appearance and **R**: Respiration.

	0 Point	1 Point	2 Point
Activity muscle tone)	Absent	Arms and legs flexed	Active movement
Pulse	Absent	Below 100 bpm	Over 100 bpm
Grimace (reflex irritability)	Flaccid	Some flexion of extremities	Active motion (sneeze, cough, pull away)
Appearance (skin color)	Blue, pale	Body pink, extremities blue	Completely pink
Respiration	Absent	Slow, irregular	Vigorous cry

- **Interpretation of score:**
  - Severely depressed: 0–3
  - Moderately depressed: 4–6
  - Excellent condition: 7–10

BIBLIOGRAPHY

1. https://www.bila.ca/2017/08/whats-an-apgar-score-and-why-is-it-important-to-my-baby/

4. PARTOGRAPH

- If alert line is crossed (the plotting moves to the right of the alert line) it indicates abnormal labor like prolonged/obstructed labor and do as indicated:
  - Note the time
  - Refer patient to FRU
  - Send partograph with patient

Annexures

- Crossing of the **action line** (the plotting moves to the right of the action line): Indicates the need for intervention
- By the time the action line is crossed the woman should ideally have reached the FRU for the appropriate intervention to take place.

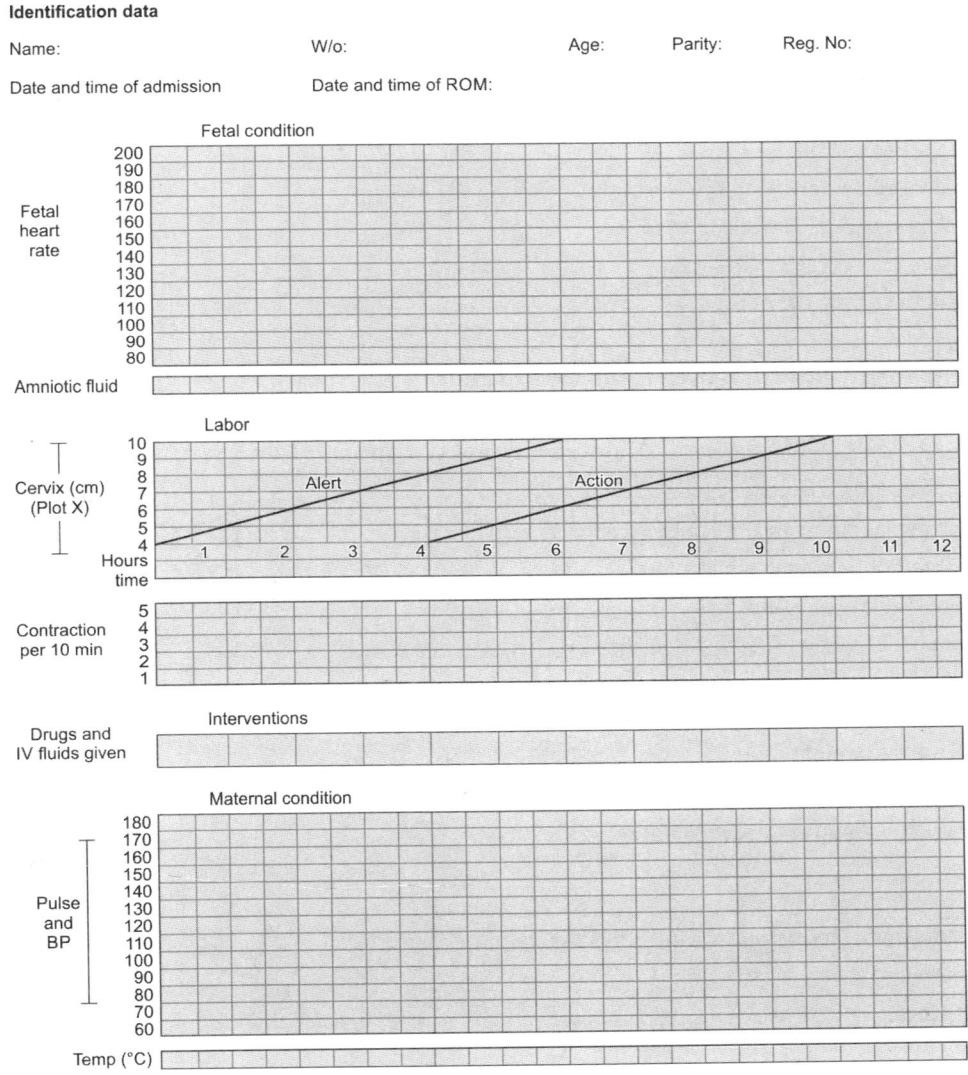

Note: Other details about partograph covered in details in the Chapter 2.

BIBLIOGRAPHY

1. https://nhm.gov.in/images/pdf/programmes/maternalhealth/guidelines/sba_guidelines_for_skilled_attendance_at_birth.pdf

5. OBJECTIVE STRUCTURED CLINICAL EXAMINATION (OSCE)

Some evaluation forms are given here for OSCE.

EDD, WEIGHT, AND BP MEASUREMENT

Equipment: Weight scale, blood pressure machine, stethoscope, chair, role player, and medical record.

	Total mark	Score	Remark
Ask to calculate EDD	2		
Explain and demonstrate the use of the weighing scales			
• Ensure scale is on flat and hard surface	1		
• Ensure scale is calibrated to zero	2		
• Read to nearest 100 g	1		
• Record on MCP card	1		
Describe and demonstrate the measurement of BP			
• Ensure patient is sitting or lying down on her left-side	1		
• Ensure sphygmomanometer is at level of heart. *Note* zero error.	1		
• Position cuff (3 cm above elbow)	1		
• Increase cuff pressure until pulse disappears + 30 mm Hg	1		
• Put stethoscope on brachial artery	1		
• Slowly release pressure	1		
• Note the BP when the sound is heard (systolic) and when it disappears (diastolic)	2		
• Record on MCP card	1		
State normal weight gain			
9–11 kg	1		
How do you diagnose pre-eclampsia?			
• Hypertension • Albumin (+2) in urine	2		
What diastolic blood pressure indicates severe pre-eclampsia?			
110 mm Hg	1		
Total score:	**20**		

Annexures

ABDOMINAL EXAMINATION

Equipment: Abdominal mannequin, fetal stethoscope, tape measure, watch with second hand.

	Total mark	Score	Remark
Please elaborate the steps before you carry out an abdominal examination/palpation			
• Ensure privacy of woman	1		
• Obtain verbal consent from woman	1		
• Check that she has emptied her bladder and instruct her to keep her legs and thighs in a semi-flexed position with thighs kept slightly open	1		
• Examine from the right-hand side	1		
• Centralize the uterus with one hand if it is tilted to one side	1		
Please demonstrate how to do an abdominal examination/palpation			
Here instructor would prompt: What do you look for on the abdomen? Visually assess:			
• Scars	1		
• Shape	1		
• Size	1		
Measure fundal height:			
• Using ulnar border of left hand, start palpating gently from xiphisternum downwards till you meet the first resistance (fundus of the uterus)	1		
• Identify symphysis pubis	1		
• Measure the distance between symphysis pubis and fundus in cm with the tape face down	1		
Here the facilitator would prompt: What is the importance of this?			
• cm = approx. gestational age in weeks	1		
Palpation:			
• Fundal grip: Keep both hands over the fundus and try to palpate the part of the fetus at the upper pole of the uterus to identify head or breech	1		
• Lateral grip: Keep hand on one side of the abdomen and palpate other side of the abdomen with other hand and repeat the maneuver to identify which side is the back of the fetus and determine the lie	1		
Pelvic pole to confirm presenting part and determine engagement:			
• First pelvic grip: With the fingers and thumb of the right hand try to hold the part of the fetus at the lower pole of the uterus just above the symphysis pubis and identify it and move it to see if it is movable or fixed	1		
• Second pelvic grip: Turn towards the feet of the woman, slightly extend the woman's legs. Keep both hands on either side of the presenting part with fingers towards the pelvis	1		

Auscultate FH on spinoumbilical line at the side identified as back			
• For 60 seconds	1		
• Record findings	1		
• Explain to mother	1		
What is the normal FH range?			
120–160 beats/min regular	1		
Total score:	**20**		

HEMOGLOBIN ESTIMATION

Equipment: Sahli's Hemoglobinometer, N/10 HCl, gloves, spirit swabs, lancet, distilled water and dropper, puncture proof container, 0.5% chlorine solution.

	Total mark	Score	Remark
Perform hemoglobin estimation with Sahli's Hemoglobinometer			
• Keep all the necessary items ready	1		
• Wash hands and wear gloves	1		
• Clean the Hb tube and pipette	1		
• Fill the Hb tube with N/10 HCl up to 2 g with the dropper	1		
• Clean tip of the person's ring finger with the spirit swab	2		
• Prick the ring finger with the lancet and discard the first drop of blood	2		
• Allow a large blood drop to form on the fingertip	1		
• Suctions it with the pipette up to 20 cu.mm mark. (Connect pipette to syringe and pull the barrel instead of mouth sucking by pipette)	2		
• Take care that air entry is prevented while suctioning the blood	1		
• Wipe the tip of the pipette and transfer the blood to the Hb tube containing N/10 HCl	1		
• Rinse the pipette 2–3 times with N/10 HCl in the Hb tube	1		
• Leave the solution in test tube for 10 minutes	1		
• After 10 minutes, dilute the acid by adding distilled water drop-by-drop and mix it with stirrer	1		
• Match with the color of the comparator	1		
• Note down the reading (lower meniscus)	1		
• Dispose of the used lancet in a puncture proof container	1		
• Immerse the used gloves in 0.5% chlorine solution	1		
Total score:	**20**		

PREGNANCY DETECTION TEST

Equipment: Pregnancy test kit with dropper, urine sample in container, watch or clock with second hand.

	Total mark	Score	Remark
How would you confirm her pregnancy?			
• Explain what you are doing and why	1		
• Ask woman to collect her urine sample in the container	1		
• Check expiry date on test kit and read instructions	2		
• Take out the test card from packaging and place on flat surface	2		
• Use dropper to put 2–3 drops of urine in the correct place on the test kit	1		
How long should you wait?			
• As per manufacturer's instructions	1		
How would you read the test?			
• 1 band = not pregnant	2		
• 2 bands = pregnant	2		
• 0 bands = test kit failed, try again with new test kit	2		
Test is positive—what would you do next?			
• Explain to the patient that she is pregnant	2		
• Encourage her to attend ANC	2		
• Register on MCP card/MCTS system	2		
Total score:	**20**		

URINE TEST

Equipment: Urine collection bottles, urine dipsticks, red disposal bin, and clock with second hand.

	Total mark	Score	Remark
Demonstrate how you would carry out a routine urine test for sugar and protein (albumin)			
• Explain to the patient what the test is for	1		
• Ask for a urine sample	1		
• Check expiry date on dipsticks and read instructions carefully	2		
• Remove one strip and close container tightly	2		
• Dip indicator side of the strip in the urine sample, remove it and tap at the edge of container to remove excess urine	2		
• Follow manufacturer's recommendations for when it is time to read the results	1		
• Compare the sugar reagent part with the sugar chart on the container	1		

Annexures

Compare the albumin reagent part with the albumin results chart on side of bottle	1		
Discard used test stick in red bin (as per GoI protocol)	1		
Explain results to the patient and record on MCP card	2		
Why is it important to test urine for the presence of protein?			
To detect pre-eclampsia	2		
Why do you test urine for glucose?			
To screen for gestational diabetes	2		
What will you do if test is positive for sugar?			
Refer to higher facility for further blood tests	2		
Total score:	**20**		

HAND WASHING

Equipment: Running water, soap, clean towel.

	Total mark	Score	Remark
Demonstrate how you would wash your hands			
Remove rings, bracelets and watches	2		
Wet hands with clean running water and apply soap	2		
Rub hands vigorously on both sides in the following order:			
• Palms, fingers and web spaces	1		
• Back of hands	1		
• Fingers and knuckles	1		
• Thumbs	1		
• Fingertips and creases	1		
• Wrist	1		
Rinse thoroughly under clean running water	2		
Dry hands using clean towel or air-dry	2		
What could you do if there was no running water available?			
Use alcohol rub	2		
How would you use this?			
Rub both sides of hands for 30 seconds or until the solution is dry	2		
When would this not be appropriate?			
If hands are soiled or bloody	2		
Total score:	**20**		

PREPARATION OF 0.5% CHLORINE SOLUTION

Equipment: Plastic bucket with cover, plastic mug, wooden stirrer, 1 L clean water, utility gloves, plastic apron, teaspoon, bleach powder in airtight container.

	Total mark	Score	Remark
What would you use to carry out the primary decontamination of the gloves and instruments?			
0.5% chlorine solution	3		
Please demonstrate how to prepare 0.5% chlorine solution			
• Put on plastic apron and utility gloves	2		
• Pour 1 L of water into the plastic bucket	2		
• Take some water in the mug from the bucket, then add 3 level teaspoons of bleaching powder to it to make a thick paste	4		
• Add the paste to the 1 L of water in the bucket and mix with the wooden stirrer	2		
• Cover bucket	3		
How would you store the bleaching powder?			
Airtight container away from sunlight	2		
When do you need to change the solution?			
At least every 24 hours or if it becomes turbid due to multiple use	2		
Total score:	20		

PERSONAL PROTECTIVE EQUIPMENT (PPE)

Equipment: Waterproof apron, gown, cap, mask, eye cover, shoe covers.

	Total mark	Score	Remark
Demonstrate how you would use PPE to protect yourself and the patient			
• Shoe covers	1		
• Waterproof apron	1		
• Eye cover	1		
• Cap	1		
• Mask	1		
• Gown	1		
• Gloves	1		
Put on the sterile gloves using the following procedure:			
• Ask assistant to open the outer package of the gloves	1		
• Open the inner wrapper exposing the cuffed gloves with the palm facing upwards	1		
• Pick up the first glove by the cuff, touching only the inside portion of the cuff	1		

• Hold the cuff in one hand and slip the other hand into the glove ensuring that the fingers enter the corresponding finger of the glove	1
• Pick up the second glove by sliding the fingers of the gloved hand under the cuff of the second glove	1
• Put the second glove on the ungloved hand by maintaining a steady pull through the cuff until the fingers reach the end of the corresponding finger of the glove	1
• Adjust the cuff until the gloves fit comfortably and cover both the wrists.	1
After the procedure, how would you remove the contaminated gloves?	
• Grasp one of the gloves near the cuff and pull downwards towards the fingers	1
• Grasp the second glove and pull downwards	1
• Pull off the two gloves at the same time, being careful to touch only the inside surfaces of the gloves with your bare hands	1
• Place them in a container of 0.5% chlorine solution	1
What precautions should you take to avoid contaminating sterile gloved hands?	
• Don't touch unsterile items with gloved hands	1
• Keep gloved hands above waist level	1
Total score:	**20**

CERVICAL DILATATION

Equipment: Cervical dilatation model, sterile, gloves, bowl with cotton swabs, antiseptic solution, sponge holder, 0.5% Chlorine solution, color coded waste disposal bins, PPE, kidney tray.

	Total mark	Score	Remark
Ask the participant to demonstrate the steps to assess cervical effacement and dilatation inform that in woman has just urinated.			
• Wash hands	2		
• Wear HLD/sterilized gloves on both hands	2		
• Take an antiseptic solution swab in a sponge holder and clean both labia from above downwards.	2		
• Repeat the step again using another swab	2		
• Discard the swabs in the yellow bucket	1		
• Separate the labia, clean with a swab from above downwards	2		
• Insert index and middle finger to perform the vaginal examination	2		
• Rotate the hand 90 degrees so that the palm faces upwards and gently stretches the fingers till the rim of cervix is felt (usually at 3–9 o'clock position)	2		

• Assess cervical dilatation and informs in cms	2
• Feel the rim of the cervix with the index and middle finger	1
• Assess the cervical effacement and informs (in %)	1
• Remove the glove inside out and put in 0.5% chlorine solution	1
Total score:	**20**

NORMAL DELIVERY

Equipment: Mannequin, baby, towels, gloves, antiseptic solution swabs, normal delivery set, and disposal bins. Plastic sheet is placed under buttocks and a clean towel on abdomen.

	Total mark	Score	Remark
How would you ensure the woman's bladder is empty?			
Palpate the suprapubic region	1		
Which aseptic techniques are important?			
• Wash hand and put on sterile gloves	1		
• Clean the woman's perineum	1		
How do you control the birth of the head?			
• Encourage the woman to make small pushes with contractions	1		
• Control the birth of the head with fingers of one hand to maintain flexion	1		
• Support the perineum with other hand using a clean pad	1		
What do you do after the head has delivered?			
• Allow the baby's head to turn spontaneously	1		
• Place hands on either side of baby's head and deliver anterior shoulder	2		
• Deliver posterior shoulder once axillary crease is seen by guiding head in an upwards direction	2		
• Once delivery complete, place the baby on the mother's abdomen	1		
• Inform mother of sex of baby	1		
• Delay cord clamping for 1–3 minutes	1		
• Note time of birth, sex of baby on partograph	1		
How would you care for the newborn baby?			
• Dry the baby and mother's abdomen with prewarmed towels	1		
• Cover the baby loosely with second prewarmed towel from head to toe	1		
• Simultaneously, check for crying/breathing–if crying/ breathing, then go ahead with ENBC	1		
If the baby is not breathing, what do you do?			
Cut the cord immediately and begin resuscitation	2		
Total score:	**20**		

ACTIVE MANAGEMENT THIRD STAGE LABOR

Equipment: Model of placenta, kidney tray, forceps, syringe of 'oxytocin', gloves, abdominal model (put placenta inside abdomen and hold until ready to deliver).

	Total mark	Score	Remark
Before attempting delivery of the placenta, what should you check for?			
• Exclude additional baby (babies) by palpating the mother's abdomen	1		
Describe and demonstrate how you should actively manage the third stage of labor			
• Administer inj. oxytocin (10 IU IM on anterolateral aspect of thigh) or misoprostol (600 mcg oral)	2		
• Palpate the uterus for contractions	1		
• Wait for the uterus to contract	1		
• Apply CCT with countertraction	1		
Following delivery of the placenta, what action should you take?			
• Massage fundus	1		
• Ensure uterus is well contracted	1		
• Examine placenta and membranes to ensure completeness	1		
• Put placenta in the yellow bag	1		
• Estimate blood loss	1		
• Complete records	1		
Postdelivery, what would you check and how frequently?			
Uterine contraction and vaginal bleeding every 15 minutes for 2 hours, maternal pulse, and BP	4		
How long would you wait to deliver the placenta before referring to a higher facility?			
30 minutes	2		
When would you not perform CCT?			
• When no contraction is present	1		
• Without applying counter traction above symphysis pubis	1		
Total score:	**20**		

POSTPARTUM HEMORRHAGE

Equipment: MamaNatalie, IV arm, drip stand, BP apparatus, stethoscope, tourniquet, catheterization model, IV set, inj. oxytocin, IV fluids, iodine solution, 0.5% chlorine solution, PPE, adhesive tape, long gloves, IV cannula, drip set.

	Total mark	Score	Remark
Describe the steps you will take in this scenario			
• Shout for help	1		
• Reassure the woman	1		

Annexures

Demonstrate management

• Insert IV cannula (wide bore)	1
• Take blood for cross-matching	1
• Start IV fluids (1L RL)	1
• Check whether oxytocin has been given in AMTSL. If not, give oxytocin 10 IU IM	1
• Start oxytocin 20 IU in 500 mL of RL at 40–60 drops per minute	1
• Wash hands	1
• Wear gloves	1
• Palpate and massage uterus to ensure well contracted	1
• If atonic, start uterine massage	1
• Check for soft-tissue trauma	1
• Catheterize the bladder	1
• Continue to massage the uterus if not contracted	1
• Check placenta and membranes complete	1
If bleeding has not stopped, what further management would you perform?	
Bimanual compression	1
How do you reassess the woman once bleeding is under control?	
• Take pulse every 30 minutes	1
• Take blood pressure every 4 hours	1
• Assess urine output every 4 hours until >30 mL/hour	1
If bleeding does not settle what will you do?	
Refer to higher facility with complete referral note	1
Total score:	**20**

INSERTION OF IV LINE

Equipment: Arm model, swabs, IV cannula, spirit swabs, adhesive tape, 2 mL N/S gloves, syringe, tourniquet.

	Total mark	Score	Remark
Describe and demonstrate what steps you would take to prepare and insert an IV cannula			
Assemble the necessary equipment:			
• Sterile cotton wool swabs and iodine/betadine	1		
• IV cannula	1		
• Saline flush	1		
• Gloves and splints/tourniquet	1		
• Blood sample bottles	1		
Identify the site of insertion	1		

Apply tourniquet proximal to vein	1
Wash hands and put on gloves	1
• Clean the site with alcohol	1
• Wait for 30 seconds	1
• Apply povidone iodine solution	1
• Remove the povidone iodine using alcohol	1
• Allow to air-dry for 30 seconds	1
Insert cannula into vein (15-degree angle)	1
When blood is seen, advance cannula whilst withdrawing the stylet	1
Flush with 2 mL of NS to check for flow of the fluid	1
Connect to IV fluids or put in stopper	1
Secure cannula with adhesive tape	1
Safe disposal of:	
• Stylet in puncture-proof container	1
• Plastic waste in red bin	1
Total score:	**20**

CATHETERIZATION

Equipment: Catheterization mannequin, Foley's catheter, 10 CC syringe, 10 mL distilled water, cotton swabs, antiseptic solution, sponge holder, kidney tray, uro bag. In the below evaluation list, both procedures carry 10 marks each.

	Total mark	Score	Remark
Steps for catheterization:			
• Check the expiry date on the pack (16/18 F Foley's catheter)	1		
• Open the pack and leave it partially drawn out on the sterile tray	1		
• Hand wash and put on sterile gloves	1		
• Clean the vulva with wet cotton swabs soaked in cetrimide solution	1		
• Separate the labia majora and insert the tip of Foley's catheter in the urinary meatus	1		
• Push the catheter and connect the other end of the catheter to the urobag	2		
• Check the flow of urine	1		
• Inflate the bulb of catheter with 10 mL normal saline	2		
Steps for removal of catheter:			
• Put on sterile pair of gloves	2		
• Take 10 mL syringe and attach the barrel of the syringe to short end of catheter	2 + 2		

Annexures

	Total mark	Score	Remark
• Deflate the bulb by withdrawing normal saline with the help of syringe	2		
• Pull out the catheter and dispose catheter and urobag as per the guidelines	2		
Total score:	**20**		

CAB APPROACH

Equipment: Sphygmomanometer, stethoscope, pulse-oximeter (if available), supplemental oxygen, oxygen face mask and tubing.

	Total mark	Score	Remark
What would you do first?			
• Shout for help	1		
• Insert 2 IV lines	1		
• Take blood and send it to lab	1		
• Start fluids at a rapid rate (1 L in 20 mins)	1		
What would you do next?			
• Assess airway patency (looking at chest movements, listening for and/or feeling air through nostrils)	1		
If the airway is not patent, what would you do?			
• Perform head tilt, chin lift and jaw thrust	1		
The woman is breathing. What would you do next?			
• Provide immediate management of shock	1		
What steps would you take to provide immediate management of shock?			
• Turn patient to left lateral position	1		
• Start oxygen @ 6–8 L/min	1		
• Keep the woman warm	1		
• Elevate her legs	1		
• Catheterize the woman	1		
• Monitor vital signs every 15 mins	1		
The woman is not breathing. Demonstrate what you would do?			
• Suction only if vomit or blood present	1		
• Positioning	1		
• Insert airway	1		
• Give 30 chest compressions followed by 2 breaths @ 100 compressions/min	1		
• Press sternum vertically to depress it by 4–5 cm	1		
• Each breath should be provided for 1 second and should raise the chest	1		
You have successfully resuscitated the woman. What would you do next?			
• Find out the cause and manage accordingly	1		
Total score:	**20**		

INTRAUTERINE CONTRACEPTIVE DEVICE (IUCD)

Equipment: Sponge-holding forceps, uterine sound, Sims, speculum, vulsellum, Cu-IUCD, bowl with cotton balls, betadine solution, PPE, scissors, bucket with 0.5% chlorine solution, kidney tray.

	Total mark	Score	Remark
Demonstrate how you will insert an IUCD			
• Check the IUCD pack for expiry date and for tears in the pack	1		
• Read the instructions	1		
• Wear PPE. Wash the hands and wear 2 appropriate-sized gloves one on top of the other on each hand	1		
• Perform bimanual pelvic examination and note the size and position of the uterus	1		
• Remove the outer gloves and discard in the appropriate bin	1		
• Perform speculum examination and check cervix and vagina for signs of infection	1		
• Clean cervix and vagina with antiseptic solution	1		
• Hold the cervix by the anterior lip using vulsellum and pass uterine sound to assess depth of uterine cavity	1		
• Remove IUCD from the opened package and load plunger rod into the insertion tube	1		
• Set length-gauge at uterine length	1		
• Align the length-gauge and folded arms of the T to horizontal position	1		
• Insert IUCD into the cervical canal observing a non-touch technique	1		
• Advance until blue length-gauge comes into contact with the cervix, keeping it in a horizontal position	1		
• While holding the plunger rod, withdraw the insertion tube and gently push the insertion tube towards the fundus	1		
• Withdraw the insertion tube from the canal and locate the strings	1		
• Cut strings at 3 to 4 cm from the cervical os	1		
• Gently remove the speculum and the vulsellum	1		
• Put all used instruments in 0.5% chlorine solution for decontamination	1		
Can you name two complications the mother may experience and report back?			
Candidate needs to provide two of the answers below: • IUCD device is expelled • Heavy vaginal bleeding • Lower abdominal pain • Fever or purulent vaginal discharge	2		
Total score:	20		

Annexures

ECLAMPSIA

Equipment: IM injection mannequin, Inj. 50% $MgSO_4$—10 ampoules, syringes (10 mL syringe and 22G needle)-2, alcohol/spirit swabs in a bowl, kidney tray, knee hammer, ampoule of 10% calcium gluconate, SS large tray-1.

	Total mark	Score	Remark
• Call for help • Check circulation • Establish and maintain airway • Check breathing • Place woman in left lateral position	1 1 1 1 1		
• Take the required number of $MgSO_4$ and check the expiry date • Prepare two 10 mL syringes of 5 g (10 mL) 50% magnesium sulfate • Wash and dry hand • Wear gloves • Clean injection site with alcohol • Administer 5 g (10 mL) by DEEP IM injection in each buttock (upper outer quadrant) • Cut the needle with hub cutter • Dispose of used syringe in a proper disposal box • Records drug administration in woman's record	1 1 1 1 1 1 1 1 1		
Before administering magnesium sulfate to a woman who is conscious, what would you warn her about?			
She may experience a feeling of warmth/irritation along IV site	2		
Here the instructor would prompt: If the mother is not stabilized, what should you do next?			
Refer to a higher facility if treatment not available	2		
When transferring a woman with suspected eclampsia, what do you need to ensure is available?			
Basic life support-Patent IV line, airway and referral slip with documentation of all medication given	2		
Total score:	**20**		

NEWBORN CARE CORNER

Equipment: Radiant warmer, bag and mask, suction machine, oxygen cylinder, newborn mannequin.

	Total mark	Score	Remark
Demonstrate how to use the radiant warmer			
• Connect plug to electricity supply • Switch on the radiant warmer • Check display for mode, air temperature and temperature bars • Check whether probe is attached to the machine • Identify servo and manual mode and select manual mode • Switch to servo mode and set temperature to 36.5°C • Identify and connect skin probe	1 1 1 1 1 1 1		

Demonstrate how to assemble bag and mask and how to use them	
• Connect mask to bag	1
• Check bag by occluding patient outlet with palm and squeezing the bag	1
• Check quick refilling of the bag	1
• Check that the pop-up valve moves up and down with a hissing sound	1
• Apply mask to mannequin—mouth and nose is covered, not the eyes	1
• Connect oxygen source if required	1
• Attach reservoir if oxygen source is connected (must be readily available/should ask for it if not, so that the skill develops to look for it)	1
What size face mask do you use for preterm newborn?	
Size 0	1
Demonstrate how to operate a foot-operated suction machine	
• Place foot suction on floor, bellows on right-side and fluid collection jar on left-side	1
• Place right foot on bellows and press the foot down	1
• Block the suction tubing, press the bellows	1
• Check for suction pressure	1
What is the maximum suction pressure that can be used safely in a newborn?	
100 mm Hg	1
Total score:	**20**

ESSENTIAL NEWBORN CARE

Equipment: Neonatal mannequin, 2 towels, cord clamp, ID band, scissors, cap, weighing machine, syringe, needle and injection of vitamin K.

	Total mark	Score	Remark
Demonstrate immediate care			
• Call out time of birth	1		
• Receive in prewarmed towels	1		
• Place on mother's abdomen in a prone position	1		
• Assess breathing	1		
• Dry baby with a prewarmed towel	1		
• Discard wet towel	1		
• Cover with another prewarmed towel and place between mother's breasts	1		
Baby is breathing normally—when would you cut the cord?			
• 1–3 minutes after birth	1		

What actions would you take now?

• Place an identity wristband on the baby	1
• Cover head with cap	1
• Record the weight	1
• Give injection of vitamin K to the baby	1
• Initiate breastfeeding	1
• Maintain skin-to-skin contact	1
• Check for any congenital malformations	1

Demonstrate the steps you would take to weigh a newborn

• Place on a flat, stable surface	1
• Place a towel on the pan	1
• Adjust the scales to zero	1
• Place baby in the weigh pan	1
• Record your findings	1
Total score:	**20**

NEWBORN RESUSCITATION

Equipment: Neonatal mannequin, neonatal bag and mask, towels (2), and stethoscope.

	Total mark	Score	Remark
Please demonstrate what you would do (Facilitator pass the baby to candidate)			
• Clamp and cut the cord immediately	1		
• Place under radiant warmer	1		
• Dry and wrap in a prewarmed towel	1		
• Position baby in slight neck extension using a shoulder roll	1		
• Do not suction, as there is no meconium	1		
• Stimulate by rubbing the back	1		
• Assess breathing and heart rate.	1		
Baby is breathing, has a heart rate of 90 bpm and is blue. What would you do next, please demonstrate?			
• Choose correct size bag and mask and position correctly covering mouth and nose	2		
• Give 5 inflation breaths of 2–3 seconds each (chest must rise)	2		
• Reassess the heart rate and breathing	2		
The heart rate is now 70 bpm with little respiratory effort. What would you do, please demonstrate?			
• Continue bagging at a rate of 40–60 breaths/min (candidate has to demonstrate)	2		
• Provide oxygen if available	1		
If oxygen and a pulse oximeter are available, what is the recommended oxygen saturation level?			
• 90–95%	1		
If baby is breathing well and HR >100, what would you do?			
• Refer him for observational care	1		

If no improvement after effective ventilation, what would you do?	
• Continue bag and mask ventilation	1
• Ask someone to prepare referral to appropriate center	1
Total score:	**20**

INHALER AND NEBULIZER

Equipment: Nebulizer and multi-dose inhaler with spacer. Normal saline, multi-dose vials, syringes and needles. Mannequin/volunteer.

	Total mark	Score	Remark
Demonstrate the correct use of the nebulizer			
• Wash hands (participant has to mention it but doesn't have to do it)	1		
• Measure the correct dose of medication to be used in the nebulized chamber (specify the dose)	1		
• Add normal saline to make the volume up to 3 mL	1		
• Connect the nebulizer tubing to the port on the compressor	1		
• Turn on compressor and check the nebulizer for misting	1		
• Connect the mouthpiece or mask to the T-shaped elbow	1		
• Hold the nebulizer in an upright position	1		
• Ensure the mask is a good fit	1		
Your patient is now stabilized, how would you teach the parents how to use the multi-dose inhaler (MDI) with spacer? Please demonstrate your teaching			
• Check expiry date	1		
• Shake the container	1		
• Remove the cap from the inhaler	1		
• Insert the inhaler mouthpiece into the slot of the spacer	1		
• Attach mask to the mouthpiece of the spacer	1		
• Instruct the mother to hold the child in the proper position	1		
• Place the mask over the child's nose and mouth so that there is a good seal with the face	2		
• Press down on the inhaler canister to spray 1 puff of medicine into the spacer	1		
• Allow the child to breathe normally for 5 breaths	1		
Here the facilitator would prompt: How do you know the medicine is dispersed? • Momentary misting of the spacer and hissing noise	1		
When to administer next dose?			
• Wait for 2–3 minutes, shake the inhaler and repeat steps	1		
Total score:	**20**		

KANGAROO MOTHER CARE

Equipment: Baby doll, baby clothes, bed sheet, blanket, volunteer mother if available.

	Total mark	Score	Remark
Demonstrate how you would perform Kangaroo Mother Care (give participant clothed baby)			
• Explain the procedure to the mother	1		
• Ensure privacy for the mother	1		
• Ensure the mother is sitting or reclining comfortably	1		
• Gently undress the baby except for cap, nappy, and socks	1		
• Place baby prone on the mother's chest	1		
• In an upright position	1		
• Between her breasts, skin to skin	1		
• In a frog-like position (arms and legs flexed)	1		
• Turn baby's head to one side so airway is open	1		
• Support baby's bottom using appropriate sling or binder	1		
• Cover mother and baby with blanket or shawl	1		
• Ensure baby is breastfed frequently	1		
What should the ideal room temperature be?			
• 26–28°C	1		
What are the two key components of KMC?			
• Skin-to-skin contact	1		
• Exclusive breastfeeding	1		
What are the benefits of KMC?			
• Reduces risk of hypothermia	1		
• Promotes lactation	1		
• Promotes weight gain	1		
• Reduces infections	1		
• Improves bonding between mother and newborn	1		
Total score:	20		

BIBLIOGRAPHY

1. https://nhm.gov.in/images/pdf/programmes/maternalhealth/guidelines/SKILLS_LAB_TRAINING_MANUAL_FACILITATOR.pdf

Index

Page numbers followed by *f* refer to figure, *fc* refer to flowchart, and *t* refer to table.

A

ABC analysis 219
ABCDE approach 11
Abdomen, acute 18
Abdominal examination 281
Abdominal palpation 281
Abdominal region 8*f*
Abhiyan Indradhanush 148
Abortion
    ratio 86
    unsafe 60
Absolute eosinophil count 215
Abstinence 123
Abuse 174
Accredited Social Health Activist
    assisting 204
    facilitator, role of 161
    incentives of 273
    role of 161, 204
    urban 208
Acquired immunodeficiency syndrome 109
Acute abdominal pain, differential diagnosis of 18*f*
Acute encephalitis syndrome 277
Adequate funding 177
Administrative work 202, 204
Adolescent
    centered counseling, principles of 132
    friendly health clinics 62
    initiatives for 63
    tips for interacting with 132
Adolescent health 30, 275
    days 63
Agoraphobia 164
Air (vayu) 223
Airway 12
Albendazole 63
Albumin 283
Alcohol 173
    dependence 174, 175
        detoxification of 175
Alimentary system examination 7
All health-related information, repository of 186
All India Women's Conference 268
Alzheimer's disease 154, 170

Amniotic fluid, color of 45
Analytic tools 198
Anaphylaxis 76
Anemia 25
    cause 25
    diagnose 25*t*
    prevalence 32
    prevention of 26
Animal bite 15
    cat 15
    categories 16
    dog 15
    monkey 15
    wild 15
Annapurna Scheme 159
Antara Program 121
Antenatal care 209
    basics of 33
    coverage 273
    essential
        components of 33
        elements of 34*f*
Antenatal check-up 205
Antenatal period 38
Antenatal visits, suggested schedule for 35
Anthracosis 142
Anthropometric measurements 3
Antidepressant medication 167
Antipsychotic medication 169
Antiseptic solution 286
Anxiety
    disorders 163
    pathological 163
Apex beat 6
Apgar score 278
Appetite, loss of 153
Application program interface 197
Arithmetic mean 105
    demerits of 106
    merits of 106
Articular disorders 153
Asbestosis 142
Aseptic techniques 287
Ashtanga yoga 224
Atal Bimit Vyakti Kalyan Yojana 149

Index

Atal Pension Yojana 160
Atal Vayo Abhyudaya Yojana 158
Atherosclerosis 153
Audit, screening methods like 174
Auditory effects 140
Auscultation 2, 6, 7
Autoclave, type of 256
Autocratic leaders, decisions of 231
Autocratic leadership 231
Auxiliary nurse midwife 202
    online application 188
    responsibilities of 76
    role of 161
Average cost method 222
Avil injections 174
Awareness generation 202, 208
Ayurveda 223
Ayush 223
Ayushman Bharat 200
    Digital Mission 186
    Health Account number 186

B

Bacterial infection 23
Bagassosis 142
Bar diagram 100
    simple 101, 101f
Barrier mehods 116
Basic health services 207f
Bed
    capacity 213
    requirement 213
    sheet, color of 149
Bellary model 179
Below poverty line family 83
Benefits under scheme 43
Beti Bachao Beti Padhao Scheme 84
Bhakti yoga 225
Bilateral agencies 261
Bilateral edema 4
Bile
    black 226
    yellow 226
Biohazard symbol 255
Biological agents 140
Biomedical research 259
Biomedical waste 246
    categories 253
    hazardous nature of 247
    management 246, 249, 251

    stage of 252
    overview of 246
    standards for autoclaving of 256
    treatment 256
    and disposal of 254
Biomedical Waste Management Act 251
Biomedical Waste Management Rules 251, 252
    and Guidelines 211
Bipolar disorder 168
Birth control
    back-up with 124
    vaccine 123
Bite 15
Bladder control, loss of 153
Bleaching powder 285
Bleeding
    internal 12
    time 215
Blind people's association 268
Blood 226
    cross matching 215
    storage units 217
    sugar 216
    urea 216
Blood pressure 5
    demonstrate measurement of 280
    diastolic 280
    machine 280
    measurement 280
Body parts, distribution of 17f
Bone strength, decrease in 153
Bowl with cotton swabs 286
Box-and-whiskers plots 104, 104f
Brachial neuritis 76
Brain
    tuberculosis of 171
    tumors 171
Breastfeeding 50, 54, 55
    exclusive 54, 55
    initiating 55
Breathing 12, 287
Budgeting, advantages of 217
Buffer stock 222
Building design 145
Bulging precordium 6
Buprenorphine injections 174
Burn 17
    area, assessment of 17f
    chemical 17
    degree of 17

Index

electrical 17
flame 17
scald 17
superficial 18
types 17
Byssinosis 142

C

Cab approach 291
Calculating beneficiaries 272
Cancer bladder 143
Cannabis 174
Cardiopulmonary resuscitation 21
Cardiovascular diseases 160
Cardiovascular system examination 6
Case fatality rate 87
Catatonic behavior 168
Catatonic schizophrenia 168
Catatonic symptoms 169
Catheter, steps for removal of 290
Catheterization 290
Central nervous system 154, 170
    examination 9
Central Social Welfare Board 268
    activities 268
    functions 268
Central surveillance unit 111
Central tendency, measure of 104
Central tuberculosis division 191
Central waste collection 211
Cerebrovascular accidents 154
Certifying surgeons 146
Cervical
    cancers 193, 212
    cap 117
    dilatation 43, 286
        model 286
    effacement 43, 286
Chemical
    agents 140
    disinfection, standards for 256
    hazards 141
    methods 118
    waste 247
Chest, shape of 7
Chhaya 122
Chikungunya 277
Child death rate 87
Child health 30, 260, 273
Child morbidity 127

Child mortality 127
    rate 32
Child nutrition 260
    interventions for 67
    status 236
Child woman ratio 86
Chlorination, water testing for 212
Chlorine solution 285
    preparation of 285
Chloroquine 205
Cholera 212
Chronic obstructive lung disease 3
Civil and criminal liabilities 245
Claustrophobia 164
Clean cord cut 38
Clean cord tie 38
Clean hands 38
Clean perineum 38
Clean surface 38
Clean umbilical stump 38
Clinical outreach teams 134
Clinical work 201, 202
Clotting factor 212
Clotting time 215
Clubbing, causes of 4
Cluster sampling 92
Code of medical ethics 215
Codeine containing cough syrups 174
Cognitive improvement, drugs for 171
Coitus interruptus 123
Collaborative leadership 232
Colloidal silver 18
Colombo plan 265
Combined injectable contraceptives 121
Combined oral contraceptive pills 119
Common childhood illnesses, management of 57
Common disorders, primary care of 22
Common emergencies, management of 11
Common medical emergencies, basics of 14
Common sampling methods 90
Common substance abuse 173
Communicable diseases 191
    preventing and controlling 242
Communication
    technology 185
    verbal 132
Community Health Center 157, 179, 199, 200, 205,
    210, 216, 217
    population norms for 217
Community health nurse, role of 1, 182, 243, 248

Index

Community Health Officer, role of 161, 201
Community health services, delivery mechanism of 199
Community mobilization 209
Community-based programs 57
Complementary feeding 55
Compliance with statutory norms 215
Comprehensive health services, development of 258
Comprehensive Primary Healthcare 200, 277
Condom 116, 205
    female 116
Congestive cardiac failure 3
Consciousness 9
Constipation 27
Consumer price index 219
Consumer Protection Act 215
Contaminated gloves 286
Contraception 50
    methods of 133, 137
Contraceptive
    injectable 120
    method, types of 123
    production of 261
Controlled cord traction 47
Copper devices, advantages of 118
Core strategies 156
Coronary artery disease 153
Correlation diagram 100
Cost-benefit analysis 218
Cost-effective analysis 218
Cost-oriented pricing method 218
Cost-plus pricing 218
Cough 23
    assessment of 24
    cause 23
    types 23
Council for Child Welfare 266
Counseling 37, 49, 131, 208
    adolescents 131
        essential steps for 132
        communication skills for 132
        tasks involved in 131
Couple counseling 131
Couple protection rate 137
COVID-19
    vaccination, evaluation of 194
    vaccine
        delivery management system 194*f*
        intelligence network 194

Cranial nerve 9
    examination 9
Creating enabling environment 130
Cross cutting issues 177
Crude birth rate 84
Crude death rate 87
Crude marriage rate 86
Crude rate 84
Cu T 380 A 119
Culturally sensitive 131
Cumulative frequency 96
    diagram 99, 99*f*
Cumulative relative frequency 96
Curative care and supplies 209
Current problem statement 178
Cyanosis 3
    causes of 3
Cyanotic heart disease 3
Cyst 212
Cytotoxic symbol 255

D

Daily feeding 190
Daily protein intake 107
Danger signs 51
Data 95
    analysis 95
    and meta data standards 198
    interpretation 95
    methods of collection 95
    presentation of 96
        methods of 96
    qualitative 95, 96
    quantitative 96
    source 95
    types of 95
    ungrouped 105, 106
Dead, care of 242
Death rate
    age specific 87
    fender specific 88
Deep burial 249
    pit 211
        layout of 250*f*
        standards for 256
Degenerative disorders 170
Dehydration, assessment of 28
Delivering assured services 129
Delivery
    after 53

Index

clean 53
home 38
kits, disposable 205
normal 287
Delusions 168
Dementia 170
Demographic burden 83
Demographic data
    methods of 95
    sources of 88
Demographic dividend 83
Demographic structure 271
Demographic transition 79
    phases of 79, 79f
Demography 78
    cycle 81
    surveillance, and data 78
Dengue 191, 212, 277
Dependency ratio 83
Depot-medroxyprogesterone acetate 120
Depression 165
    mild 166
    moderate 166
    severe 166
Development care, support for 57
Diabetes 160
    test for 212
Diaphragm 117
Diarrhea 27
    treatment of 28
    types 27
Different family planning measures 115
Digi doctor 187
Digital health ecosystem 186
Diphtheria 212, 261
    throat swab for 216
Disability 13
Disablement benefit 148
Disaster 238, 242, 243
    biological 239
    general effects of 239
    impact and rescue 241
    manage 243
    man-made 239
    mitigation 243
    morbidity related to 240
    natural 239
    preparedness 243
    prone zones 245
    related legislations 245

risk 239
    types of 239
    wise nodal ministry list 240
Disaster management 238, 240
    Act 243
    cycle 241
    organogram for 244f
    sequence 241f
Disinflation 218
Disorders identification test, alcohol used 174
Distribution, types of 98f
District De-addiction Center 176
District Mental Health Program 179
District surveillance unit 111
Donepezil 171
Drinking water and sanitation 277
Drowning victim
    signs of 19
    symptoms of 19
Drug
    expired 246
    logistics information and management system 195
Drug Deaddiction Programs 175
Drugs and Cosmetics Act 215
Dwarfism 3
Dyspnea 24
    causes 24

E

Early neonatal mortality rate 87
Early warning signals 110
Ears 5
Earth (prithvi) 224
E-aushadhi 195
Eclampsia 293
Economic problems 154
Edema 4
    unilateral 4
Education 268
Effective couple protection rate 138
Effective Food Relief Program, steps for 242
E-Health 185, 188, 191, 192
    basics of 185
    global observatory for 185
    innovations 185
Electrocardiogram 166
Electroconvulsive therapy 167
    usage of 180
Electrolytes 166

Electronic medical record 187
Electronic vaccine intelligence network 194
Emergency and common disorders, management of 1
Emergency contraception 124, 125
    use of 124
Emergency contraceptive pills 124
Emergency oral contraception 125
Emotional maturity 230
Employees State Insurance Act 147, 149
    benefits under 147*t*
Employees' State Insurance Corporation, hospitals of 149*t*
Employer, benefits for 148
Endocrine
    cause 171
    system 154
Ensuring commodity security 130
Environment, preparation of 2
Environmental health 258
E-pharmacy and telemedicine services 186
Epidemiologic surveillance and disease control 242
Episiotomy 46
Epistaxis 24
    causes 24
Equipment 280, 282, 283, 284, 286
    preparation of 2
Ergonomics 139
Esophagus, foreign body in 20
Essential newborn care, elements of 47
Ethical leadership 232
Eugenic condition 125
Exegetical tantra 228
Eyes 5, 153

F

Face and skull 5
Factory Act 145
False perception 168
Family and child welfare 260
Family health 258
    initiative 264
Family planning 48, 115, 133, 136, 196, 267, 274
    basics of 115
    logistic management information system 196
    measures 115
    method 116, 124
Family Planning Program 134*f*, 264
    advent of 133*f*
    evolution of 126*f*
    strategies of 135*f*
Farmers lung 142
Febrile seizures 76
Fecal contamination, water testing for 212
Fertility rate
    age specific 85
    general 84
        marital 85
Fertility, measures of 84
Fetal condition 45
Fetal death ratio 87
Fetal heart rate 35
Fetal lie 36
Fever 22
Field care 241
Financial management 217
Fire (tejas) 223
First-aid 11, 241
    psychological 184
First referral unit 216
First stage of labor, management of 45
Fits
    focal 19
    generalized 19
Fixed order
    interval system 221
    size system 221
Flattened precordium 6
Food and Agricultural Organization 262
Food safety 243
Foreign body ingestion 19
Foundation's program 265
Fracture 14, 153
    common signs of 14
Frequency curve 98
Frequency distribution table 97
Frequency polygon 98, 98*f*
Frontline healthcare workers, role of 161
FSN analysis 221
Functional psychosis 168
Fundal grip 281

G

General marriage rate 86
General packet radio service 185
Generalized anxiety disorder 164
Genitourinary system 154
Genotoxic waste 247
Geriatric clinic 157

Index

Geriatric health 152, 161
Geriatric population, problems of 153
Geriatric unit 157
Geriatric ward 157
Global positioning system 185
Glucose
    test urine for 284
    tolerance test 212, 216
Glucose-6-phosphate dehydrogenase enzyme
    deficiency, screening test for 212, 215
Glycosylated hemoglobin 212, 216
Good attachment, signs of 54
Good house-keeping 145
Good leader, qualities of 230
Gram panchayat 205, 212
Graph 98, 99f
Grievance redressal platform 212
Grinder's disease 142
Gross domestic product 218
Gross national
    income 218
    product 218
Gross reproduction rate 85
Ground glass appearance 142
Grouped data 105
    median for general 107
    of continuous type, arithmetic mean of 105
Growth monitoring 190
Guillain-Barre syndrome 76
Guru-Shishya tradition 229
Gyana yoga 224

H

Hair 4
Hallucinations 168
Hand washing 284
Hanging drop, stool for 216
Harvard School of Public Health 265
Hazard 140, 238, 247
    biological 141
Hazardous chemicals, exposure to 144
Hazardous processes, employment in 146
Head and neck, examination of 5
Health
    camps 246
    care setting 232
    data consent manager 187
    education and counseling 144
    facility registry 187
    ID 186
    literature and information 259
    Management Information System 185, 196
    resources 110
    safety and welfare 145
    service delivery, sustainability of 185
    statistics 259
Health and Wellness Centers 200, 210, 212
    primary health center, population norms for 213
    sub health center, population norms for 210
Health assessment
    and examination, fundamentals of 1
    preparation for 1
    purposes of 1
Health information 187
    use of 95
Health problems 153
    of older adults 152
Healthcare
    delivery system 199, 207, 207f
    professionals registry 187
    providers 186
Hearing impairment 153
Heart, functions of 153
Hebephrenic schizophrenia 168
Height, measurement of 3
Heimlich maneuver 20f
Hemoglobin 212
    estimation 282
    levels 25t
Hemorrhage 11
Hepatitis B surface antigen test 216
Heroin 174
Hilly and tribal areas 213
Hind Kusht Nivaran Sangh 267
    activities of 267
Histogram 97f
Home visit scheduler 190
Homeopathy
    medicine 227
    principles of 227
Hormonal contraception 119, 120
Hospital waste, overview of 247, 247f
Hospitals and doctors, voluntary for 187
Household management 190
Human body
    core components of 226
        aaza (organs) 226
        afaal (functions) 226
        aklat (humors) 226

arkan (elements) 226
arwah (spirit) 226
mijaz (temperament) 226
quwa (power) 226
system, age-related changes in 153
Human chorionic gonadotropin 216
Human immunodeficiency virus 212
Human resource 213
    development 110
Humanitarian condition 125
Humanitarian supplies, managing 242
Hypertension 193
Hypothermia, prevention of 53
Hypothyroidism 171

I
Ideal contraceptive, characteristics of 115
Illicit Traffic in Narcotic Drugs and Psychotropic Substances Act, prevention of 175
Illness
    nature of 169
    progresses 170
Immunization 274
    complete 76
    full 76
    services, information for 195
Incineration, standards for 256
Income Tax Act 160
Indian Nursing Council Act 215
Indian Public Health Standards, objectives of 210
Indian Red Cross Society 265
    Act 266
Indira Gandhi National Old Age Pension Scheme 159
Infant and young child feeding 57
Infant deaths, number of 273
Infant morbidity 127
Infant mortality 127
    rate 32, 87
Infection
    control 1
    prevention of 53
    signs of 18
Inflation 218
Influence of Ayurveda 229
Information 209
    technology 198
Informed consent 131
Infrastructure 197, 211
Inhaler 296
Insect bites 16
Institutional delivery, cash assistance for 40

Instructional tantra 228
Integrated Disease Surveillance Program 110, 112
Integrated health information platform 112, 198
Integrated program for older persons 159
Integrated rehabilitation centers, maintenance of 176
Intramuscular injection 121
Intranatal care, basics of 43
Intrauterine contraceptive device 118, 292
    advantages of 119
Intrauterine devices 118
Inventory carrying cost 221
Inventory control, role of nurse in 222
Inventory management 219
Iodine 212
Ionic silver cream 18
Ionizing radiation 141
Iron
    deficiency anemia, treatment of 25
    folic acid tablet 205
Iron folic acid supplementation 63
    regime for 26t
Isolation 145

J
Jan Arogya Samiti 212
Janani Suraksha Yojana 38, 40
Janani-Shishu Suraksha Karyakram 41
Janganana Se Jan Kalyan 88
Jansankhya Sthirata Kosh 127
Japa yoga 224
Japanese encephalitis 277
Jaundice 3

K
Kala azar 212, 216
    elimination 277
Kangaroo mother care 53, 297
    benefits of 54
Karma yoga 224
Ketone 216
Kidney function 153
    test 212
Kilkari 189
Knowing your population 271

L
Labor 45
    assessment of progress of 44
    second stage of 46
    stages of 44
    third stage of 288

Index

Lactation amenorrhea method 123
Laissez-Faire leadership 232
Laparoscopic sterilization 124
Laparoscopic tubal occlusion 122
Law of minimum dose 227
Lead poisoning 143
Lead time 222
Leader
    and manager, difference between 231
    types of 231
Leadership 230
    distributed 232
    participative type of 231
    style 231
    supervision, and monitoring, fundamentals of 230
    transactional type of 232
    type of 231
Leave with wages 146
Legislative measures 145
Leukemia 143
Leukocyte esterase 216
Life, expectation of 87
Lifestyle modification diet post trauma 204
Line chart 98, 99*f*
Lipid profile 212
Liquid waste, standards for 256
List of schemes 158
Live births, number of 272
Liver function test 212
Local exhaust ventilation 145
Local government directory compliance 197
Logistic management
    cycle 221*f*
    information system 196
Longitudinal Ageing Study in India study, findings of 154
Lung
    cancer 143
    collapse of 3
    fibrosis of 3
    functions of 153
    shadow, mottling in 142
Lymphadenopathy 3
Lymphatic filariasis 276

M

Mahila Arogya Samiti 209
Malaria 276
    rapid test 216
    test 212
Malignancy 154
Man and machine 140
Man and physical, chemical and biological agents 140
Mantoux 216
Map diagram 103
Marital fertility rate, age specific 85
Mark up pricing 218
Market-oriented pricing method 218
Maternal and child health 30, 42
    current status of 32
Maternal condition 46
Maternal health 30, 273
    interventions 66
Maternal mortality ratio 86
Maternal symptoms 50
Maternity benefit 148
M-cessation 192
M-diabetes initiative 193
Measurement scales quantitative data 96
Mechanical hazards 141
Medical benefit 147
Medical college libraries, development of 265
Medical Council Act 215
Medical measures 144
Medical services 144
Medical termination of pregnancy 126
    Act 125, 215
Medicine, systems of 109
Medroxyprogesterone acetate 127
Memantine 171
Menstrual hygiene scheme 63
Mental health 163, 182
    Act 215
    establishment, maintaining 181
Mental Healthcare Act 180, 215
Mental illness 180
Mental state examination 183
Mera Aspataal 198
Metabolic cause 171
mHealth 185
Micro-birth planning 38
Micronutrient supplementation and deworming 57
Micro-pill 120
Mifepristone 125
Miner's phthisis 142
Minilap operation 122
Mini-pill 120
Ministry of Environment Forest and Climate Change 251
Ministry of Health and Family Welfare 152, 175, 191, 193

Ministry of Social Justice and Empowerment 175
Mirena 118
Mission Parivar Vikas 128, 275
   campaigns 129, 275
Mitigation 241
Mobile academy 189
Modern contraceptive methods, prevalence of 136*f*
Morbidity indicators 88
Morning after pill 124
Morphine 174
Mortality indicators, important 86
Mortality rate 87
Mother newborn care unit 56
Mothers Absolute Affection Program 57
Motivation 175
Motivational style 231
Mouth and throat 6
Multiphase sampling 92
Multiple bar diagram 101, 101*f*
Multipurpose worker
   female, role of 202
   male, role of 201
Multistage sampling 92
Muscle strength, decrease in 153

N

Nails 4
Narcotics and Psychotropic Substances Act 215
Narcotics Control Bureau 176
Nasha Mukt Bharat Abhiyaan 176
National AIDS Control Organization 109
National and International Agencies Related to Health 257
National Centers of Aging 156
National Digital Health Mission 185, 186, 188
National Disaster Management Authority 244
National Disaster Response Force 244
National Executive Committee 244
National Family Planning Indemnity Scheme 130
National Family Planning Program 121
National Family Welfare Program 126
National Health Agencies 265
National Health Authority 186
National Health Mission 179
National Identification Number 197
National immunization schedule 70*t*
National Informatics Centre 191
National Institute of Disaster Management 244
National Institute of Mental Health and Neurosciences 178

National Institute of Occupational Health 150
National Iodine Deficiency Disorders Control Programme 277
National Leprosy Eradication Programme 276
National Level Important Entities 244
National Mental Health Policy 177
National Mental Health Program 160, 178, 179
National Oral Health Programme 160
National Population Policy 109
National Program for Control and Treatment of Occupational Diseases 150
National Program for Health Care of Elderly 155
   activities under 157
   specific objectives of 155
National Program for Tobacco Control and Drug Addiction Treatment 176
National Programme for Control of Blindness and Visual Impairment 160
National Programme for Health Care of Elderly 155
National Programme for Palliative Care 160
National Programme for Prevention and Control of
   Cancer 160
   Deafness 160
National Programs Related to Nutrition 57
National Sociodemographic Goals 109
National Tele Mental Health Programme 180
National Tuberculosis Control Programme, revised 276
National Tuberculosis Elimination Programme 191
National Vector Borne Disease Control Programme 276
Natural growth rate 83
Naturopathy 225
   features of 225
   modalities of 225
Nausea 26
Navjaat Shishu Suraksha Karyakram 56
Near drowning 19
Nebulizer 296
Neck 6
Neonatal and childhood illness, integrated management of 236
Neonatal deaths, number of 273
Neonatal mortality rate 86
Neosporin 18
Nerve deafness 153
Net reproduction rate 85
Neuritis, peripheral 154

Index

Neurological assessment 9
Newborn
　baby 287
　care of 47
　criteria, high risk 55
　estimated 272
　health 30
　home-based 56
　resuscitation 295
　stabilization unit 55
Newborn and child
　care, basics of 52
　health interventions 57, 67
Newborn care
　continuum of 55
　corner 55, 293
　essential 294
　immediate 47
Newborn Care Program, facility-based 55
NHP Swasth Bharat Mobile Application 192
Nikshay 191
　patrika 192
　sampark 192
Nishchay pregnancy test kit 34f
No mortality, assumption of 85
Nodal agency 244
Nodular fibrosis 142
Non-auditory effects 140
Non-communicable diseases 156, 192, 193
　common 272
Non-communicable disorders 178
Non-first referral unit community health centers 216
Non-government Organizations 176
Nonhormonal contraception 122
Non-probability sampling 90, 93
Nonverbal cues 132
Norethisterone enanthate 121
Normal delivery, stages of 45
Normal newborn, care of 52
Normal pressure hydrocephalus 171
Nose 6
Nutrition 50, 242
Nutritional deficiencies 153
Nutritional excess 153
Nutritional status 32

O

Obsessive compulsive disorder 164
Occupational cancer 143
Occupational dermatitis 143
Occupational diseases 141, 146
　prevention of 144
Occupational environment 140
Occupational hazards 140
　in health sector 144
Occupational health 139
　global strategy for 150
　hazards 139
　nurse, role of 151
　services, role of nurse in 151
Occupational infections 144
Occupational lung diseases 141
Occupational Safety, Health and Working Conditions Code 147
Occupational stress and fatigue 144
Offences and penalties 181
Offences by companies 182
Ongoing Disease Control Programs, monitor progress of 110
Opioids 174
Oral cavity 7
Oral pills 205
Oral rehydration therapy 205
Ordering costs 221
Organic psychosis 168
Organization of Geriatric Health Services 156, 156f
Organizational structure of Integrated Disease Surveillance Program 111
Orientation training centers 264
Orientation-based style 231
Oxygen delivery systems 211, 213

P

Pain, responsive to 11
Pallor 3
Palpation 6, 7, 281
　types of 2
Panchakarmas 224
Panic disorder 163, 164
Pap smear 216
Paralytic polio, vaccine-associated 76
Paranoid schizophrenia 168
Parkinson's disease 154
Participatory learning and action 276
Partograph 278
Patient
　health questionnaire 166
　preparation of 2
Pearl index 138
Peer Education Program 62

Pelvic grip
  first 281
  second 281
Percussion, types of 2
Perform heimlich maneuver, steps to 20
Perinatal mortality rate 86
Periodical examination 144
Peripheral blood film 215
Peripheral health workers 205
Persistent delusional disorder 169
Personal digital assistants 185
Personal health records 187
Personal integrity 230
Personal protective equipment 285
Persons with Disability Act 215
Pertussis 261
pH 216
Pharmacy Act 215
Phlegm 226
Phobias 163, 164
Physical agents 140
Physical assessment, methods of 2
Physical disorders 164
Physical methods 116
Pictogram 102, 103*f*
Pie diagram 102, 102*f*
Pill
  ezy 125
  male 120
Placenta 288
  delivery of 288
Planning evaluation cycle 235*f*
Pneumoconiosis 142*t*
Polio 261
  virus, vaccine derived 76
Poor general medical status 169
Population
  and family welfare 113
  control 114
  decadal growth of 79*f*
  density 83
  explosion
    impact of 114
    reason for 114
  pyramid, concept of 81
  sex ratio, and population density, Statewise data of 80*t*
  stabilization 127
    fund 127
  target 61

Post-abortion family planning 123
Postcoital contraception 124
Postnatal care 209
  basic of 48
Postnatal check-up 205
Postneonatal mortality rate 87
Postpartum 123
  care
    and hygiene 49
    immediate 48
  hemorrhage 288
  visit, first 50
Post-traumatic stress disorder 164
Potentized remedy 227
Poverty 83
Power-based style 231
Pradhan Mantri Matru Vandana Yojana 42
Pradhan Mantri Shram Yogi Maan Dhan 278
Pradhan Mantri Surakshit Matritva Abhiyan 39
Pradhan Mantri Vaya Vandana Yojana 160
Pre-Conception and Pre-Natal Diagnostic Techniques Act 215
Pre-eclampsia
  diagnose 280
  severe 280
Pregnancy
  confirmation of 34
  detection test 283
  duration of 125
  early registration of 35, 202
  late 36
  prophylaxis during 37
  rate 86
  urine test for 216
Prehospital stroke management 16*f*
Preplacement examination 144
Pricing method, types of 218
Primary Health Center 157, 179, 200, 205, 213, 215
  facility, type of 213
Primary Health Facility 213
Primary health-care system and community 199
Probability sampling 90, 91
Producer price index 219
Progestasert 118
Progestogen
  only injectables 120
  only pill 120
Prohibited disposables 246
Promotional schemes 129
Prophylactic dose 26*t*

Index

Proportional bar diagram 102, 102f
Proportional mortality rate 87
Protective devices 145
Protein 216
  presence of 284
Psychiatric disorders 163
Psychiatric illnesses, management of 184
Psychiatric patients, assessment of 182
Psychoeducation 165
Psychological problems 154
Psychosis 167
  acute 168
  affective 168
  basics of 167
  nonpharmacological management of 169
  types of 168
Psychosocial factors 164
Psychosocial hazards 141
Psychosocial interventions comprise 184
Psychotherapy 167
Public health
  facilities 217
  institutions 269
  work 202, 203
Pulmonary AV fistula 3
Pulse 5
Purchasing power parity 218

Q

Qualitative data, measurement scales of 95
Quota sampling 94

R

Radiation, exposure to 144
Radioactive waste 247, 251
Raja yoga 225
Rare serious adverse events 76t
Rashtriya Kishor Swasthya Karyakaram 61
Rashtriya Varishth Jan Swasthya Yojana 158
Records, maintenance of 144
Regional Geriatric Center 156, 157
Registration of birth 50
  and Deaths Act 215
Rehabilitation 242
  services 157
Relapse, prevention of 175
Reordering system 221
Reporting mechanism 111f
Reproductive and child health 188
Reproductive and sexual health problems 131

Reproductive health 30, 127
  interventions for 67
Reproductive tract infection 205
  management of 109
Rescue 241
  breaths 22
Research 145
  cum-action projects 264
Residual schizophrenia 168
Respiratory rate 5
Respiratory system 153
  examination 7
Reticulocyte count 215
Revitalizing postpartum family planning 127
Rhythm method 123
Right paramedian episiotomy 46
Right to Information Act 215
Rights of Person with Mental Illness 181
Rivastigmine 171
Rockefeller foundation 264
Root tantra 228
Routine immunization session 76
  types of 77
Routine recurrent activities, incentive for 275
Running water 284
Rural health
  infrastructure, coverage of 206
  statistics 205
Rural healthcare delivery system 199

S

SAARTHI 130
Saas Bahu Sammelan 130, 275
Saathiya 62
Safety officers 146
Saheli 122
Sahli's hemoglobinometer 282
Salt with iodine, enrichment of 260
Sampling techniques 90
  classification of 90
Sanitation and hygiene 243
Scabies 29
Scalpel vasectomy 124
Scatter diagram 100, 100f
Schemes for Welfare of Older Adults 158
Schizophrenia 167, 168
  simple 168
  subtypes of 168
Schools and Anganwadi Centers, intervention in 63

Scorpion bite 15
SDE analysis 220
Second stage of labor, management of 46
Sector diagram 102, 102*f*
Seismic safety guidelines 215
Seizures 19
Self-confidence 230
Self-efficacy 175
Serum
　calcium 216
　creatinine 216
Service delivery framework 184
Service guarantee enablers 42
Sex ratio at birth 84
Sexual function, decrease in 153
Sexually transmitted infections 109, 205
Sharp pit 250
Sharp tank 250
Short message service 198
Sick newborns 272
Sickle cell anemia
　blood test for 212
　screening of 215
Sickle cell test 215
Sickling test 215
Sickness benefit 147
Siddha system of medicine 228
Siderosis 142
Silicosis 142
Silver
　nitrate cream 18
　sulfadiazine 18
Similia similibus curentur 227
Skin 4
　cancer 143
　wrinkling of 153
Skin-to-skin contact 54
Sleep, disturbed 153
Smack 174
Small family norm 115
Snake-bite 16
Snow storm appearance 142
Snowball sampling 94
Social Awareness and Action to Neutralize
　　Pneumonia Successfully campaigns
　　requires 56
Social condition 125
Social emergency response volunteers 266
Social phobia 164
Social problems 154

Sodium 166
Soframycin 18
Sounds 2
　heard 2
Sowa-Rigpa 228
　practice of 229
Spasmoproxyvon capsules 174
Special newborn care unit 56
Specific cost method 222
Specific death rate 87
　cause 88
Specific diseases, prevention and control of 258
Speech, disorganized 168
Sputum 216
Stakeholders 110
State normal weight gain 280
State surveillance unit 111
Statistical and environmental monitoring 145
Sterile gloved hands, contaminating 286
Sterilization, female 122
Stethoscope 280
Stigma 177
Stillbirth rate 86
Stomach, foreign body in 20
Stool examination 212
Stores accounting, flow of 222
Strategic information management system 197
Strategic priorities 137
Stratified random sampling 91
Stress tolerance 230
Stroke 16, 160
Subdermal implant 121
Subdistrict Hospitals and District Hospitals 199
Subsequent tantra 228
Sucking, effective 54
Sugar
　and protein, routine urine test for 283
　positive for 284
Suicide 171
　management of 172*fc*
　protective factors for 173
　risk factors for 172*fc*
　warning signs of 172
Supervision
　advantages of 235
　and monitoring, differences between 233
　types of 234
Supervisor, qualities of 233
Supervisory methods 235
Supplementary strategies 156

Index

Support system 169
Supportive supervision 234
    steps of 234
Surakshit Matritva Aashwasan (Suman) 41
Sustained release system 121
Swara yoga 225
Swedish International Development Agency 265
Syphilis 171
    tests for 212
Systematic sampling 91
Systemic examination 6

T

Take home ration 190
Tantras 228
Target couple 115
Target-returning pricing 218
Taste, change in 153
TB Arogya Sathi 192
Teenage pregnancy 59, 60
Teeth, loss of 153
Temperature 5, 256
Tenderness 8
Termination of pregnancy 125
Thalassemia, blood test for 212
Therapeutic condition 125
Third stage of labor, management of 47, 288
Thrombocytopenia 76
Thyroid function tests 166
Total fertility rate 85
Total marital fertility rate 85
Traditional supervision 234
Transformational leadership 232
Trauma and accidents 14
Treatment, nature of 169
Triage 241
Troponin 216
Tuberculosis
    Association 267
    tests for 212
Typhoid 212
    test 216

U

Ultraviolet radiation 141
Umbilical cord, care of 52
Unani system of medicine 226
Under 5 mortality rate 87
Unemployment allowance 148
United Nations Development Program 194, 262
United Nations Fund For Population Activities 261
United Nations General Assembly and Economic and Social Council 260
United Nations International Children's Emergency Fund 259
    administration of 260
United Nations Population Fund 83, 261
Universal Immunization Program 68, 195
    objectives of 69
Unsafe patient handling 144
Urban Health and Wellness Center
    population norms for 210
    role of staff nurse of 208
Urban local bodies 212
Urine test 212, 216, 283
Urobilinogen 216
Uterine massage 48
Uterotonic drug 47
U-WIN 195

V

Vaccination 242
Vaccine 70
    contraindication of 76
    reaction, common 76
Vaginal sponge 117
Vasectomy 123
Vayoshreshtha Sammans 159
VED analysis 220
Venn diagram 103, 104f
Ventilation 145
Verbally responsive 11
Vertigo 153
Vibrio cholera 216
Vision 158, 177, 268
    impairment 153
Visual inspection acetic acid 216
Vital statistics
    indicators, important 84
    sources of 88
Vitals sign 5
Vitamin
    A 57, 73
    B_{12} 3
        deficiency 92, 171
    C 25
    D_3 37
    deficiency 171
    K 52

Vocational training 148
Voluntarism 131
Voluntary organizations 176
Vomiting 26
Vulnerability 238
Vulnerable populations 177

W

Wash 261
   your hands 284
Waste
   infectious 247
   management 211
   pharmaceutical 247
   type of 253
Water 224
   supply 242
Wholesale price index 219
Withdrawal symptoms 174
Woman during labor, supportive care to 44
Woman's bladder 287

World Bank 262
World Health Assembly 258
World Health Organization 257
Wound
   bleeding 14
   management 15*f*
   minor 14
Writing prescriptions 187

X

Xerophthalmia prevalent areas 260

Y

Yoga 223, 224
   sutras 224
   types of 224
Young child, home-based care for 56
Young persons, employment of 146
Yuzpe's regimen 125